PD Dr.med. AXEL LAUTEN
Internist / Kardiologe
Mühlburgweg 49
99094 ERFURT

Clinical Atlas of Transesophageal Echocardiography

by

Martin E. Goldman, MD

Director of Echocardiography
Associate Professor Medicine
Mt. Sinai Medical Center
New York, NY

With Contributions by

Bruce P. Mindich, MD
Allen Mogtader, MD
Theresa Guarino, RN

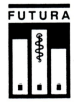

Futura Publishing Company, Inc.
Mount Kisco, New York

Library of Congress Cataloging-in-Publication Data

Goldman, Martin E., 1953–
    Clinical atlas of transesophageal echocardiography / by Martin E.
  Goldman, with contributions by Bruce P. Mindich . . . [et al.].
      p.   cm.
    Includes bibliographical references and index.
    ISBN 0-87993-539-1 (alk. paper)
    1. Transesophageal echocardiography—Atlases. I. Title.
    [DNLM: 1. Heart Diseases—ultrasonography—atlases.   WG 17
G619c
  1993]
    RC683.5.T83G65   1993
    616.1′207543—dc20
    DNLM/DLC
    for Library of Congress   93-3794
                              CIP

Copyright 1993
Futura Publishing Company, Inc.

Published by
Futura Publishing Company, Inc.
2 Bedford Ridge Road
Mount Kisco, New York 10549

LC #: 93-3794
ISBN #: 0-87993-539-1

Every effort has been made to ensure that the information in this book is as up to date and as accurate as possible at the time of publication. However, due to the constant developments in medicine, neither the author, nor the editor, nor the publisher can accept any legal or any other responsibility for any errors or omissions that may occur.

All rights reserved.
No part of this book may be translated or reproduced in any form without written permission of the publisher.

Printed in the United States of America.

This book is printed on acid-free paper.

*This book is dedicated to the long, healthy, happy lives of my beautiful daughter, Sarah Shifra, and my father, Hirsh,
and to my beloved mother, Shirley Shifra Goldman, a woman of valor, of blessed memory.*

Contributors

Theresa A. Guarino, RN
Clinical Coordinator, Cardiothoracic Surgery, St. Luke's/Roosevelt Hospital Center, New York, New York

Bruce P. Mindich, MD, FACS, FACC
Director Cardiothoracic Surgery, The Valley Hospital, Ridgewood, New Jersey, and Senior Cardiothoracic Surgeon, St. Luke's/Roosevelt Hospital Center, New York, New York

Allen H. Mogtader, MD, FACC
Assistant Professor of Clinical Medicine, Columbia University, College of Physicians and Surgeons, and Director of Echocardiography Laboratory, St. Luke's/Roosevelt Hospital Center, New York, New York

Preface

Echocardiography has had a dramatic impact in clinical cardiology because of its ability to provide immediate, on-line information that can significantly alter patient care. Over the past 10 years, echocardiography has expanded into diverse areas including transesophageal echocardiography, exercise and pharmacological stress echocardiography, 3-dimensional reconstruction, tissue characterization, and intravascular imaging. Echocardiography remains a relatively inexpensive diagnostic tool competing with more invasive and expensive technologies such as cardiac catheterization, rapid cine computerized tomography, and magnetic resonance imaging for evaluation of cardiac and thoracic pathology. Uniquely, transesophageal echocardiography expands the horizons of cardiac imaging by providing a rapid, safe modality for interrogation and evaluation of chambers and structures not easily accessible by routine transthoracic echocardiography (TEE).

In the early 1980s, Dr. Bruce Mindich, a gifted cardiothoracic surgeon, and Theresa Guarino, RN, and I began to explore the clinical utility of intraoperative echocardiography with routine M-mode and 2-dimensional equipment provided to us by Advanced Technology Laboratories through Mr. Bill Doherty, Bothell, WA. We were gratified by the dramatic impact echocardiography had in the management of valvular heart disease, particularly mitral valve repair procedures, and in difficult coronary bypass procedures. We explored the utility of contrast intraoperative echocardiography, atrial pacing to detect intraoperative ischemia before and after bypass surgery, and myocardial perfusion imaging. However, in 1984, when we had the opportunity to utilize the first elementary color-flow Doppler transesophageal echocardiography machine manufactured by Aloka (provided to us by Ms. Joan Main, then with Johnson & Johnson) its potential for intraoperative and ambulatory applications were immediately apparent. Subsequently, transesophageal echocardiography has become routine state-of-the-art technology for cardiothoracic surgery and for the high-risk cardiac patient undergoing noncardiac surgery.

Over the last few years, the introduction of less expensive equipment and smaller, more flexible transesophageal echocardiographic probes with multiplane imaging capability has facilitated the use of transesophageal echocardiography as a routine procedure in the echocardiographic laboratory and in the private office. With appropriate patient selection and in experienced hands, TEE should have much fewer complications than routine stress testing. As with any technology, transesophageal echocardiography requires specialized training, experience, and expertise to provide a safe, rapid, and cost-effective examination.

This book is a picture atlas of routine as well as esoteric TEE cases intended for the novice as well as those already experienced. The purpose of this text is to provide a pictorial reference to those interested in or performing transesophageal echocardiography in the echo laboratory, the office, or in the operating room, for cardiologists, anesthesiologists (both cardiothoracic and general), and cardiac surgeons. This book can be opened during a TEE exam to compare real-time images on the screen to over 500 pictures contained within. The spectrum of TEE incorporated in this book includes biplane and multiplane imaging, B-color technology, automated border detection, and intraoperative echo. Hopefully, this text will provide a practical introduction and reference for those interested in transesophageal echocardiography.

Martin E. Goldman, MD

Acknowledgment

I would like to acknowledge the influence of those people who have been invaluable in my training in both medicine and subsequently cardiology: Drs. Eugene Braunwald, Joseph Alpert, and Marshall Wolf at Peter Bent Brigham of Harvard University: Drs. Simon Dack, Valentin Fuster, Richard Gorlin, José Meller, and Louis Teichholz at Mount Sinai Hospital; Drs. James Seward, Jamil Tajik and Arthur Weyman, leaders in the field of echocardiography whose laboratories I visited numerous times.

I am very grateful for the skill and patience of Dr. Bruce Mindich and Theresa Guarino, RN, with whom I worked very closely in expanding my knowledge of intraoperative and transesophageal echocardiography.

Credit for success of our current facility for ambulatory transesophageal echocardiography is due to the diligence and dedication of Drs. Edward Fisher and Jeffrey Stahl who as fellows assisted in the initiation of our program; Drs. Edward Fisher and Stacey Rosen expert TEE attendings; Ms. Maureen Baker, supervisor, who also taught me M-mode echo; current and past fellows; and Ms. Jacqueline Budd, senior clinical nurse, whose extraordinary bedside manner and clinical acumen is invaluable on a daily basis.

I finally express my deepest gratitude to my co-workers: physicians, technologists, and staff; without their patience this book could not be possible and who continue to teach me everyday. Also to Ms. Karen O'Farrell, my assistant, and Ms. Marcy Leoncini for their secretarial assistance.

I also would like to thank the efforts of Steven E. Korn and Jacques G. Strauss of Futura Publishing Company, as well as Linda Shaw, senior editor, who helped shape this book into its final form; and both Ms. Ellen Selten and Nancy Kriebel who provided the art work.

Most importantly, I would also like to acknowledge the tremendous impact my parents had in attempting to instill in me the moral and ethical values which are as important to a physician as are his clinical skills: my mother, Shirley, of blessed memory who would have had tremendous *nachas*, satisfaction, upon reading this book; and my father, Hirsch.

Contents

Introduction		vii
1	Examination Techniques, Anatomy, and Basic Views: Monoplane, Biplane, and Multiplane Transesophageal Echocardiography	1
2	Mitral Valve Disease	33
	Mitral Stenosis	33
	Mitral Regurgitation	43
	Mitral Valve Prolapse	60
	Mitral Valve Endocarditis	63
	Mitral Valve Replacements	72
	Ball Valves	72
	Disc Valves	78
	Heterografts	89
	Mitral Valve Repair	101
3	Aortic Valve Disease	105
	Normal Variants and Aortic Valve Stenosis	105
	Aortic Regurgitation	113
	Aortic Valve Endocarditis	121
	Aortic Valve Prostheses	128
	Bicuspid Aortic Valve	137
4	Tricuspid Disease	147
	Tricuspid Regurgitation	147
	Tricuspid Valve Endocarditis	155
5	Aortic Dissection	159
6	Aortic Plaque	183
7	Left Ventricular Outflow Obstruction (Nonvalvular)	203
8	Coronary Artery Disease	209
	Coronary Artery Anatomy	209
	Ischemic Heart Disease	220
9	The Left Atrium	233
	Left Atrial Myxomas	233
	Left Atrial Appendage and Left Atrial Thrombi	244
	Pulmonary Veins	266
	Interatrial Septal Aneurysms	272
10	The Right Atrium	277
11	Pericardial Disease	297
12	Congenital Heart Disease	303
	Atrial Septal Defects	303
	Patent Foramen Ovale	327

Ventricular Septal Defect 336
Ebstein's Anomaly 341
Endocardial Cushion Defect 343
Cor Triatum 344
Transposition of the Great Arteries 346

13 Intraoperative Application of Transesophageal
   Echocardiography 349
   Allen Mogtader, MD, Theresa Guarino, RN,
   Martin E. Goldman, MD, Bruce P. Mindich, MD

   Intraoperative Transesophageal Procedure 350
   Mitral Valve Evaluation 354
   Tricuspid Valve Evaluation 360
   Prosthetic Valve Evaluation 360
   Aorta, Aortic Valve, Left Ventricular
      Outflow Tract Evaluation 363
   Intracardiac Shunts 363
   Impact of Intraoperative Echocardiography 366

Index 371

1

Examination Techniques, Anatomy, and Basic Views: Monoplane, Biplane, and Multiplane Transesophageal Echocardiography

Transesophageal echocardiography (TEE) is a modification of routine transthoracic echo technology, consisting of a small transducer mounted on the tip of a modified flexible gastroscope that facilitates imaging of cardiac structures not easily accessible by routine transthoracic echocardiography. The first transesophageal probe was introduced in 1976 and acquired only M-mode images; subsequently, two-dimensional TEE imaging was introduced in 1977.

Intraoperative color flow TEE was introduced in 1984 by Goldman and Mindich. Transesophageal echocardiography is utilized extensively in the operating room for cardiac monitoring, evaluation of valvular and congenital heart surgery, as well as in the ambulatory setting or intensive care unit. Presently, due to improved technology and imaging capacity, TEE is an integral part of the diagnostic approach to the patient with cardiac or thoracic aortic disease.

Methods

In the anesthetized unconscious patient undergoing a TEE exam, the airway is already protected from aspiration from gastric contents. The conscious nonintubated patient requires adequate topical anesthesia and sedation to facilitate transducer intubation and promote patient cooperation during the procedure. However, the basic imaging planes for all applications of TEE are similar.

Though techniques may vary from institution to institution, our protocol is to introduce the probe into the esophagus and lower it into the fundus of the stomach and begin imaging at that level since manipulation of the probe at the aortic arch level may not be well tolerated, causing premature termination of the exam. Therefore, we prefer to begin the examination in the stomach, slowly raising the scope to the base of the heart, then examining the origin of the great vessels, rotating and lowering the scope to view the descending aorta, and finally interrogating the arch. A complete thorough study is done on all patients. However, if the patient is very unstable or uncooperative, the imaging should begin focusing immediately on the area of interest, completing the study as time allows.

Patient Preparation (Table 1)

The equipment required to perform TEE includes: medications for topical anesthesia (viscous lidocaine and Cetacaine aerosol spray), intravenous medications for sedation, lubricating jelly, a pulse oxymeter, suction apparatus, manual or automatic sphygmomanometer, oxygen by nasal cannula, crash

Table 1

Setting Up a TEE Laboratory

Personnel
- Physician (1 or 2)
- Nurse
- Technologist (optional if physician is proficient with technical aspects of the machine)

Lab Equipment
- ECG monitor (single lead or echo machine)
- Sphygmomanometer (automatic or manual)
- Pulse oxymeter
- Oxygen via nasal cannula
- Suction apparatus
- Cardiopulmonary resuscitation cart (equipped with defibrillation, intubation apparatus, emergency drugs, etc.)

Performance of a TEE: Step by Step
- Brief history and physical
- Transthoracic echo
- Informed consent
- Intravenous access established
- (ECG, blood pressure and oxymeter monitoring)
- Anesthesia (topical) of mouth and oral pharynx
- Intravenous sedation—slow titration
- Insertion of mouthpiece
- Suction just prior to tube insertion
- Lubricate transducer well
- Tube insertion over tongue
- Patient swallows as tube enters esophagus
- Complete TEE study
- Remove probe in neutral position
- Narcan (optional)
- Wash off secretions
- Sterilize in 2% glutaraldehyde solution

cart, and glycopyrollate (a secretion-drying agent). We routinely obtain formal informed consent on all patients prior to the procedure. The patient then gargles three times with the viscous lidocaine, swallowing the last mouthful. Cetacaine spray provides more complete anesthesia. Begin spraying the front of the tongue moving posteriorly to the back of the tongue, reaching the posterior pharynx; this method may reduce a coughing spasm that is sometimes induced by the jet spray. Most importantly, "mental anesthesia" is essential for successful transesophageal imaging; the patient needs to be educated about the purpose of the procedure and the exact protocol to be used during the performance of the study. Patient cooperation is vital for success of the procedure. Patients are then given intravenous sedation with a varying combination of Demerol and Versed. The dosage is individualized to the patient's needs and medical condition. For example, Versed may induce excessive respiratory depression in an elderly patient. Therefore, particularly in older patients, we utilize very low doses of Versed or none at all and rely primarily on Demerol, which can be reversed quickly by Narcan. An antidote is now available for diazepam-type medications, but it may have limited effectiveness for respiratory depression. Parenthetically, all patients are monitored by a pulse oxymeter (placed on a fingertip, toe, or earlobe), which has been invaluable in extremely ill patients, alerting us to early signs of respiratory depression. Patients are given oxygen by nasal prongs. The patient is reassured that the oxygen is entering the "breathing tubes," which are unimpeded by the transducer which slides down the esophagus or their "food pipe."

The patient is usually placed in the left lateral decubitus position with a dental suction hook inserted into the angle of the mouth. If the person has excessive oral secretions, glycopyrollate may be used to reduce the need to suction and the risk of aspiration. The mouthguard is positioned and the well-lubricated tube introduced as the patient is instructed to take deep swallows. If the tube is not swallowed independently, a finger is put in the mouth alongside the mouthguard to assist in directing the transducer. If intubation is difficult in the decubitus position, the patient can sit at a 45° angle or upright. We have even resorted to using a laryngoscope to direct the probe. Rarely, if the patient is very reluctant to swallow the tube, has a severe gag reflex, or is hypotensive and cannot receive premedication, we have an anesthesiologist administer a superior laryngeal nerve block. The injection of lidocaine at the appropriate location in the neck can induce anesthesia of the oral pharynx for up to 2 hours. Following the TEE, patients are advised not to swallow hot or cold liquids for up to 2 hours after the procedure to avoid damage to the oral pharynx, which may still be anesthetized.

Imaging Planes (Table 2)

Currently, transesophageal probes are "monoplane," "biplane," or "multiplane." *Monoplane* imaging utilizes a single transducer mounted at the distal end of a routine gastroscope to obtain *horizontal* or *transverse* cross-section cuts of the heart. *Biplane* imaging has a second transducer positioned on the scope tip imaging at a 90° angle to the horizontal plane, providing longitudinal cross-sections (Fig. 1-1). Because of the limited maneuverability of the TEE probe once lowered into the esophagus, the biplane probe provides additional windows not available by monoplane imaging (Figs. 1-2A,B). The *multiplane probe* will provide up to a 360° window by electronically rotating the transducer (Fig. 1-3). Current AHA guidelines recommend that antibiotic prophylaxis is not necessary for endoscopy. We suggest that you conform

Table 2
TEE Imaging Protocol: View by View

Transgastric Transverse (T, or Horizontal) Five-Chamber View
- Aortic gradient (CW Doppler aligned parallel to valve or prosthesis)
- LV function
- Ventricular side of mitral prosthesis
- Aortic regurgitation
- LV outflow (subvalvular obstruction)

Transgastric Longitudinal (L) Five-Chamber View
- Aortic gradient
- LV outflow

    [raise probe]

Transgastric, T Short Axis
- LV function (midpapillary)

Transgastric, L Long Axis
- LV function (mitral plane to apex)

    [raise probe]

Transgastric (T) Mitral Short Axis
- Mitral valve orifice
- Mitral regurgitation
- Mitral vegetation
- Prosthetic valve function

    [raise probe above diaphragm]

RV Inflow, T View
- Inferior vena cava
- Eustachian valve
- Chiari network
- Coronary sinus
- Tricuspid valve

    [raise probe]

Interatrial Septum, T Plane
- RA and LA
- Patent foramen ovale (contrast injection)
- Tricuspid valve
- Atrial septal defect (primum and secundum)

RA Inflow, L Plane
- Inferior and superior vena cava
- Tricuspid valve
- RA appendage
- PFO (contrast injection)
- ASD

    [rotate probe]

Great Vessels, L Plane
- Pulmonic valve
- Pulmonary artery
- Aorta (evaluate cusps)
- RV outflow

    [raise probe]

- Aortic valve
- Aortic regurgitation

    [rotate]

LV 2 Chamber View, L Plane
- Anterior and posterior/inferior walls
- LV function from base to true apex
- Left atrium
- Mitral valve
- Mitral regurgitation

    [rotate]

LA, L View
- LA appendage
- Left pulmonary veins

    [lower slightly]

Four-Chamber, T View
- LV, LA, RA, RV chamber sizes
- Mitral and tricuspid valves (Doppler for stenosis or regurgitation)
- ASD
- VSD

    [raise slightly]

LVOT, T View
- Aortic regurgitation
- LVOT obstruction

Aortic and Pulmonic Valves, T View
- Aortic valve (all cusps)
- Pulmonic valve (all cusps)

    [anteflex probe tip raise slightly]

LA Appendage, T View
- LA appendage
- Left pulmonary veins

    [raise slightly]

Coronary Arteries, T View
- Left coronary artery
- Right coronary artery (slightly higher)

    [raise slightly]

Superior Vena Cava, T View
- SVC
- Sinus venosus ASD
- Right pulmonary veins
- Back wall LA

    [raise slightly]

Pulmonary Artery, T View
- Bifurcation
- Right PA

    [rotate probe 90° to aorta lower probe to diaphragm]

Descending Aorta, T and L Views
- Aortic plaque
- Aortic dissection

Table 2. (Continued)	
TEE Imaging Protocol: View by View	
Ascending Aorta, L Plane (5–9 cm length)	[raise probe and rotate]
Aortic aneurysm	*Aortic Arch, T and L Views*
Aortic dissection	Aortic plaque
Aortic prosthesis	Aortic dissection
Aortic stenosis	Carotid and subclavian arteries
Aortic vegetation/abscess	[rotate and retroflex tip]
[rotate and lower slightly]	*Ascending Aorta and Arch Junction*
LV Outflow Tract, L Plane	Aortic plaque
LVOT obstruction	Aortic dissection

to guidelines of your local infectious disease experts for studying patients with prosthetic valves.

Transducer Manipulation

The typical TEE transducer is fitted with two wheel controls that facilitate anterior, posterior, and side-to-side manipulation of the probe tip (Fig. 1-4). Additionally, the physician can rotate the transducer by rotating the entire probe as done with a catheter during cardiac catheterization. The scope is raised and lowered in the esophagus as it is being rotated and the wheels turned to maximize and idealize imaging planes. The transducer is introduced into the mouth with the imaging tip facing downward toward the tongue to position it facing anteriorly in the esophagus to image cardiac structures. Rotating the scope 180° directs it posteriorly, to image the descending aorta.

Image Orientation

As with transthoracic echo, the structures closer to the transducer are seen at the top of the video screen. TEE images from a retrocardiac position

Fig. 1-1.

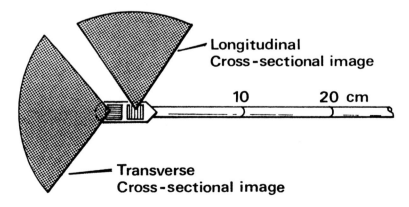

Figure 1-1: Biplane probe tip demonstrating the two transducer heads.

6 • Clinical Atlas of Transesophageal Echocardiography

Fig. 1-2.

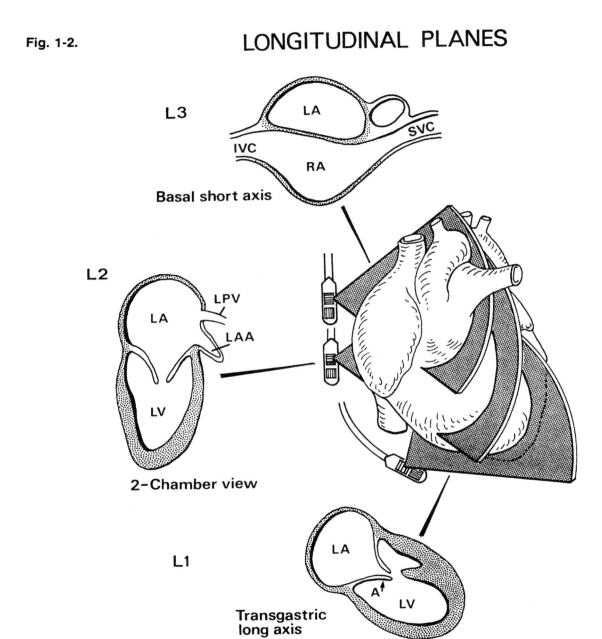

Figure 1-2A: TEE: standard longitudinal planes. L1–3 refer to specific imaging planes mentioned in text.

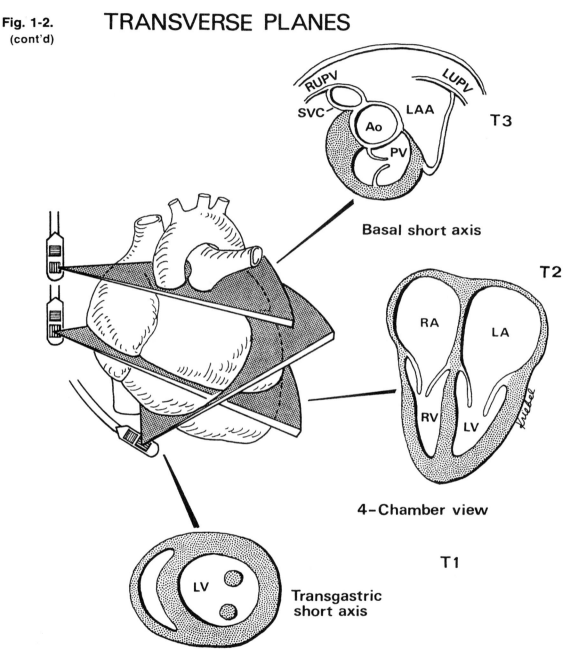

Figure 1-2B: TEE: standard transverse planes. T1–3 refer to specific imaging planes mentioned in text.

Fig. 1-3.

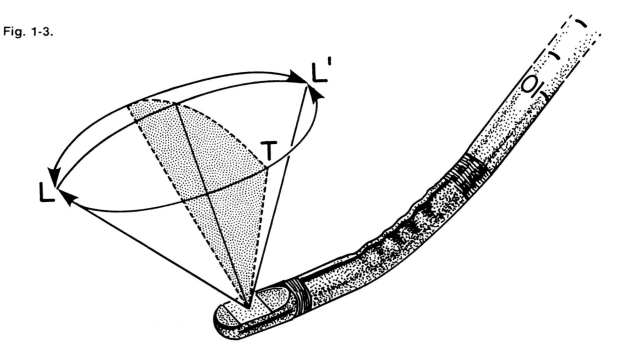

Figure 1-3: Multiplane probe tip with 360° imaging capability. T and L represent standard transverse and longitudinal planes.

and structures presented anterior on the screen are those through which the transducer beam transverses first. Thus, in a *transthoracic apical* view, the ultrasonic beam courses through the LV apex first and the apex is presented at the top of the screen and the atria at the bottom. However, with TEE, the left atrium is closer to the transducer and is presented at the top of the video screen.

Fig. 1-4.

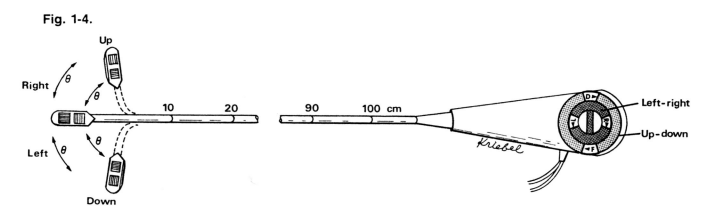

Figure 1-4: Transducer probe tip (on the left) can be manipulated by rotary dials and switches on the probe handle (on the right).

Standard Views

Subxiphoid

With the probe in the fundus of the stomach, several views are possible. The *horizontal* plane images the midpapillary muscle short axis plane (Figs. 1-2B,T1, 1-5), which facilitates cross-sectional evaluation of ventricular function similar to the corresponding transthoracic short axis plane (Fig. 1-6). However, TEE orientation is different from transthoracic because the transducer beam is emanating from a retrocardiac position; thus, the posterior and inferior walls of the heart are closer to the probe and are presented at the top of the screen. The anterior wall is more distant from the transducer and presented lower on the screen. The posteromedial papillary muscle is imaged at the bottom of the screen. The two papillary muscles and the right ventricle can be used as landmarks. The right ventricle is to the left and superior on the image compared to the routine transthoracic plane; the TEE short axis is rotated 90° counterclockwise from the transthoracic plane. A 2-D directed M-mode echocardiogram taken at this plane to measure ventricular contractility is a nonconventional plane since it is directed anteroinfero/laterally while the routine transthoracic M-mode beam tracks the septal to posterior walls (Fig. 1-7).

The ventricle can be divided into thirds at this level corresponding to the usual coronary artery distribution. The "clock face" has to be rotated appropriately using the papillary muscles as landmarks to determine coronary circulation in a transesophageal study (Fig. 1-5). The *left anterior descending* (LAD) artery supplies the anterior wall and septum (9:00 to 2:00 on a routine transthoracic echo and 6:00 to 12:00 by TEE). The *left circumflex circulation*

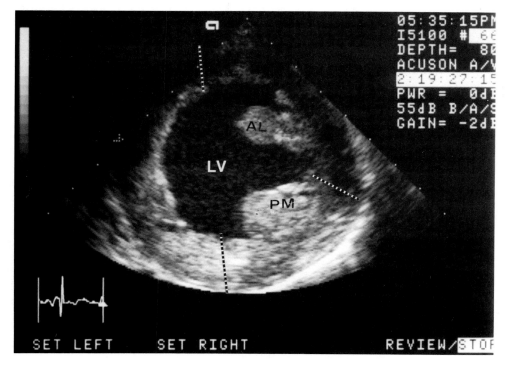

Figure 1-5: Subxiphoid transverse plane, midpapillary muscles. LV = left ventricle; AL = anterolateral papillary muscle; PM = posteromedial papillary muscle.

Fig. 1-6.

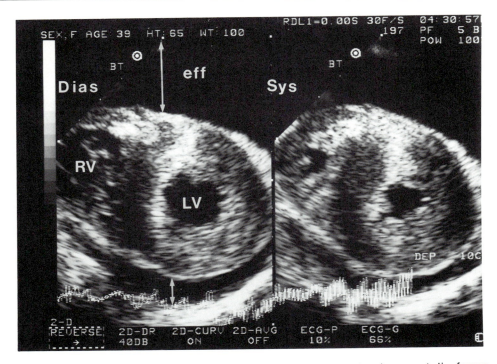

Figure 1-6: Subxiphoid transverse plane, midpapillary muscle view, systolic frame (Sys), and diastolic frame (Dias). There is a small pericardial effusion anteriorly and a large effusion posteriorly (closer to transducer, at top of screen marked by arrows. RV = right ventricle; LV = left ventricle.

Fig. 1-7.

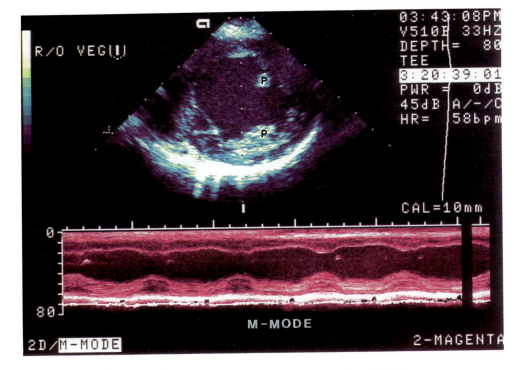

Figure 1-7: Subxiphoid transverse plane, M-mode view.

supplies the myocardium (from 2:00 until 6:00 by TTE, and 6:00 to 3:00 by TEE) and the *right coronary* artery supplies the inferior wall, (6:00 until 9:00 by TTE and 12:00 to 3:00 by TEE).

The TEE biplane longitudinal image at the subxiphoid level (Fig. 1-2A,L1) gives a different orientation: the left ventricle and left atrium are seen in a two-chamber foreshortened apical view with the anterior wall most distant from the transducer (lower on screen); both leaflets of the mitral valve (anterior leaflet is lower) and the papillary muscles and chordae are seen (Figs. 1-8A–C, 1-9). Rotating the transducer may bring the right ventricle and the true apex of the heart into view so that an apical aneurysm or thrombi can be seen.

If the transducer is lowered slightly further into the stomach, a four- and five-chamber view in the subxiphoid *transverse* plane are obtained (Fig. 1-10). This view may be particularly valuable for evaluating ventricular function in patients with aortic stenosis or aortic prosthetic valves. The left ventricular and aortic outflow tracts, mitral valve, and right ventricle can also be assessed in this plane.

Mitral Short Axis

As the probe is raised to the level of the diaphragm, the mitral valve is seen in short axis in the horizontal cross-section plane (Figs. 1-11, 1-12). This plane is useful to assess the motion of the anterior leaflet and the middle, medial, and lateral cusps of the posterior leaflet. The specific location and pathophysiological mechanism of mitral regurgitation can be identified in this plane before and immediately following valve repair. Mitral prosthetic valves can be imaged evaluating possible paravalvular leaks and vegetations as well as dehisced sutures.

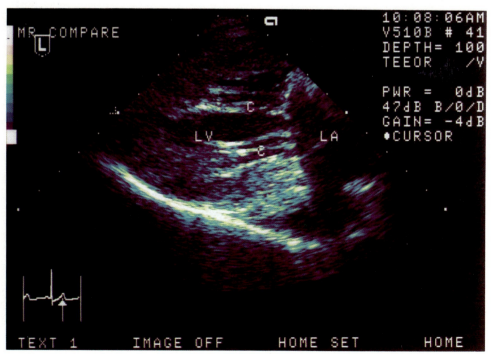

Figure 1-8A: Subxiphoid longitudinal plane. C = chordae tendineae; LA = left atrium; LV = left ventricle.

Fig. 1-8. (cont'd)

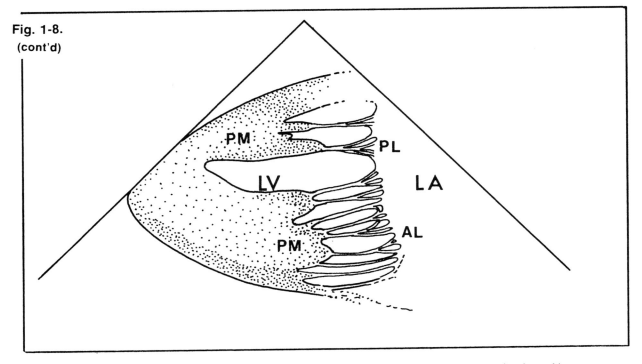

Figure 1-8B: Corresponding drawing of longitudinal transgastric long axis view. AL = anterior leaflet mitral valve; PL = posterior leaflet mitral valve; PM = papillary muscle.

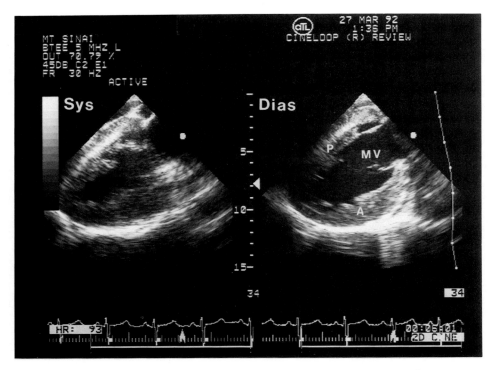

Figure 1-8C: Subxiphoid longitudinal plane. Diastolic frame (Dias) and systolic frame (Sys) demonstrate ventricular contractility from base to apex. A = anterior wall; MV = mitral valve; P = posterior wall.

TEE Examination Techniques • 13

Fig. 1-9.

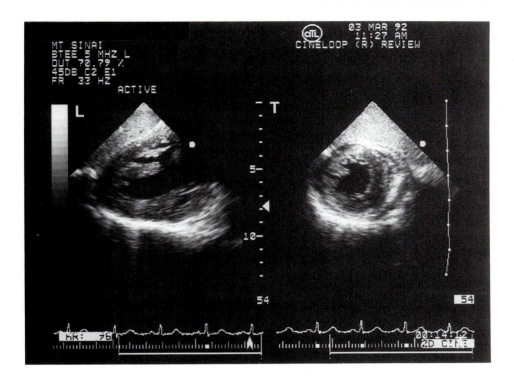

Figure 1-9: Corresponding subxiphoid transverse plane (T) and longitudinal long axis view (L).

Fig. 1-10.

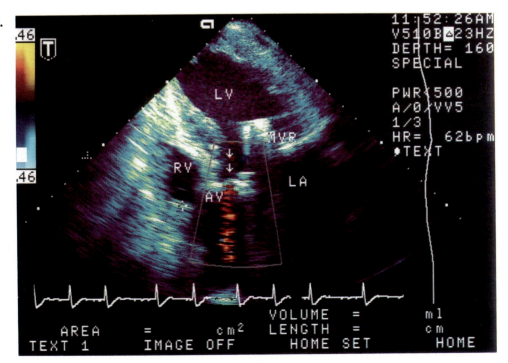

Figure 1-10: Subxiphoid five-chamber view, transverse plane. LV = left ventricle; RV = right ventricle; LA = left atrium; AV = aortic valve; MVR = mitral ball valve replacement.

14 • Clinical Atlas of Transesophageal Echocardiography

Fig. 1-11.

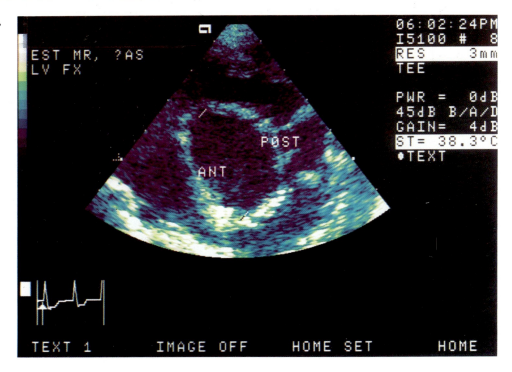

Figure 1-11: Mitral short axis, transverse plane. Both the anterior and posterior leaflets are seen. The commissures are marked by diagonal lines.

Fig. 1-12.

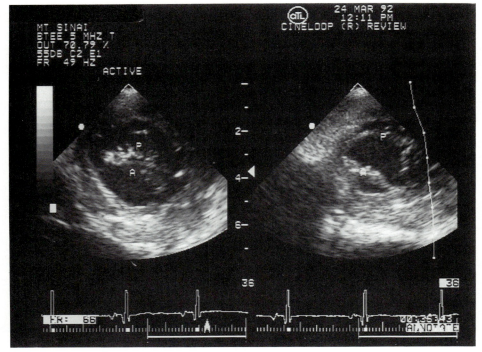

Figure 1-12: Mitral short axis, transverse plane. Mitral orifice can be measured in diastole (right side) and assessed in systole (left side).

Right Ventricular Inflow

As the probe is raised just above the diaphragm and rotated counterclockwise, to the right of the patient, the right ventricular inflow view is seen in the *horizontal* plane (Fig. 1-13). The septal and anterior leaflets of the tricuspid valve are seen with the coronary sinus entering superiorly and to the middle of the screen. The severity of tricuspid regurgitation can be assessed. The *eustachian valve* at the junction of the inferior vena cava and the atrium is a vestigial valve or flap that is nonobstructive (Figs. 1-14A,B). A frequent source of problems in interpretation is the *Chiari network*, a filamentous nonobstructive membrane in the right atrium that does not obstruct and may undulate with blood flow (Fig. 1-15). The right atrium frequently has small pectinate muscles that must be differentiated from thrombus or mass (Fig. 1-16). A thrombus may develop in a dilated atrium and will protrude from the free wall and have a different videodensity from the underlying endocardium. The atrial appendage is sometimes seen posterior to the tricuspid annulus. The longitudinal plane images the great veins (Fig. 1-2A,L3). As the probe is raised, the tricuspid valve can be seen in the longitudinal plane (Fig. 17).

As the probe is raised higher, the transverse three-chamber view is seen with very good visualization of the atrial septum. In the *transverse* plane, the relative size of the right and left atria can be evaluated and atrial septal defects (ASD) (secundum or primum) can be detected. We routinely inject "contrast" in the horizontal and longitudinal planes to determine the presence or absence of a patent foramen ovale (PFO), which may not be readily visualized even with color flow Doppler. A contrast injection can be performed by rapid injection of hand-agitated saline or dextrose water (5–10 cc), which generates microbubbles that ordinarily enter the right atrium and exit out the right ven-

Fig. 1-13.

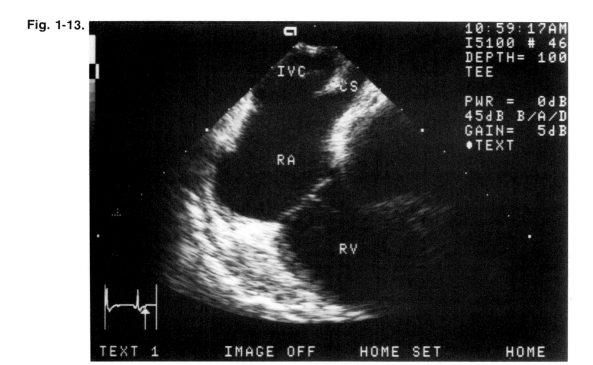

Figure 1-13: Right atrium, transverse plane. The coronary sinus (CS), inferior vena cava (IVC), right atrium (RA), and right ventricle (RV) are seen, with the anterior and septal leaflets of the tricuspid valve.

16 • Clinical Atlas of Transesophageal Echocardiography

Fig. 1-14.

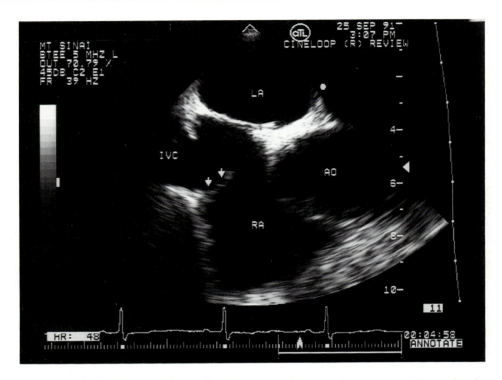

Figure 1-14A: Right atrial (RA) inflow view, longitudinal plane: eustachian valve (arrows). IVC = inferior vena cava; AO = aorta; LA = left atrium.

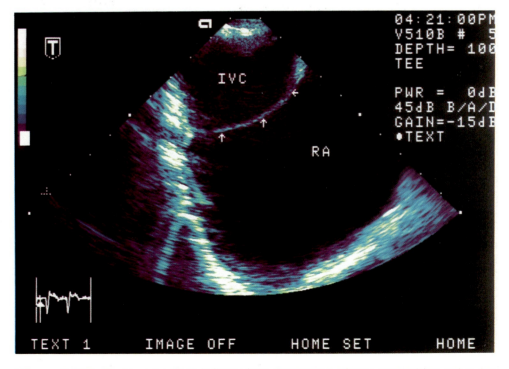

Figure 1-14B: Right atrial (RA) inflow view, transverse plane: eustachian valve (arrows). IVC = inferior vena cava.

Fig. 1-15.

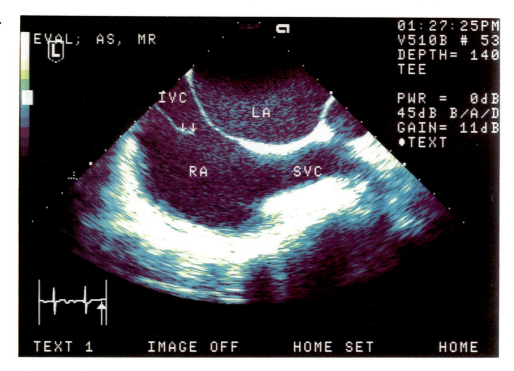

Figure 1-15: Right atrial (RA) inflow, longitudinal plane: Chiari network (arrows). IVC = inferior vena cava; LA = left atrium; SVC = superior vena cava.

Fig. 1-16.

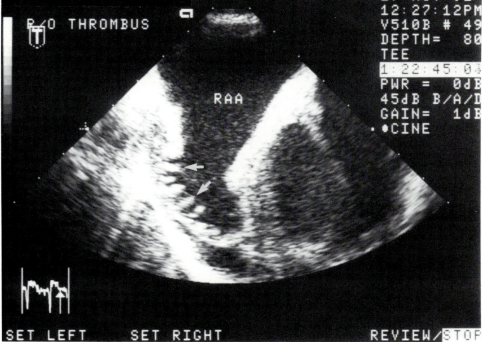

Figure 1-16: Right atrial appendage (RAA), transverse plane: pectinate muscles (arrows).

Fig. 1-17.

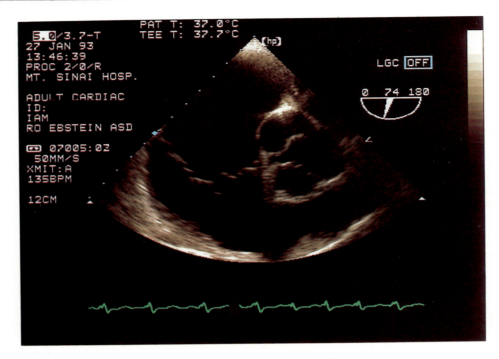

Figure 1-17: Tricuspid valve, longitudinal plane.

tricle and pulmonary artery (Figs. 1-18A,B). In the presence of a left-to-right shunt through an atrial septal defect, blood entering from the left atrium creates negative contrast against the opacified right atrium. If a patent foramen ovale is present, just a few microbubbles may traverse the atrial septum from the right to the left atrium during the first few cardiac cycles, which can be enhanced if the patient coughs or by performing a Valsalva manuever during the injection (the later is frequently difficult if the patient has been heavily sedated) (Figs. 1-19A,B). Color flow Doppler will usually demonstrate an ASD, but may not detect a PFO because of its small orifice and intermittent flow.

Four-Chamber View

Rotating the transducer to the left of the patient while raising slightly presents the transverse four-chamber view with the anterior and posterior leaflets of the mitral valve easily seen (Figs. 1-2B,T2, 1–20). By rotating the transducer, the entire left atrium can be visualized. Color Doppler can assess mitral regurgitation and the coaptation plane of the mitral leaflets (Fig. 1-21), valvular vegetations, the basal ventricular septal thickness, and membranous ventricular septal defects are imaged at this level. Transmitral pulsed Doppler can be obtained to assess the early (E wave) and atrial contraction (A wave) flow velocity integrals (Figs. 1-22A–C). The five-chamber apical view demonstrates the aortic valve and left ventricular outflow tract in the *transverse* plane (Fig. 1-23). This view will detect systolic anterior motion of the mitral valve (SAM in HCOM or IHSS), aortic regurgitation, and basal septal hypertrophy.

text continues on p. 24

Fig. 1-18.

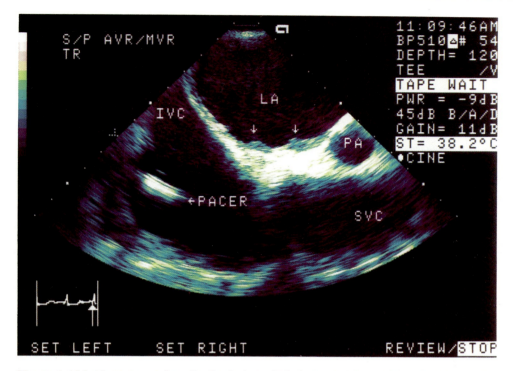

Figure 1-18A: Vena cavae, longitudinal plane. Inferior vena cava (IVC), left atrium (LA), pulmonary artery (PA), and superior vena cava (SVC) are seen. A pacemaker (PACER) is present in the right atrium. Two arrows in left atrium point to sutures and pledgets following atrial septal defect repair.

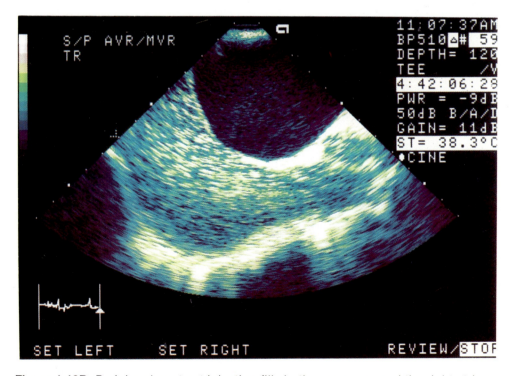

Figure 1-18B: Peripheral contrast injection fills both vena cavae and the right atrium with echogenic microbubbles while the left atrium remains echo-free.

20 • Clinical Atlas of Transesophageal Echocardiography

Fig. 1-19.

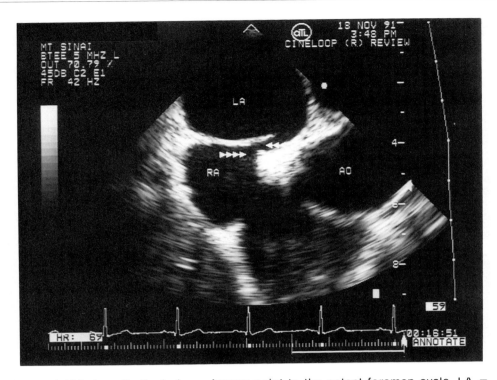

Figure 1-19A: Longitudinal plane. Arrows point to the patent foramen ovale. LA = left atrium; RA = right atrium; AO = aorta.

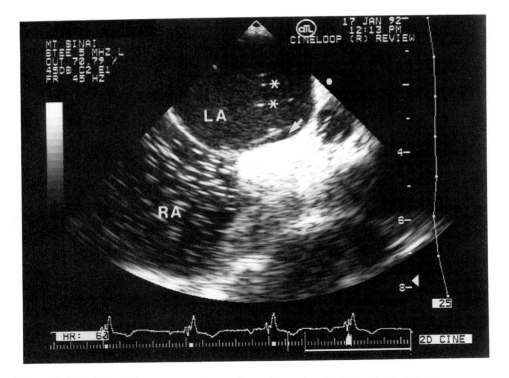

Figure 1-19B: Patent foramen ovale confirmed by microbubbles (asterisks) transverse from the right atrium (RA) through the patent foramen ovale (arrow) into the left atrium (LA).

Fig. 1-20.

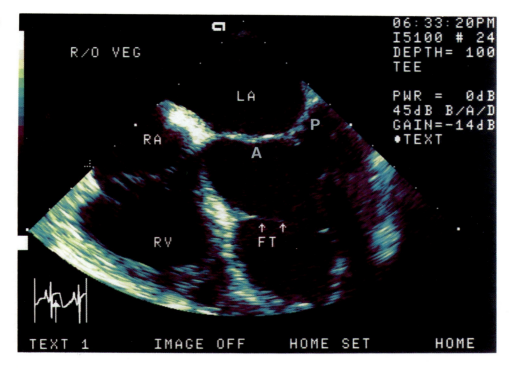

Figure 1-20: Four-chamber view, transverse plane. A false tendon (FT) is seen in the left ventricle. Anterior (A) and posterior (P) leaflets of the mitral valve are seen. LA = left atrium; RA = right atrium; RV = right ventricle.

Fig. 1-21.

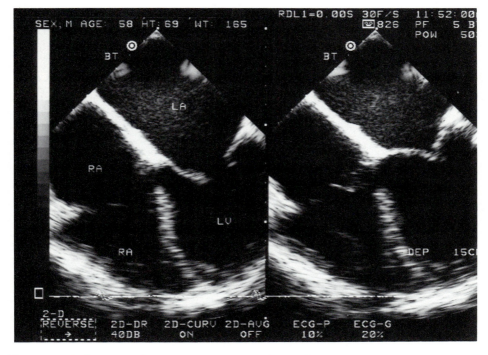

Figure 1-21: Four-chamber view, transverse plane. Diastolic (left side) and systolic motion of the mitral valve. LA = left atrium; LV = left atrium; LA = left atrium; LV = left ventricle.

Fig. 1-22.

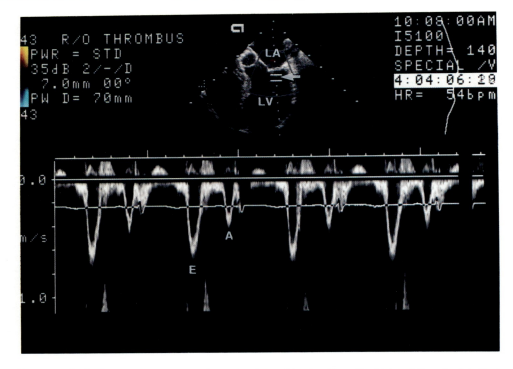

Figure 1-22A: Transmitral pulsed Doppler flow. Since transmitral blood flow is moving away from the transducer, the waveform is negative. The early peak (E wave) is taller than the atrial contraction "A" wave, yielding a "normal" E/A ratio, suggesting normal diastolic inflow. Arrow = Doppler sample volume; LA = left atrium; LV = left ventricle.

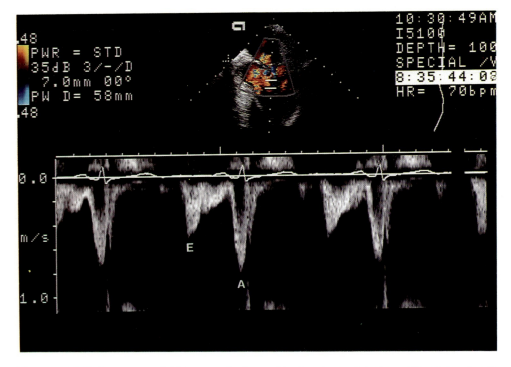

Figure 1-22B: Reversal of E/A wave forms, with the A wave being taller than the E wave, suggesting abnormal diastolic compliance.

Fig. 1-22.
(cont'd)

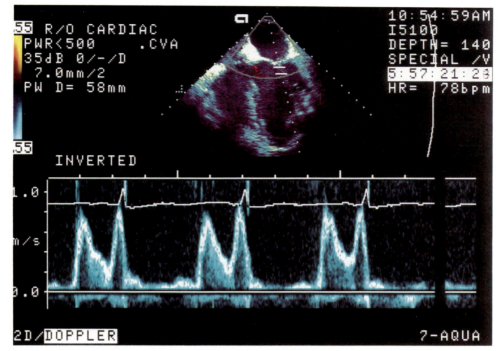

Figure 1-22C: The transmitral Doppler tracings can be inverted automatically on most machines.

Fig. 1-23.

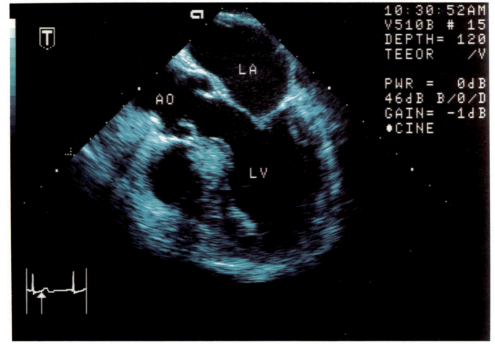

Figure 1-23: Transverse plane, five-chamber view. Basal septal thickness and aortic excursion can be assessed. AO = aorta; LA = left atrium; LV = left ventricle.

Longitudinal Plane

The two-chamber longitudinal view (Fig. 1-2A,L2) images the anterior and inferior walls whereas the transverse plane four-chamber view visualizes the septal and lateral walls (Fig. 1-24A). The true apex can frequently be seen in the transverse two-chamber view, as well as a good view of the left atrial appendage (LAA) and the left upper pulmonary vein separated from the LAA by a dense ridge of tissue with a bulbous tip (Fig. 1-24B). Ventricular contractility can be assessed in this plane (Fig. 1-24C).

Basal Views

Raising the transducer from the esophagus with slight anteflexion generates a *horizontal* plane basal short axis view of the aorta (in the middle of the screen), left atrium (anterior), and pulmonary artery (posterior and to the right of the aorta) (Fig. 1-2B,T3). M-mode imaging will demonstrate the excursion of both the aortic and the pulmonic valves (Figs. 1-25A,B). The corresponding *longitudinal* section demonstrates a long axis of the right ventricular outflow tract and the aortic valve (Fig. 1-26). Further rotation of the tranducer in the longitudinal plane provides an ideal view to assess aortic vegetations and dilatation of ascending aorta (Fig. 1-27A,B).

text continues on p. 28

Fig. 1-24.

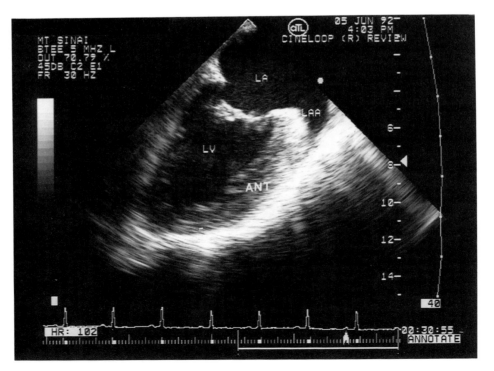

Figure 1-24A: Longitudinal two-chamber LV plane. The anterior (ANT) and inferior walls of the left ventricle (LV), as well as the left atrial appendage (LAA) can be seen.

Fig. 1-24. (cont'd)

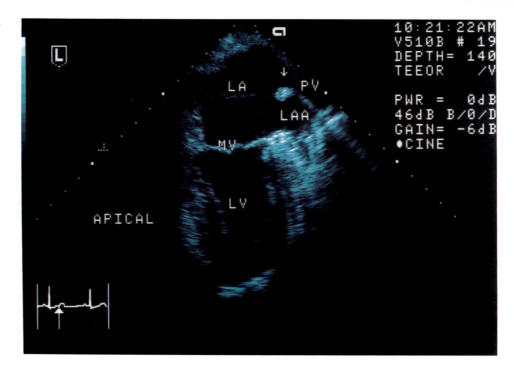

Figure 1-24B: The left atrial appendage (LAA) and pulmonary vein (PV) are separated by a septum with a bulbous tip (arrow) which could be confused with a vegetation. MV = mitral valve.

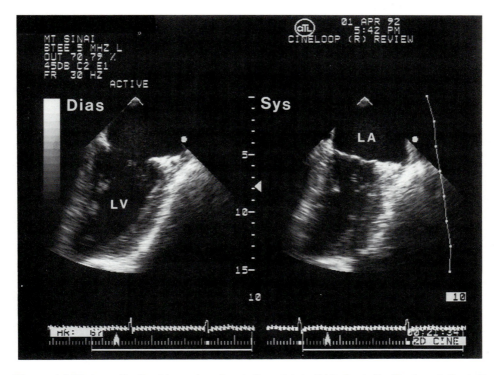

Figure 1-24C: Longitudinal two-chamber left ventricle (LV). Systolic (Sys) and diastolic (Dias) frames facilitate assessment of ventricular function.

Fig. 1-25.

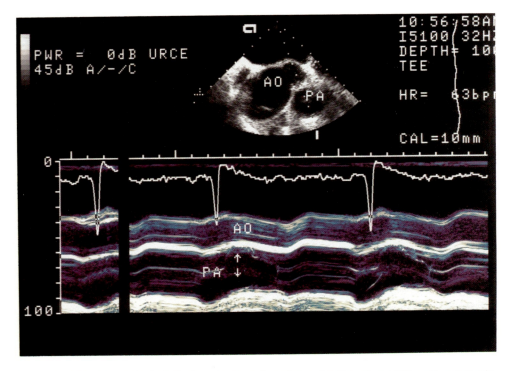

Figure 1-25A: M-mode, basal view, transverse plane. Aortic valve (AO) and pulmonic valve (PA) excursion can be identified.

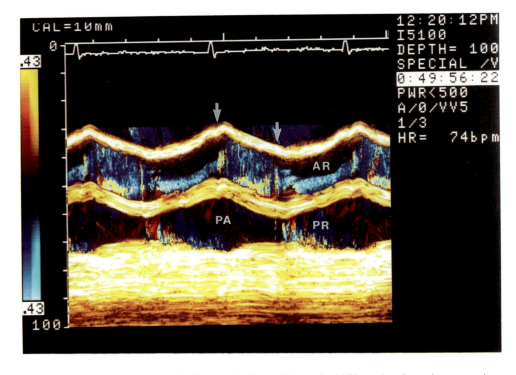

Figure 1-25B: Color M-mode demonstrates mild aortic (AR) and pulmonic regurgitation (PR) during diastole. Arrows delineate systolic aortic flow. PA = pulmonary artery.

Fig. 1-26.

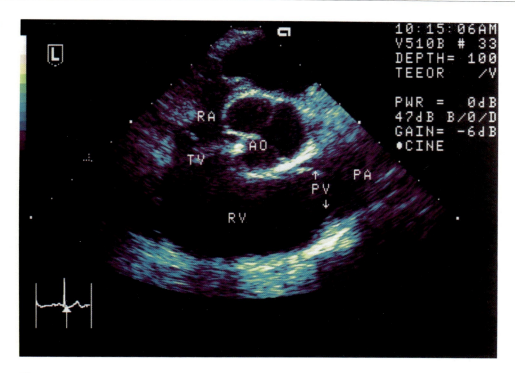

Figure 1-26: Basal view, longitudinal plane. The aortic (AO) pulmonic (PV, arrows), and tricuspid (TV) valves are seen. RA = right atrium; RV = right ventricle; PA = pulmonary artery.

Fig. 1-27.

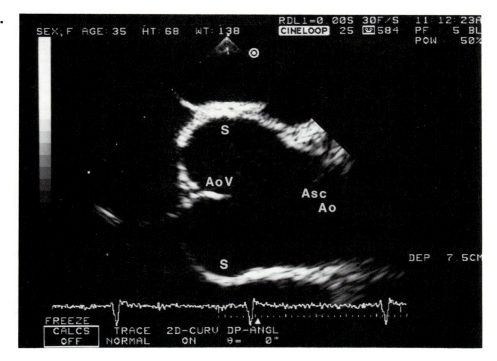

Figure 1-27A: Basal view, longitudinal plane. Aortic valve (AoV), sinuses of Valsalva (S), and proximal ascending aorta (Asc Ao) can be seen.

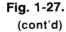Fig. 1-27. (cont'd)

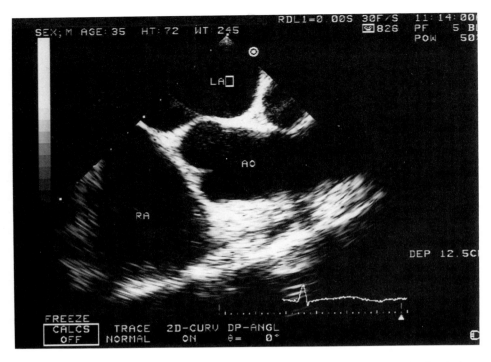

Figure 1-27B: The ascending aorta and aortic valve (diastole) in the longitudinal plane. LA = left atrium; RA = right atrium.

Basal View: Left Atrial Appendage, Aortic Leaflets, Coronary Arteries

Raising the transducer higher in the esophagus and rotating to the left of the patient and anteflexing will image the left atrial appendage, pulmonary artery, aorta, and coronary arteries (Figs. 1-2T3, 1-28) in the basal transverse plane.

Pulmonary Artery

If the probe is raised higher in the *horizontal* plane, the superior vena cava, aorta, and left atrium are seen. As the probe is directed towards the left of the patient, the bifurcation of the pulmonary artery can be imaged at the right pulmonary artery directly over the aorta and the left pulmonary artery branching off away from the aorta (Figs. 1-29A,B).

Thoracic Aorta

We then rotate the probe 180° to image the descending aorta. The *transverse* plane yields cross-sectional, round slices of the aorta (Fig. 1-30A), whereas the *longitudinal* plane will provide long axis sections of the tube (Fig. 1-30B). The visualization of the descending aorta is essential in the evaluation of patients with possible aorta dissection (and its pathognomonic inti-

text continues on p. 31

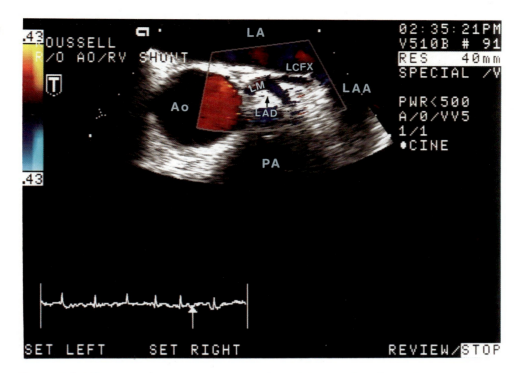

Figure 1-28: Coronary arteries, transverse plane. LAD = left anterior descending artery; LCFX = left circumflex; LM = left main artery; LAA = left atrial appendage.

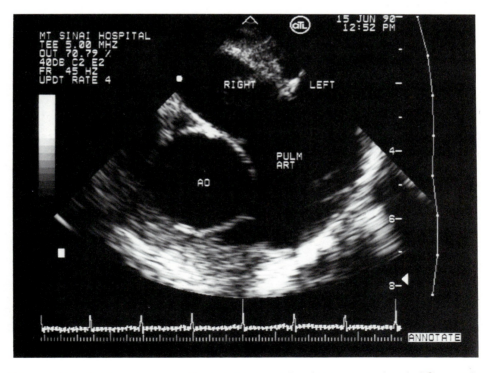

Figure 1-29A: Pulmonary artery (Pulm Art) bifurcation (transverse plane). AO = aorta.

Fig. 1-29. (cont'd)

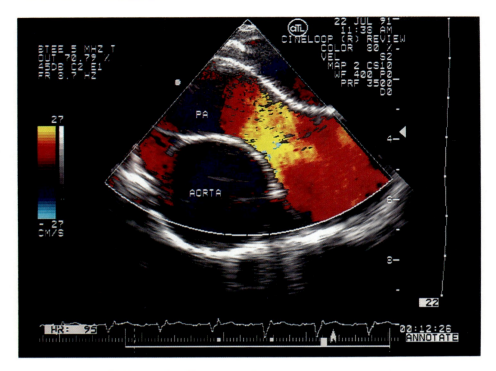

Figure 1-29B: Color flow Doppler of the pulmonary artery (PA) and aorta.

Fig. 1-30.

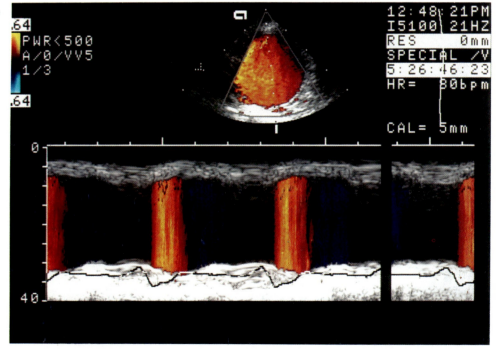

Figure 1-30A: Descending aorta (transverse plane) with corresponding M-mode below, demonstrating foward systolic flow (orange/red) and minimal negative reversal of flow (blue).

Fig. 1-30. (cont'd)

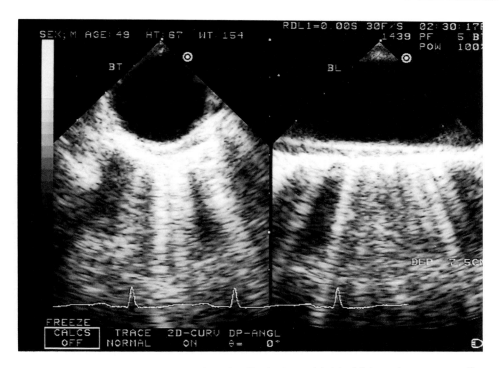

Figure 1-30B: Descending aorta: longitudinal plane (right side) and corresponding transverse plane (left).

mal flap) or aneurysm. As the probe is raised to approximately 25 cm from the mouth, the aortic arch is brought into view and is identified in the *horizontal* plane by the loss of the left side of the aorta. If the probe is then rotated to the right of the patient, the transverse and ascending aorta can be visualized. The probe can be lowered following the ascending aorta and pulmonary arteries (Fig. 1-31).

There may be a 2–3 cm ultrasound blind spot in the ascending aortic at the level of the trachea. Rarely, an aortic dissection may originate and be isolated to this location. The longitudinal plane may facilitate imaging the blind spot.

Multiplane probe imaging utilizes the basic transverse (0° axis) and longitudinal planes (90° axis). However, since the best longitudinal plane may be at 75° or 85°, the multiplane probe may provide a better image than a biplane probe. Additionally, structures can be interrogated more completely by focusing on an abnormality (i.e., mass in the atrial appendage) and rotating the probe from 0° to 180°.

Additional comments on the anatomy seen in the different planes will be discussed in specific pathological sections. Mastering image orientation is vital to successful TEE. The preparation and intubation of the patient are important; both are easily learned from observing gastroenterologists or anesthesiologists. However, learning how to manipulate the probe to acquire specific planes and images is essential for maximizing diagnostic information from the transesophageal echocardiogram. To gain experience in intubation techniques, a gastroenterologist or a cardiologist skilled in TEE can give invaluable guidance. Experience in manipulation of the probe can be gained in the operating suite or intensive care unit where patients are intubated and sedated. When the technique is mastered, a thorough transesophageal echocardiogram can be peformed in 10 to 20 minutes, providing invaluable information on cardiac function.

Fig. 1-31.

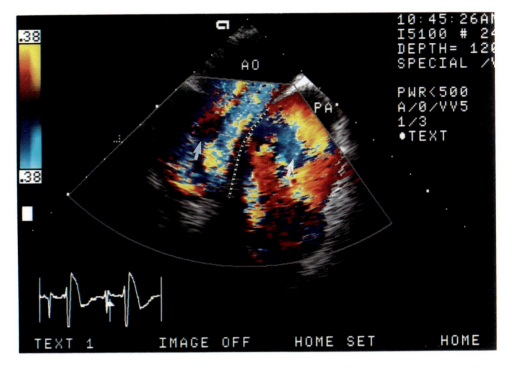

Figure 1-31: Ascending aorta (AO) and pulmonary artery (PA) in the transverse plane interrogated by color flow Doppler.

Bibliography

1. Hisanaga K, Hisanaga A, Nagata K, Yoshida S: A new transesophageal real time two-dimensional echocardiographic system using a flexible tube and its clinical application. *Proc Jpn Soc Ultason Med* 32:43–44, 1977.
2. Seward JB, Khandheria BK, Oh JK, Abel MD, Hughes RW Jr, Edward WD, Nichols BA, Freeman WK, Tajik AJ: Transesophageal echocardiography: technique, anatomic correlations, implementation and clinical applications. *Mayo Clin Proc* 63:649–680, 1988.
3. Matsuzaki M, Toma Y, Kusukawa R: Clinical applications of transesophageal echocardiography. *Circulation* 82:709–722, 1990.
4. Fisher E, Stahl J, Budd J, Goldman ME. Transesophageal echocardiography: Clinical application. *JACC* 18:1333–1348, 1991.
5. Khandheria BK. Prophylaxis or no prophylaxis before transesophageal echocardiography? *J Am Soc Echo* 5:285–287, 1992.
6. Seward JB, Khandheria BK, Edwards WD, et al: Biplanar transesophageal echocardiography: anatomic correlations, image orientation and clinical application. *Mayo Clinic Proc* 65:1193–1213, 1990.
7. Daniel WG, Erbel R, Kasper W, et al: Safety of transesophageal echocardiography: A multicenter survey of 10,419 examinations. *Circulation* 83: 817–821, 1991.
8. Pearson AC, Castello R, Labovitz AJ: Safety and utility of transesophageal echocardiography in the critically ill patient. *Am Heart J* 119:1083–1089, 1990.
9. Seward JB, Khandheria BK, Oh JK, Freeman WK, Tajik AJ: Critical appraisal of transesophageal echocardiography: limitations, pitfalls and complications. *J Am Soc Echo* 5:288–305, 1992.

2

Mitral Valve Disease

One of the most important applications of transesophageal echocardiography (TEE) is the evaluation of mitral valve pathology. Ordinarily, the mitral valve is well seen by routine transthoracic echocardiography (TEE). However, TEE is essential under certain circumstances, such as technically difficult transthoracic studies, prosthetic valves, or for more accurate evaluation of the severity of mitral regurgitation. The mitral valve can be imaged in several planes (see Chapter 1, Basic Views).

Mitral Stenosis

Mitral stenosis is due to rheumatic fever following a streptococcal infection with subsequent fibrosis and calcification of the mitral valve. During this process, the mitral valve orifice begins to narrow and there is restriction to blood flow into the left ventricle. The process is usually gradual with varying degrees of involvement of the other valves. Beginning in the subxiphoid longitudinal plane, the anterior and posterior leaflets of the valve can be appreciated in a classic view similar to the parasternal long axis view. As the transducer is raised, the short axis subxiphoid plane at the mitral leaflet level is visualized: relative mobility and fibrosis of the leaflet can be assessed, leaflet mobility, commissural fusion can be identified, and orifice size planimetered. As the transducer is raised above the diaphragm, the tricuspid valve can be visualized quickly to determine if there is tricuspid stenosis with restriction of leaflet motion. In the four- (transverse) and two-chamber views (longitudinal plane), the mitral leaflet doming secondary to fibrosis, and leaflet restricted motion can be seen.

The severity of mitral stenosis can be quantified by planimetry, or more precisely by continuous wave Doppler. Color flow echo can localize the direction of the left ventricular inflow jet and the Doppler sample volume can be aligned within the region of highest velocity. Because the blood flow is moving away from the transducer, from the left atrium to the left ventricle, the Doppler spectral display is negative or below the zero line. Some machines allow inversion of the tracing so the velocity flow appears positive. Pressure half-times can be measured by pulsed or continuous wave Doppler. Doppler flow measurements should be obtained as parallel as possible to left ventricular inflow by raising or lowering the probe to maximize flow velocity. Additionally, the left atrium should be interrogated to evaluate the possible mitral regurgitation that may accompany mitral stenosis. The left atrial appendage should be imaged to exclude thrombus. Occasionally, mitral regurgitation accompanies the mitral stenosis because the leaflets do not coapt well due to the retraction, fibrosis, and calcification of the leaflets. The rheumatic process and fibrosis may involve the supporting apparatus of the mitral valve including the chordae tendineae and papillary muscles.

A semiquantitative echocardiographic assessment of mitral valve morphology to predict successful percutaneous mitral valve balloon valvotomy has been described (*British Heart Journal* 60:299–308, 1988). The severity score evelutes four aspects of the mitral valve and scores them on the basis of a 0–4+ scale; the higher the number, the more severe the pathology:

1. valve mobility;
2. calcification and fibrosis of the valve;
3. valve thickening;
4. involvement of the subvalvular apparatus.

Generally, a score greater than 9–10 predicts a poorer outcome following balloon valvuloplasty. Mitral regurgitaiton usually increases after valvotomy. The procedure produces a small atrial septal defect because the catheters are advanced through the atrial septum to be positioned into the mitral valve plane. This may affect subsequent hemodynamic and echo Doppler assessment of valve area.

Bibliography

1. Fraser AG, Stumper OFW, van Herwerden LA, et al: Anatomy of imaging planes used to study the mitral valve: advantages of biplane transesophageal echocardiography. *Circulation* 82:III-668, 1990.
2. Casale PM, Whitlow P, Currie PJ, Stewart WJ: Transesophageal echocardiography in percutaneous balloon valvuloplasty for mitral stenosis. *Cleve Clinic J Med* 56:597–600, 1989.
3. Wilkins GT, Weyman AE, Abascal VM, et al: Percutaneous balloon dilatation of the mitral valve: an analysis of echocardiographic variables related to outcome and the mechanism of dilatation. *Br Heart J* 60:299–308, 1988.

Fig. 2-1.

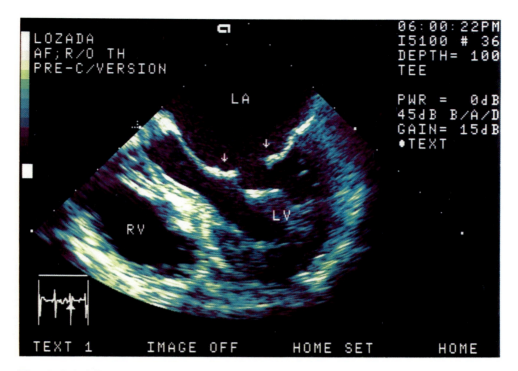

Figure 2-1: Mild mitral stenosis with doming of the valve is seen in the transverse four-chamber view. B-color accentuates the mild fibrosis of the leaflet tips (arrows).

Fig. 2-2.

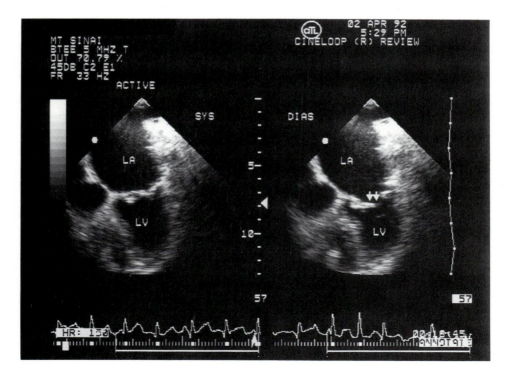

Figure 2-2: The diastolic frame (right) demonstrates a thick, calcified valve with limited excursion (arrows) and a markedly dilated left atrium. The systolic frame (on the left) is emphasized the limited leaflet mobility.

Fig. 2-3.

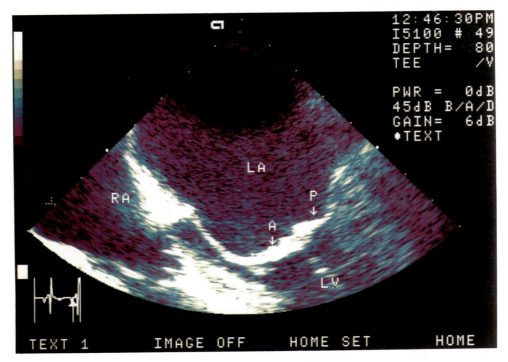

Figure 2-3: The mitral valve has extremely limited diastolic motion; the anterior (A) and posterior (P) leaflets are virtually fused and domed.

Fig. 2-4.

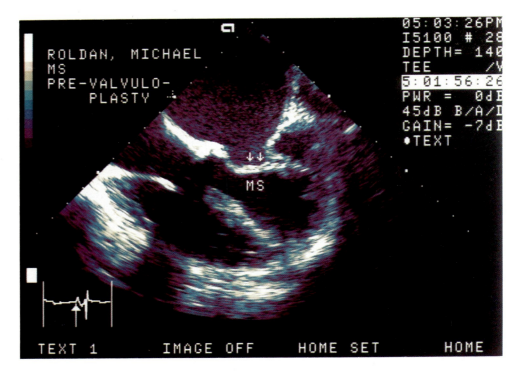

Figure 2-4A: B-color demonstrates the extent of involvement of the leaflets and the subvalvular apparatus. Only the anterior leaflet domes (arrows) while the posterior leaflet is immobile.

Fig. 2-4. (cont'd)

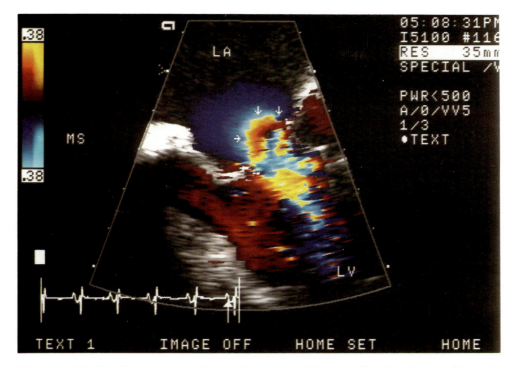

Figure 2-4B: This figure demonstrates the proximal isovelocity velocity area (arrows) which is generated from the blood converging on the atrial side in its attempt to enter into the left ventricle. This connotes a more significant degree of mitral stenosis.

Fig. 2-5.

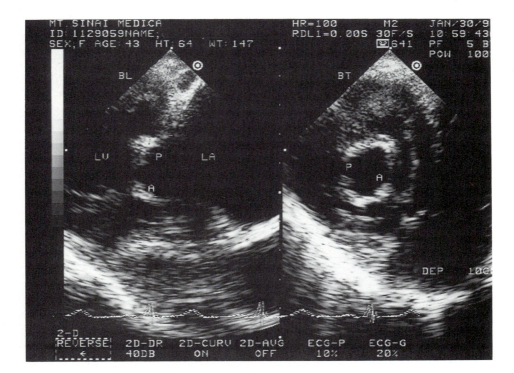

Figure 2-5: In biplane imaging, the subxiphoid position. The thickening of the anterior and posterior leaflets in the longitudinal plane (left side) with subvalvular apparatus involvement; the corresponding transverse plane (right side) demonstrates thickening of the leaflets with fibrosis and typical fishmouth orifice in a short axis view.

Fig. 2-6.

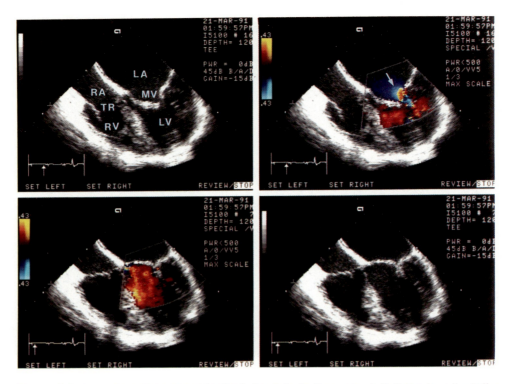

Figure 2-6: A multiple sequence of mitral stenosis. In the upper left, there is a diastolic doming with marked reduced excursion of the posterior leaflet. In the upper right, restricted inflow with proximal isovelocity area is demonstrated (arrow). The systolic frames in the lower left and lower right demonstrate mild prolapsing of the anterior leaflet into the left atrium. There is no mitral regurgitation.

Fig. 2-7.

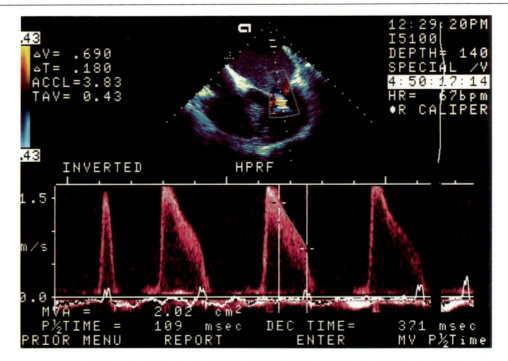

Figure 2-7: Quantification of mitral stenosis can be performed using pulsed or continuous wave Doppler in the four- or two-chamber view. B-color Doppler facilitates differentiation of the fine feather Doppler edge occasionally seen in stenotic and regurgitant lesions. For this particular valve area, high pulsed repetition Doppler was utilized: pressure half-time of 109 ms, with a valve area of 2.02 cm^2.

Fig. 2-8.

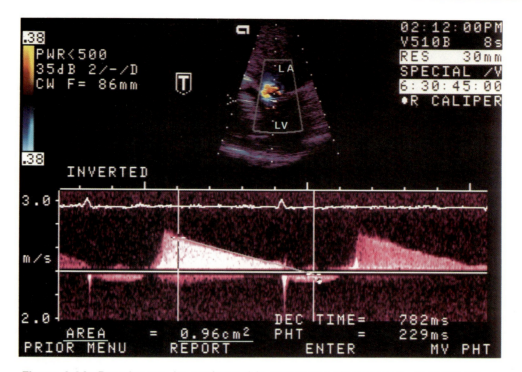

Figure 2-8A: Doppler can be performed in transverse (A) or longitudinal (B) plane. The valve area was approximately 1 cm² in both planes. Note the variation in Doppler velocity with atrial fibrillation.

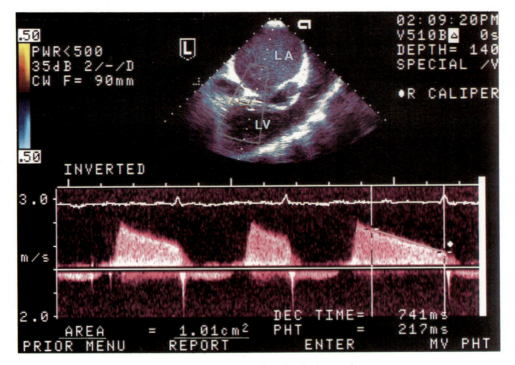

Figure 2-8B: The longitudinal plane view.

40 • Clinical Atlas of Transesophageal Echocardiography

Fig. 2-9.

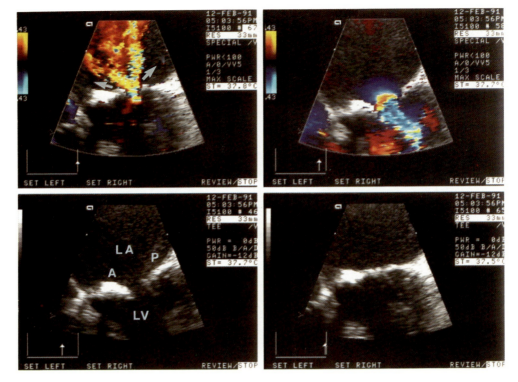

Figure 2-9: Patients with mitral stenosis may have mitral regurgitation because the leaflets are fibrosed and do not coapt well. In this sequence, a stenotic mitral valve with calcified leaflets is demonstrated in the lower left; in the lower right, systolic valve closure is demonstrated. In the upper right, diastolic inflow with an isovelocity area is demonstrated; The upper left shows multiple jets of mitral regurgitation.

Fig. 2-10.

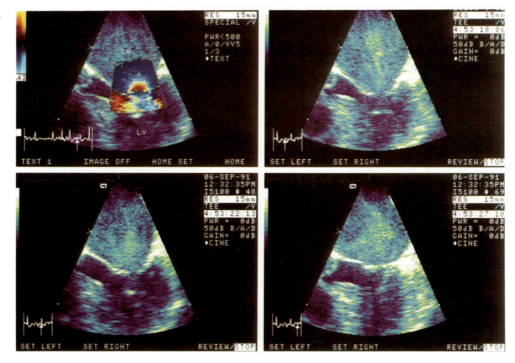

Figure 2-10A: As a consequence of mitral stenosis and atrial fibrillation, there is a large left atrium with stasis of blood documented by echogenic contrast or "smoke" seen as a dynamic, swirling, whitish haze in the left atrium.

Fig. 2-10.
(cont'd)

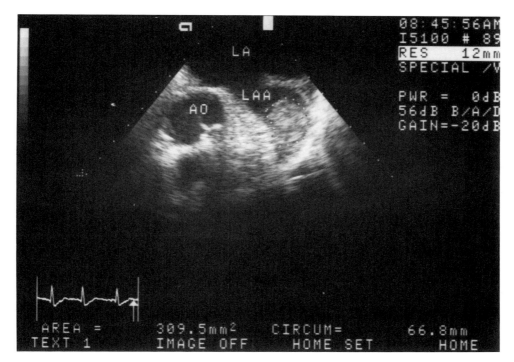

Figure 2-10B: Because of blood stasis, a left atrial appendage (LAA) thrombus developed (outlined by the circle).

Fig. 2-11.

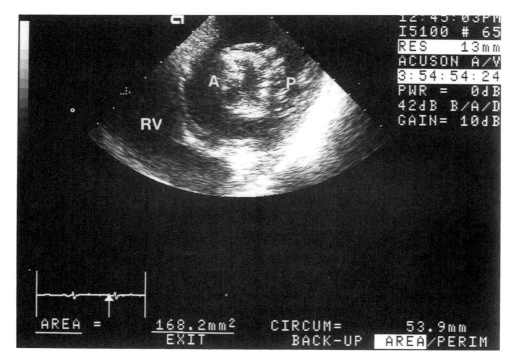

Figure 2-11A: The planimetry of the valve (see dotted outline) in the short axis subxiphoid plane yields a valve area of 1.68 cm^2. A = anterior leaflet; P = posterior leaflet.

Fig. 2-11. (cont'd)

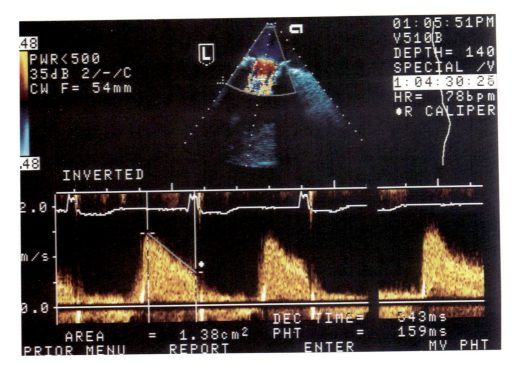

Figure 2-11B: Pressure half-time yields a valve area of 1.38 cm².

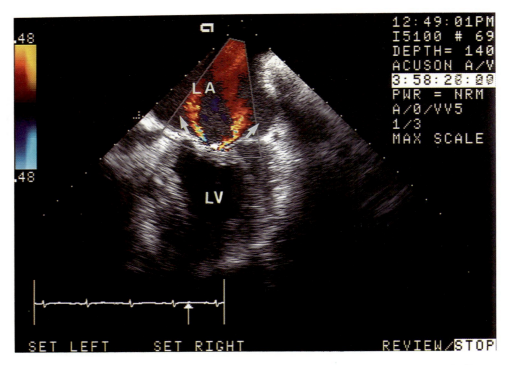

Figure 2-11C: This figure demonstrates two jets of mitral regurgitation from this fibrosed poorly coapting valve.

Mitral Regurgitation

Mitral regurgitation is one of the applications of TEE application in which a clear benefit over transthoracic echocardiography (TTE) can be demonstrated. The pathoanatomy, etiology, and severity of regurgitation can be assessed more accurately by TEE. The general approach to mitral regurgitation by either TTE or TEE echo should be to initially identify the pathophysiology causing the regurgitation by 2-D imaging. Subsequently, the amount of regurgitation should be quantified by color Doppler. Frequently, initial identification of the mechanism results in a more accurate color flow interrogation of the regurgitant jet. For instance, if in mitral valve prolapse the posterior leaflet hammocks more than the anterior leaflet, the expected regurgitant jet would be directed toward the interatrial septum. However, if the anterior leaflet prolapses more, the jet will be directed to the free wall of the left atrium.

The major etiologies of mitral regurgitation are:
1. mitral valve prolapse;
2. redundant mitral valve without prolapse;
3. ruptured chordae;
4. flail leaflet;
5. rheumatic thickened leaflets with varying degrees of mitral stenosis;
6. vegetation/abscess;
7. papillary muscle dysfunction;
8. annular dilatation (cardiomyopathy);
9. congenital cleft mitral valve;
10. calcified mitral annulus;
11. "physiological" regurgitation.

Quantification of mitral regurgitation severity is based on the length and width of the regurgitant jet compared to the size of the left atrium (similar to TTE). Because transesophageal imaging has excellent resolution, many normal mitral valves have minimal regurgitation depicted as a small low-velocity (dark red) jet emanating from the closure point of the valve leaflets. This "physiological regurgitation" may be seen more frequently in hypertensive patients with increased left ventricular pressure. This benign regurgitant jet is distinguished from pathological mitral regurgitation, by its thin small jet, short duration, and low velocity.

As valve pathology increases, causing more regurgitation, the jet becomes larger, wider, and more turbulent. Frequently, the jet may be angled anteriorly, posteriorly, laterally, or medially into the left atrium.

Importantly, though a regurgitant jet has three dimensions, echocardiography obtains only a single plane at any one time. Therefore, it is imperative to interrogate the left atrium in as many planes as possible by moving the transducer, rotating, raising, and lowering the scope to obtain a stereoscopic appreciation of the full extent of the regurgitant jet. Since color flow Doppler is a velocity map and not actual blood volume, it has limitations in quantifying valvular regurgitation. An analogy can be made to a bowling ball sent caroming down a bowling lane at high velocity impacting one, two, or three pins directly but the force imparted to those pins will knock down all 10 pins, even including those not hit directly. However, a bowling ball sent down the lane very slowly may hit the same one, two, or three pins but the energy imparted to those pins is not adequate to knock down neighboring pins. Therefore, a high velocity jet may actually recruit more color pixels, creating a regurgitant jet that is longer and wider than the same reguritant blood volume at a lower velocity. The velocity of the regurgitant jet will be determined by the force of left ventricular contractility and the pressure gradient between the left ventricle and left atrium. The orifice size will also influence jet size. For the same driving force, a small orifice will generate a longer and higher velocity jet than a wider, larger regurgitant orifice. Thus, color flow Doppler jet size is not always equivalent to the true regurgitant volume determined by cardiac catheterization. For example, a patient with cardiomyopathy and severe ventricular dysfunction may have a smaller color jet of mitral regurgitation for a given regurgitant volume than a patient with normal ventricular function. The diseased ventricle contracts less forcefully, there may be ventricular dilation and subsequent annular dilation producing a wide orifice, and left atrial pressures may be higher and left ventricular systolic presure lower, all yielding a smaller color jet.

Notwithstanding these limitations, color flow Doppler usually provides an accurate noninvasive estimate of the relative severity of mitral regurgitation. Patients with very large left atria may have underestimation of the severity of their mitral regurgitation by cardiac catheterization due to dilution of the radiopaque dye in a large left atrium. Additionally, patients may be too ill to tolerate the additional dye load during a cardiac catheterization ventriculogram and TTE may not be adequate. Thus, color flow Doppler may be invaluable in clinical decision making.

Not infrequently mitral regurgitation may reflux into the left atrium with multiple jets due to multiple sites of poor leaflet coaptation.

Another potential error in mitral regurgitation estimation is the laterally directed jet that for the same volume is depicted with a smaller color Doppler map than a central jet.

Color M-mode can also be used to determine if the jet is holosystolic, early, or midsystolic, which assists in determining lesion severity.

Rheumatic mitral regurgitation is diagnosed by the presence of a thickened valve with fibrosis or calcification causing leaflet doming and decreased mobility. Because the anterior leaflet has more free tissue than the posterior leaflet, the doming and restricted motion is more evident in the anterior leaflet, though the posterior leaflet may be more immobile. Leaflet retraction may also affect leaflet coaptation causing mitral regurgitation.

Use of the videocassette machine frame-by-frame slow motion feature or on-line cine-loop capacity facilitate better appreciation of the relative severity and origin of the jet of regurgitation which may be missed in *real* time.

Severity of regurgitation secondary to mitral valve endocarditis depends on the extent of leaflet damage: if the leaflets still coapt well, there may be only mild regurgitation. As the leaflets become more affected by the disease process, there may be more destruction and distortion of the leaflets, causing a larger regurgitant jet. Frequently, acute mitral regurgitation may generate larger jets because of hyperdynamic ventricular contractility.

Mitral regurgitation is a potential complication of balloon dilatation of mitral stenosis occurring in 25–32% patients (McKay CR, *Circulation* 77: 113–121, 1988). Since the transseptal approach is used during balloon valvuloplasty, the catheter can be guided safely (and potentially even more accurately than by fluoroscopy) through the atrial septum. The TEE can assess mitral regurgitation during the TEE procedure as well. Possibly, every premitral valvotomy patient should undergo echocardiography to exclude the presence of a thrombus in the left atrial appendage that could potentially embolize if dislodged by the catheter.

Since the color sector is narrow, it must be directed to interrogate the entire left atrium. Important features of mitral regurgitation to remember are:

1. The jets may be multiple.
2. A laterally directed jet or one that traverses along the atrial septum may be underestimated compared to a central jet.

3. Multiple planes of interrogation are required to maximize the regurgitant jet size.

4. The pathophysiology will often assist in determining the direction of the jet.

5. Studies have shown that downgrading the estimated transesophageal severity of mitral regurgitation by one full grade will better correlate the severity of mitral regurgitation depicted by TEE with the corresponding transthoracic echo.

6. The area of only the turbulent component of the color flow jet may be a better estimate of regurgitation than the entire color flow area.

Fig. 2-12.

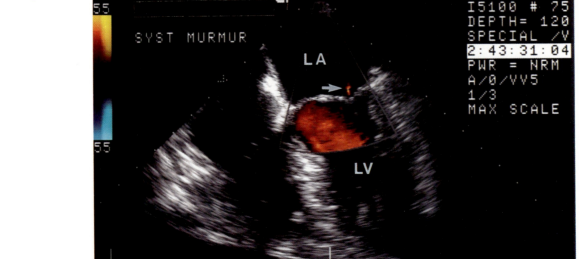

Figure 2-12: A trace amount of physiological mitral regurgitation, barely noticeable, detectable only by the sensitive TEE (transverse four chamber). LA = left atrium; LV = left ventricle.

46 • Clinical Atlas of Transesophageal Echocardiography

Fig. 2-13.

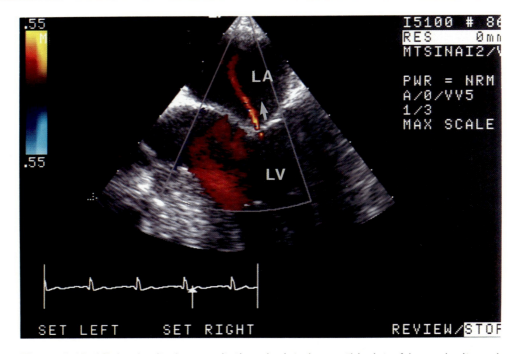

Figure 2-13: Minimal mitral regurgitation depicted as a thin jet of low-velocity red which extends and tapers into the left atrium (transverse five chamber). LA = left atrium; LV = left ventricle.

Fig. 2-14.

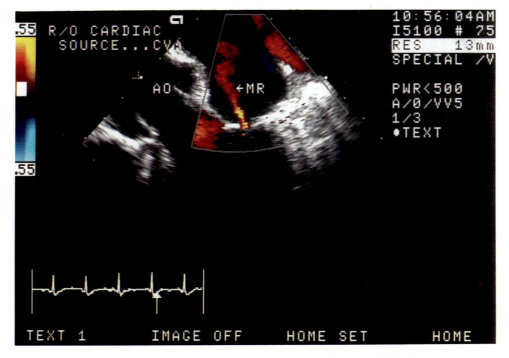

Figure 2-14: Another example of minimal mitral regurgitation (MR) (transverse five chamber). AO = aorta.

Fig. 2-15.

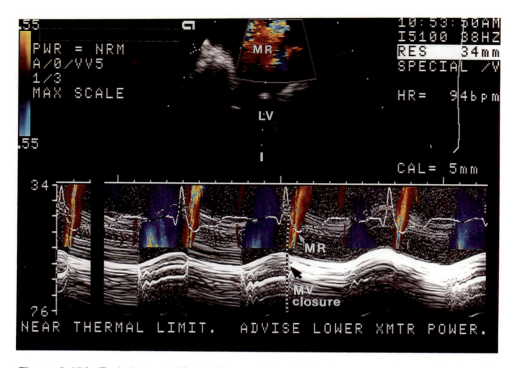

Figure 2-15A: To help quantify relative severity of mitral regurgitation, utilize the M-mode color technique which allows temporal quantification. The forward flow in blue is followed by a very brief regurgitant mitral jet seen as a reddish flame. Timing with the QRS denotes that the regurgitant jet begins with systole immediately following mitral valve closure. LV = left ventricle.

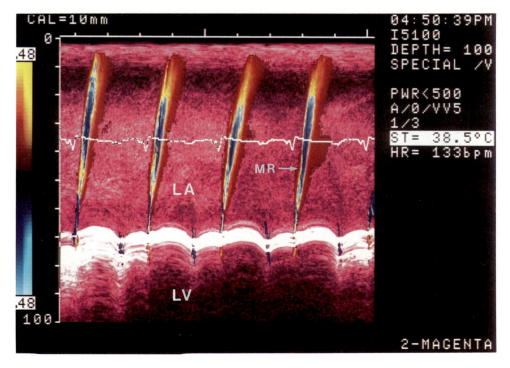

Figure 2-15B: The regurgitant jet is seen as a longer red jet into the left atrium. LA = left atrium; LV = left ventricle; MR = mitral regurgitation.

Fig. 2-16.

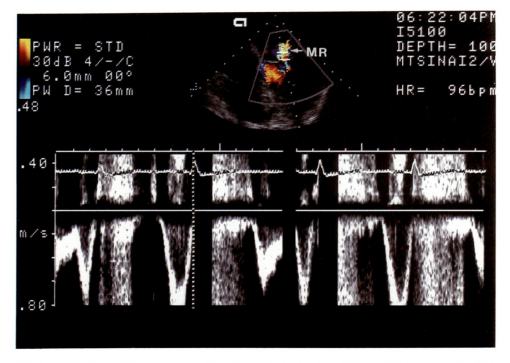

Figure 2-16: Pulsed Doppler can time the onset of regurgitation. Mitral regurgitation (MR) is seen to begin in midsystole in a patient with mitral valve prolapse (dotted line marks systolic closure of the mitral valve).

Fig. 2-17.

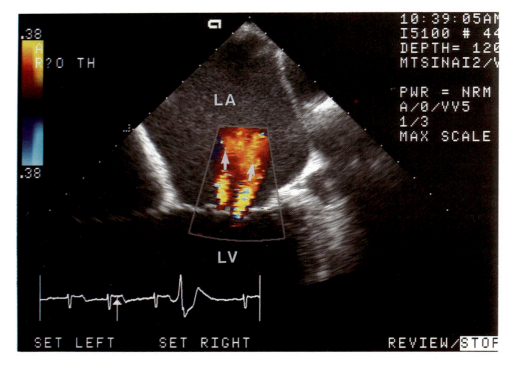

Figure 2-17: Occasionally, there may be several distinct small jets seen; this patient with mild mitral regurgitation had two distinct jets (transverse four chamber). LA = left atrium; LV = left ventricle.

Fig. 2-18.

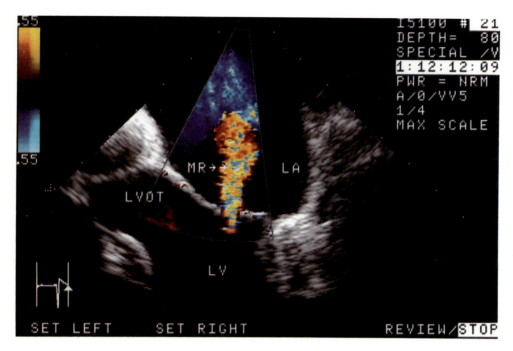

Figure 2-18: Mild mitral regurgitation (MR): the area of the mosaic jet compared to a wider jet the left atrial (LA) size, as well as it absolute length and duration determine mitral regurgitation severity (transverse five chamber). LV = left ventricle; LVOT = left ventricular outflow tract.

Fig. 2-19.

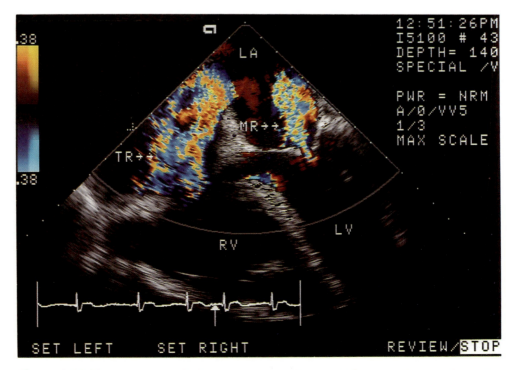

Figure 2-19: The patient has 1–2+ mitral regurgitation (MR) as well as 3+ tricuspid regurgitation (TR) (transverse four chamber). LA = left atrium; LV = left ventricle; RV = right ventricle.

Fig. 2-20.

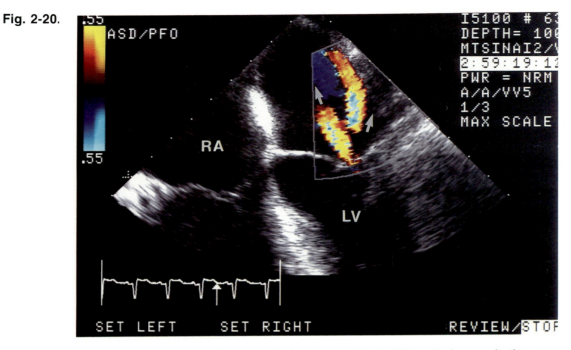

Figure 2-20: This figure demonstrates two separate jets of 2+ mitral regurgitation, one central and one extending laterally along the free wall of the left atrium. Importantly, thorough interrogation of the left atrium facilitates detection of both the origin and extent of all separate regurgitant jets. RA = right atrium; LV = left ventricle.

Fig. 2-21.

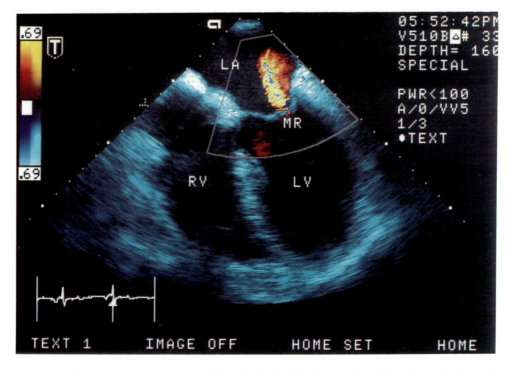

Figure 2-21: Isolated mild-moderate jet (1–2+) mitral regurgitant jet along the lateral wall of the left atrium.

Fig. 2-22.

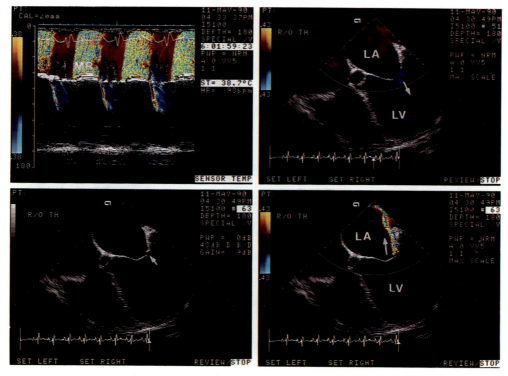

Figure 2-22: Four frames of 1–2+ mitral regurgitant jet in a patient with congestive cardiomyopathy; in the upper right, diastolic dark blue mitral inflow is seen. In the lower right, a thin jet of mitral regurgitation extends all the way to the back of the left atrium. The lower left demonstrates poor coaptation of the leaflets due to annular dilatation; the upper left color mode M-mode demonstrates that the mitral regurgitant jet is holosystolic. LA = left atrium; LV = left ventricle.

Fig. 2-23.

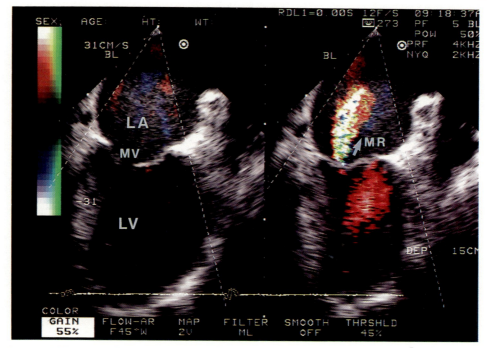

Figure 2-23: Diastolic frame on the left and a systolic regurgitant frame on the right demonstrating the origin of the mitral regurgitant jet (two-chamber longitudinal plane). LA = left atrium; LV = left ventricle; MV = mitral valve.

Fig. 2-24.

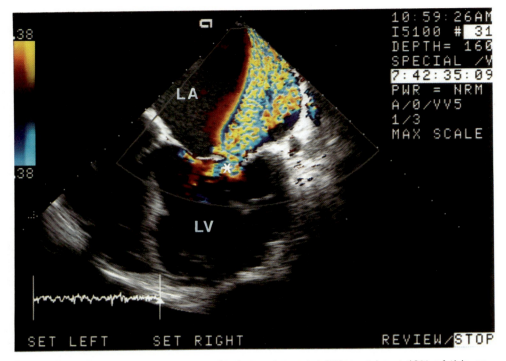

Figure 2-24: Moderate mitral regurgitation: a large jet filling at least 40% of this enlarged left atrium (LA). Importantly, the color map is turbulent and there is a proximal isovolumetric jet on the left ventricular (LV) side of the mitral valve (asterisk) consistent with a significant regurgitant volume (transverse four chamber).

Fig. 2-25.

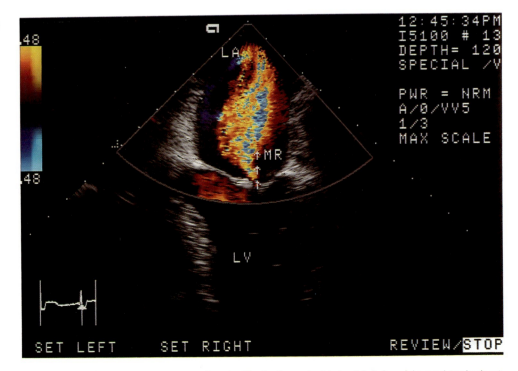

Figure 2-25: Demonstrates a moderate (3–4+) central jet which is wide and turbulent and extends to the back of the left atrium (LA), almost completely filling it. LV = left ventricle; MR = mitral regurgitation.

Fig. 2-26.

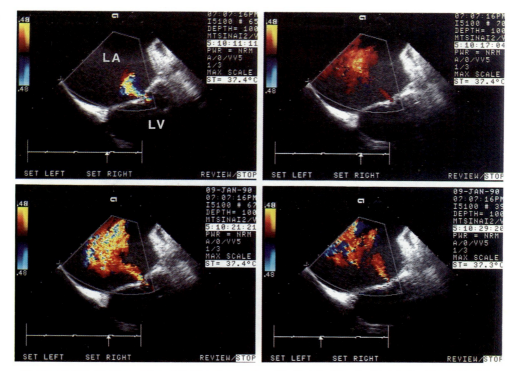

Figure 2-26: Phases of a mitral valve regurgitant jet: The upper left demonstrates onset of systole with the jet seen just behind the mitral valve; in the lower left, the jet is seen to mushroom in the middle of the left atrium (LA) filling a large part of it; in the latter part of systole the jet is seen dissipating as seen in the lower and upper right. The jet becomes smaller, less turbulent and becomes lower velocity red/orange (upper right). LV = left ventricle.

Fig. 2-27.

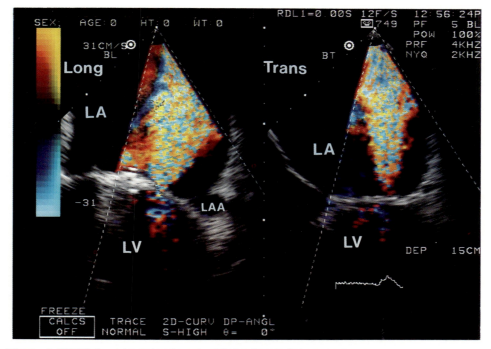

Figure 2-27: Biplane imaging is valuable in determining the full extent of mitral regurgitation. This moderate jet of mitral regurgitation is seen in both the transverse plane (Trans) (right) as well as the longitudinal plane (left). LA = left atrium; LV = left ventricle; LAA = left atrial appendage.

Fig. 2-28.

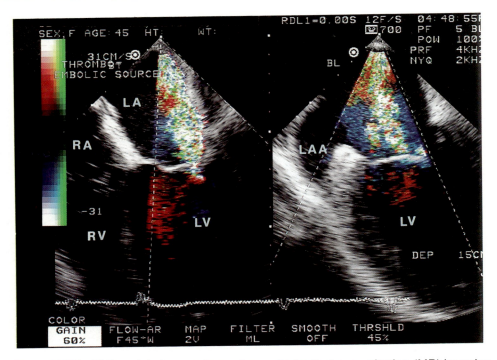

Figure 2-28A: Biplane jet shows a larger amount of mitral regurgitation (MR) by color mapping on the transverse (Trans) (left) than the longitudinal (Long) (right) plane.

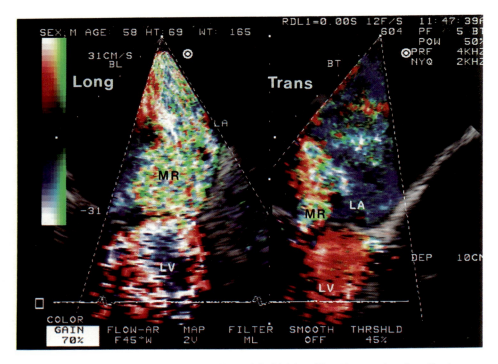

Figure 2-28B: The longitudinal plane (Long) (left) identifies the moderate mitral regurgitant jet which is only mild in the transverse plane (Trans) (right). LA = left atrium; LV = left ventricle.

Fig. 2-29.

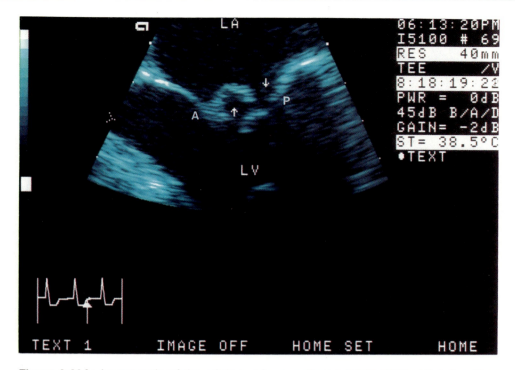

Figure 2-29A: An example of the etiology of regurgitant jet determining the direction of flow. The anterior mitral leaflet (A) does not coapt well (arrows) with the posterior leaflet (P) due to ruptured chordae; the expected moderate jet is directed along the lateral free wall of the left atrium (LA) (Fig. 2-29B). LV = left ventricle.

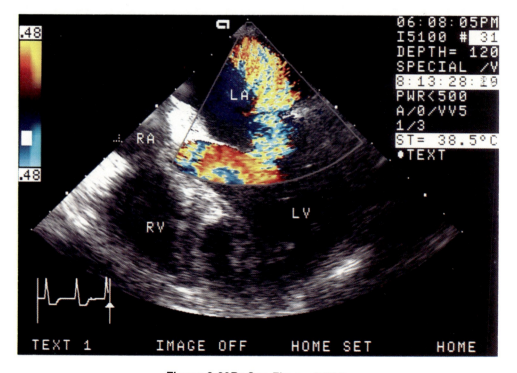

Figure 2-29B: See Figure 2-28A.

Fig. 2-30.

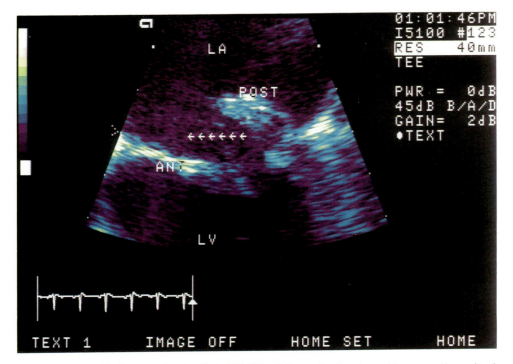

Figure 2-30A: Flail posterior leaflet (POST) of the mitral valve will cause the mitral regurgitant jet to be directed towards the interatrial septum. LA = left atrium; LV = left ventricle; ANT = anterior leaflet.

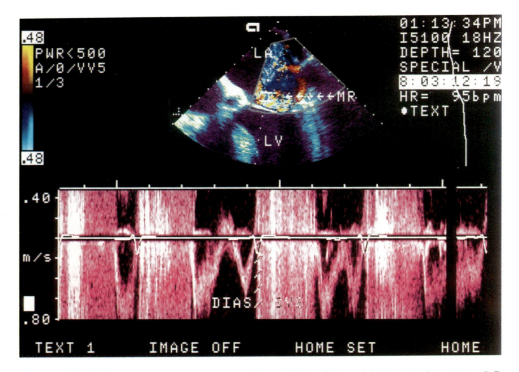

Figure 2-30B: The mitral regurgitant jet is medially directed (seen on the upper 2-D frame). The M-mode below depicts the normal biphasic diastolic mitral inflow and the holosystolic mitral regurgitant jet. LA = left atrium; LV = left ventricle.

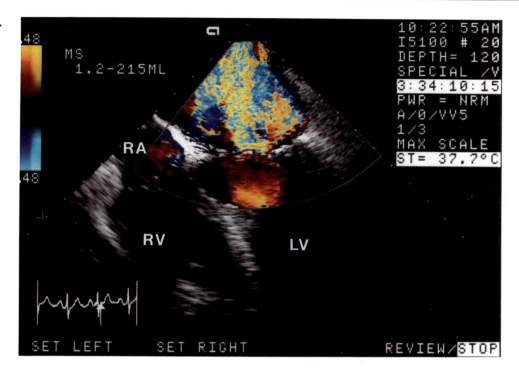

Figure 2-31A: Severe mitral regurgitation: the mitral regurgitation fills almost the entire left atrium (transverse four chamber view). RA = right atrium; RV = right ventricle; LV = left ventricle.

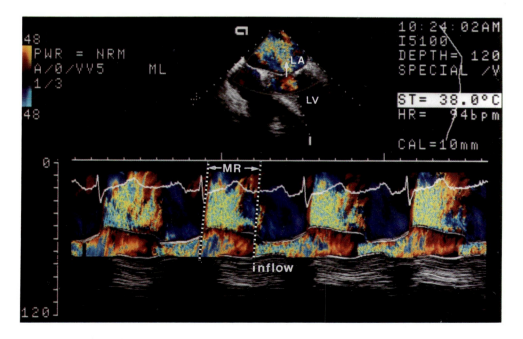

Figure 2-31B: Color M-mode (bottom) demonstrates this mitral regurgitant jet to be holosystolic (the first dotted line marks the closure of the mitral valve. Mitral regurgitation (MR) begins immediately after the valve closes and continues until the mitral valve reopens (mitral inflow is turbulent as seen on the 2D inset above). LA = left atrium; LV = left ventricle.

Fig. 2-32.

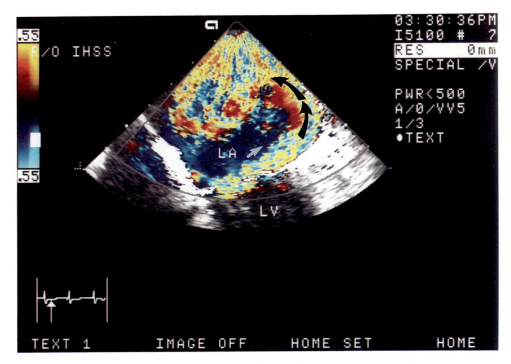

Figure 2-32: The severe mitral regurgitant jet is directed laterally and wraps around the entire left atrium (LA). LV = left ventricle.

Fig. 2-33.

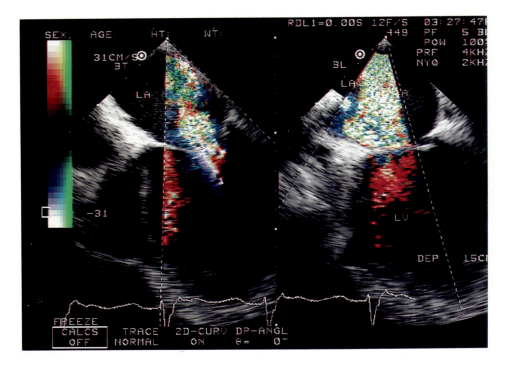

Figure 2-33: The longitudinal plane (right) demonstrates the severe mitral regurgitation better than the transverse image (left). LA = left atrium; LV = left ventricle.

Fig. 2-34.

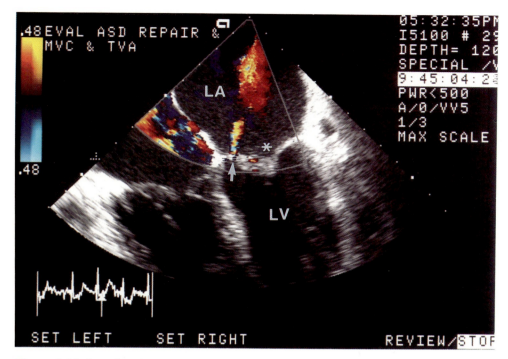

Figure 2-34: A perforation in the anterior leaflet (arrow) generates a small mitral regurgitant jet in the middle of the leaflet, not at the coaptation point (*) asterisk. LA = left atrium; LV = left ventricle.

Fig. 2-35.

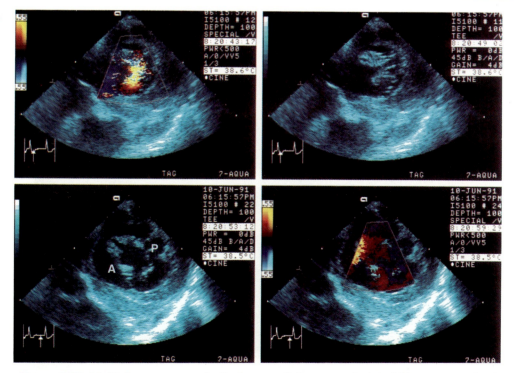

Figure 2-35: Multiple sequence of mitral regurgitation on subxiphoid transverse short axis: the lower left shows the mitral valve anterior (A) and posterior (P) leaflets open during the diastole; lower right, transmitral flow in diastole; upper right, the redundant leaflets are closed during systole; the upper left demonstrates moderate central mitral regurgitation. The ECG facilitates timing of events and frame-by-frame viewing provides more accurate analysis.

Mitral Valve Prolapse

Mitral valve prolapse is probably the most common cardiac abnormality, occurring in up to 7% of all women and 5% of all men. Valves that are thicker with more myxomatous tissue and prolapse more dramatically are usually those that develop the most significant complications, including severe mitral regurgitation, endocarditis, heart failure, and emboli. Mitral valve prolapse is usually defined by both auscultation and hammocking of either leaflet by 2 mm or more behind the annular plane as seen in the parasternal transthoracic long axis view. The exact criteria for defining prolapse in the transesophageal planes have not been established yet.

Fig. 2-36.

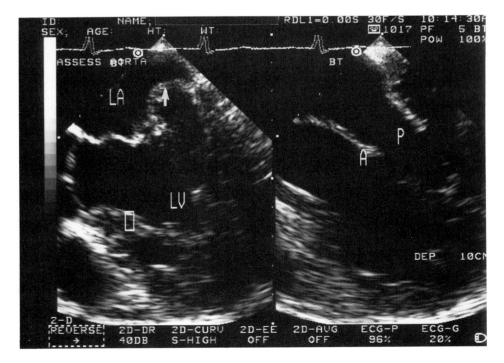

Figure 2-36: Mitral valve with normal diastolic excursion (right side) but the posterior (P) leaflet prolapses back (arrow) in systole (left side). LA = left atrium; LV = left ventricle; A = anterior leaflet.

Fig. 2-37.

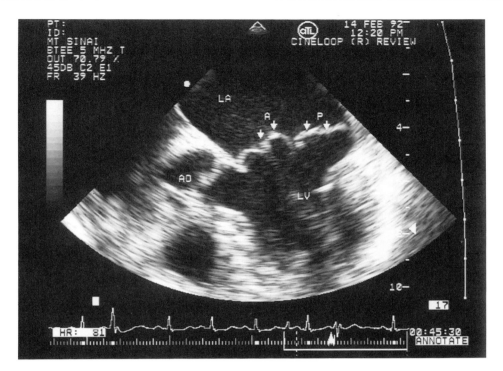

Figure 2-37A: Redundant, myxomatous valve, transverse plane: multiple hammocking segments of both the anterior (A) and the posterior (P) leaflets. LA = left atrium; LV = left ventricle; AO = aorta.

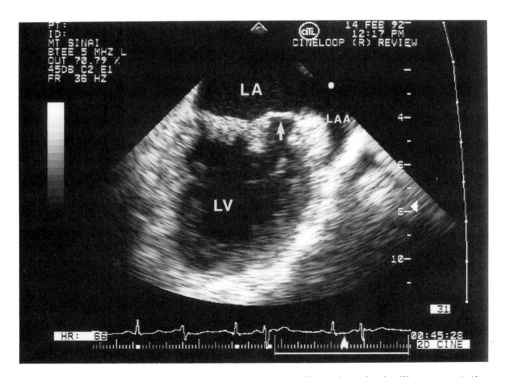

Figure 2-37B: The same floppy valve in the longitudinal plane looks like a vegetation due to the myxomatous tissue (arrow points to hammocking segment of the anterior leaflet). LA = left atrium; LV = left ventricle; LAA = left atrial appendage.

Fig. 2-38.

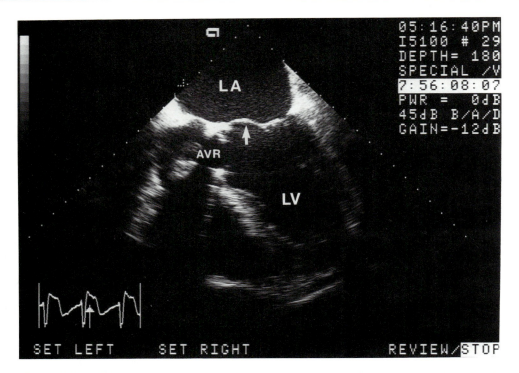

Figure 2-38A: The anterior mitral leaflet prolapses (arrow) in the transverse five-chamber view (the patient had prior aortic valve replacement, AVR). LA = left atrium; LV = left ventricle.

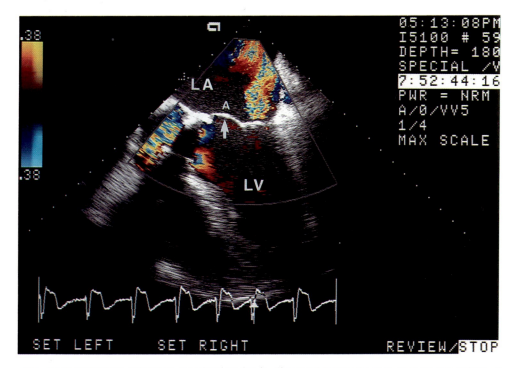

Figure 2-38B: The mitral regurgitation jet is directed laterally due to hammocking of the anterior leaflet (A). LA = left atrium; LV = left ventricle.

Mitral Valve Endocarditis

Endocarditis can have multiple clinical manifestations; it can masquerade as an insidious smoldering illness, present with severe congestive heart failure or a devastating embolic event. TTE can frequently detect a mitral vegetation. The criteria for defining a vegetation include: an echogenic density distinct from the valve leaflets, which has an amorphous fluffy appearance ("cotton ball") though it may appear more consolidated and denser in the more chronic stages. There may also be varying degrees of destruction of the valve, including torn leaflets with perforations as well as ruptured chordae and abscess formation. The mitral valve can be seen in multiple planes and should be interrogated in all views (particularily in the four- and two-chamber views) to detect small vegetations prolapsing back into the left atrium. Endocarditis usually develops on an abnormal valve, with the most common predisposing factor being mitral regurgitation. Thus, according to pathophysiological principles, the vegetation will develop in the area of turbulence, which in the case of mitral regurgitation is on the left atrial side of the mitral valve.

Sensitivity of Transesophageal Echocardiography (TEE) Versus Transthoracic Echocardiography (TTE) in Detecting Endocarditis

Author	Reference #	# of Patients	TEE	TTE
Daniel	9	69	94%	40%
Erbel	4	96	82%	44%
Mugge	6	80	90%	58%
Shiveley	2	62	94%	44%

Bibliography

1. Sanfilippo AJ, Picard MN, Newell JB, et al: Echocardiographic assessment of patients with infectious endocarditis: prediction of risk for complications. *J Am Coll Cardiol* 1:1191–1199, 1991.
2. Shively BK, Gurule FT, Roldan CA, et al: Diagnostic value of transesophageal compared with transthoracic echocardiography in infective endocarditis. *J Am Coll Cardiol* 18:391–397, 1991.
3. Daniel WG, Mugge A, Martin RP, et al: Improvement in the diagnosis of abscesses associated with endocarditis by transesophageal echocardiography. *N Engl J Med* 324:795–800, 1991.
4. Erbel R, Rohman S, Drexler M, Mohr Kahaly S, Gerharz CD, Iverson S, Olert H, Meyer J: Improved diagnostic value of echocardiography in patients with infective endocarditis by transesophageal approaches: A prospective study. *Eur Heart J* 9:43–53, 1988.
5. Taams MA, Gussenhoven EJ, Bos E, deJaegre P, Roelandt JR, Sutherland GR, Bom N: Enhanced morphological diagnosis in infective endocarditis by transesophageal echocardiography. *Br Heart J* 63:109–113, 1990.
6. Mugge A, Daniel WG, Gunter F, Lichtlen P: Echocardiography in infective endocarditis: Reassessment of prognostic implications of vegetation size determined by tranthoracic and the transesophageal approach. *J Am Coll Cardiol* 14:631–638, 1989.

7. Rohmann S, Seifer T, Erbel R, Jakob H, et al: Identification of abscess formation in native valve infective endocarditis using transesophageal echocardiography: Implications for timely surgical treatment. *Thorac Cardiovasc Surg* 39:273–280, 1991.
8. Gussenhoven EJ, Van Herwerden LA, Roelandt TC Jr, Bos E, de Jong N: Detailed analysis of aortic valve endocarditis: comparison of precordial, esophageal and epicardial two-dimensional echocardiography with surgical findings. *J Cardiac Ultrasound* 14:209–211, 1986.
9. Daniel WG, Shroder RE, et al: Conventional and transesophageal echocardiography in the diagnosis of infective endocarditis. *Eur Heart J* 8(Suppl): 287–292, 1987.

Fig. 2-39.

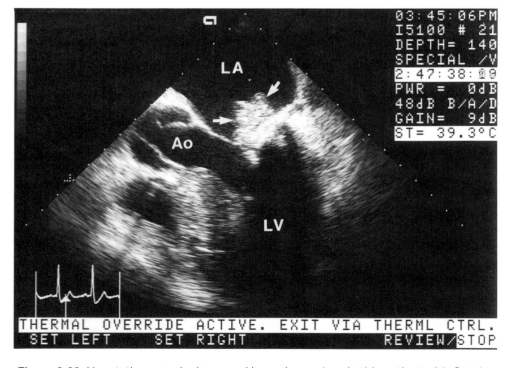

Figure 2-39: Vegetations can be large and irregular such as in this patient with *Staphylococcus aureus* mitral endocarditis (transverse five-chamber view). The vegetation is on the left atrial side of the posterior leaflet. LA = left atrium; LV = left ventricle; Ao = aorta.

Fig. 2-40.

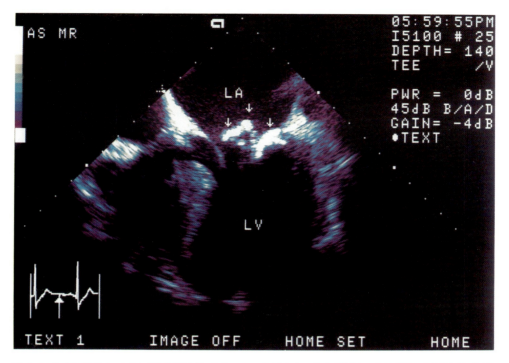

Figure 2-40: Color echo highlighting the posterior leaflet with vegetations prolapsing (arrows) into the left atrium. LA = left atrium; LV = left ventricle.

Fig. 2-41.

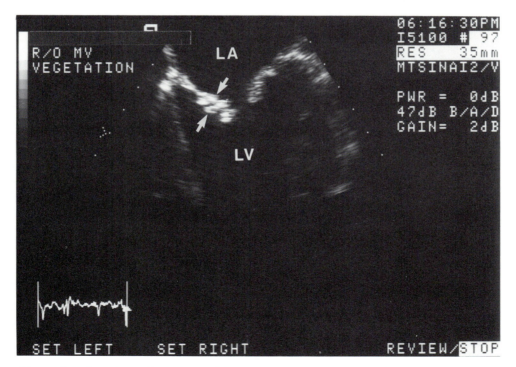

Figure 2-41A: Anterior leaflet vegetation appears irregularly lobulated or nodular (arrows) compared to the posterior leaflet. LA = left atrium; LV = left ventricle.

Fig. 2-41.
(cont'd)

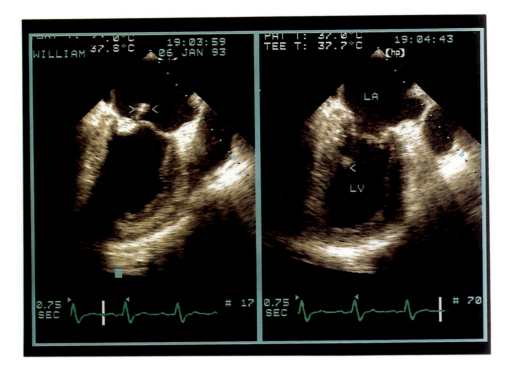

Figure 2-41B: Mitral valve vegetation on the posterior leaflet (right side, arrowhead), prolapses back into the left atrium in systole (left side, arrowheads) (longitudinal plane). LA = left atrium; LV = left ventricle.

Fig. 2-42.

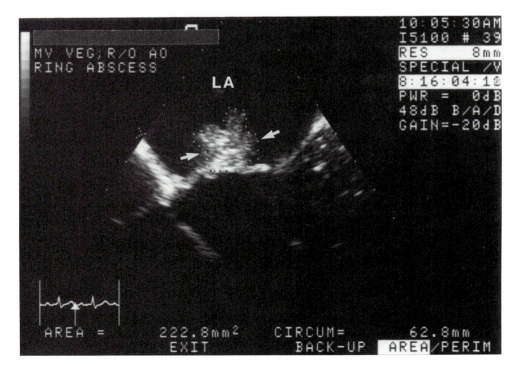

Figure 2-42A: A large fungal vegetation (arrows) on the anterior leaflet of the mitral valve, measuring 2.2 cm^2 with consequent significant mitral regurgitation. LA = left atrium.

Fig. 2-42.
(cont'd)

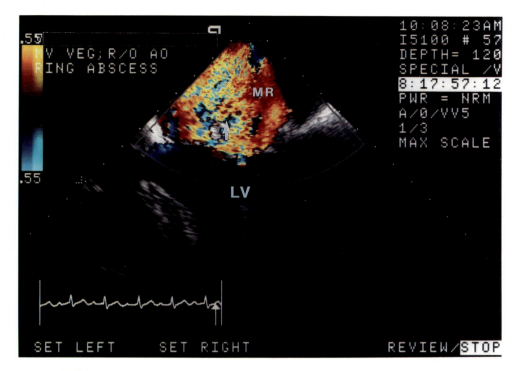

Figure 2-42B: The large mass causes poor coaptation of the leaflets, producing severe mitral regurgitation (MR). LV = left ventricle.

Fig. 2-43.

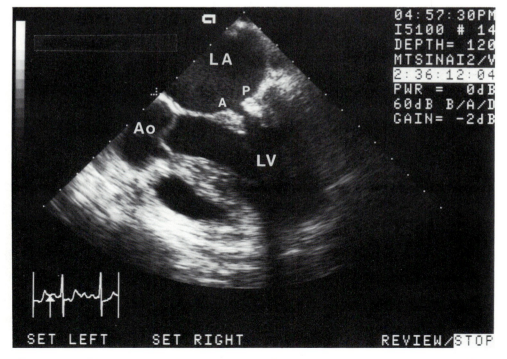

Figure 2-43: Both anterior (A) and posterior (P) leaflets are infected (transverse five-chamber view). LA = left atrium; LV = left ventricle; Ao = aorta.

Fig. 2-44.

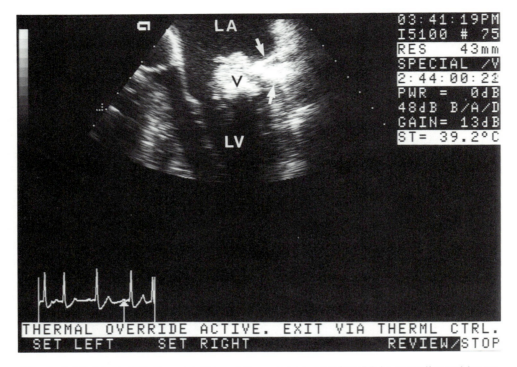

Figure 2-44: Large mitral vegetation of the posterior leaflet (V) is complicated by an abscess of the posterior annulus, seen as a dense white mass (arrows) with a lucent center. LA = left atrium; LV = left ventricle.

Fig. 2-45.

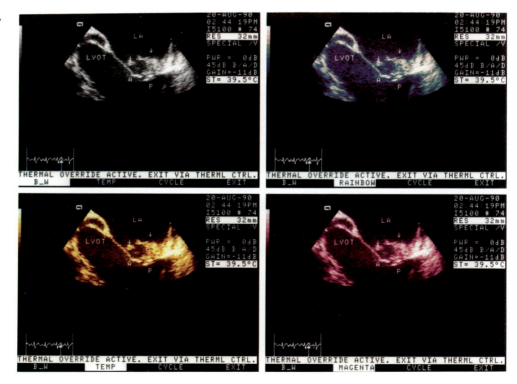

Figure 2-45: B-color can occasionally help outline vegetations and abnormalities of the valve. Several different B-color maps are used to highlight a large vegetation on the posterior leaflet (P) and two pedunculated segments which prolapse into the left atrium (LA). A = anterior leaflet; LVOT = left ventricular outflow tract.

Fig. 2-46.

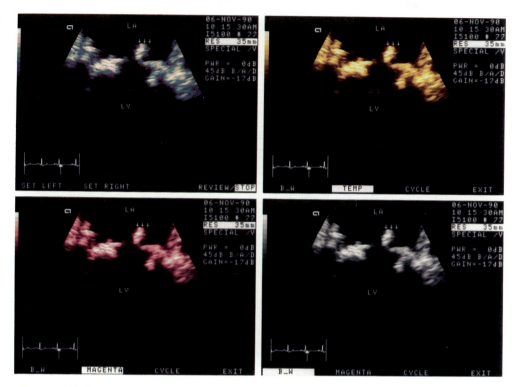

Figure 2-46: B-color image of dense vegetations on both anterior and posterior leaflet with a segment of the posterior leaflet flailing into the left atrium (LA, arrows). LV = left ventricle.

Fig. 2-47.

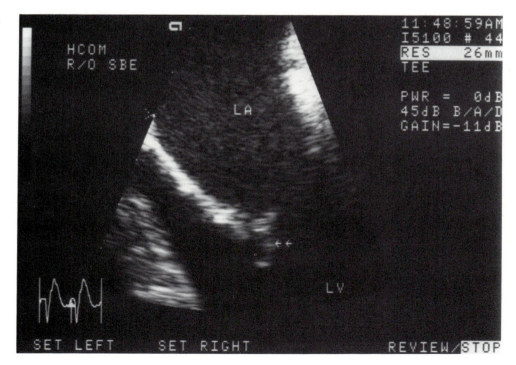

Figure 2-47A: A very small vegetation on the anterior leaflet causes (arrows) prolapse creating a regurgitant jet along the lateral wall of the left atrium (LA) (Fig. 2-47B). LV = left ventricle.

Fig. 2-47. (cont'd)

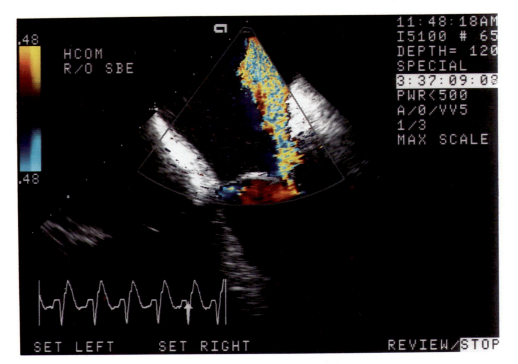

Figure 2-47B.

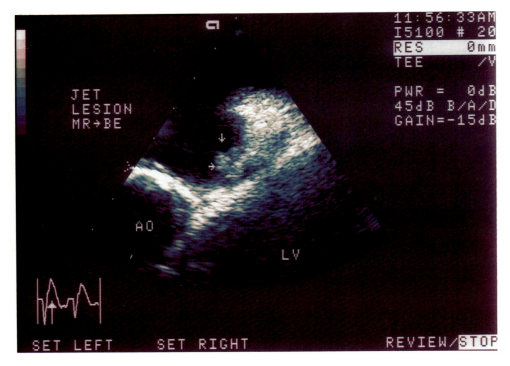

Figure 2-47C: As a complication of this lateral jet, a vegetation developed along the left atrial free wall, distant from the valve (the arrows point to a small pedunculated segment). A complete, comprehensive exam is important to detect these unusual complications. LA = left atrium; LV = left ventricle; AO = aorta.

Fig. 2-48.

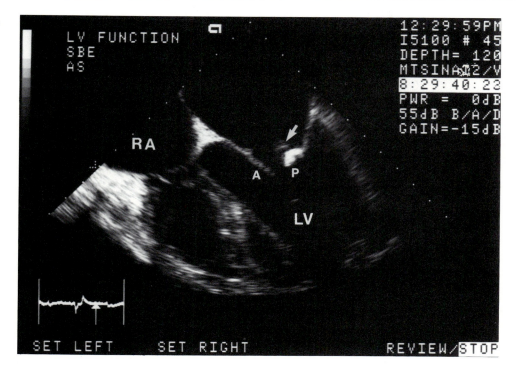

Figure 2-48A: A 43-year-old woman with several weeks of fever presented with congestive heart failure. The transesophageal echocardiogram demonstrates posterior leaflet (P) density with a pedunculated mass at its tip, consistant with a vegetation (arrow). RA = right atrium; LV = left ventricle; A = anterior leaflet.

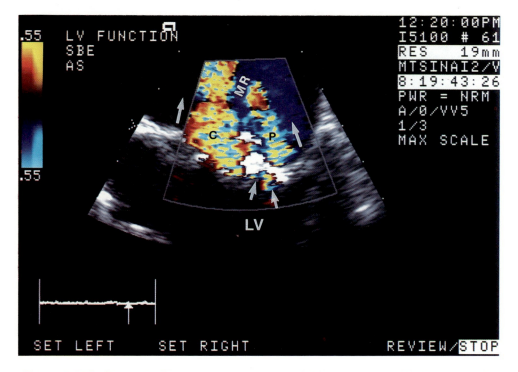

Figure 2-48B: The color Doppler demonstrates mild to moderate mitral regurgitation (MR), with a central MR jet (C), as well as a smaller lateral jet due to a perforation (P) on the posterior leaflet (P, two small arrows). LV = left ventricle.

Mitral Valve Replacement: Ball Valves

The ball-valve-in-cage prosthetic device first introduced by Starr in the early 1960s is still utilized though it is implanted much less commonly than the lower profile disc valves. The ball prosthesis consists of a ball suspended in a cage formed by the three struts. The ball prosthesis cage protrudes into the left ventricle and has a distinct Doppler flow velocity profile: the blood has to circumnavigate around the ball, creating two distinct jets as the blood enters into the left ventricle. Potential prosthetic valve problems include thrombosis, endocarditis, paravalvular leak, and dehiscence.

Fig. 2-49.

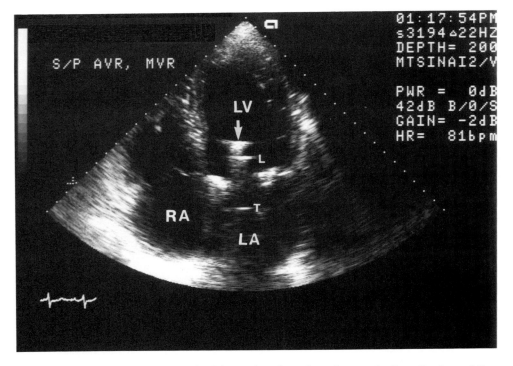

Figure 2-49A: Transthoracic apical four-chamber view demonstrating the top of the cage (arrow) projected into the left ventricle (LV) and the leading (L) and trailing (T) edges of the ball valve. Note extra echoes in the left atrium (LA) due to shadowing from the ball valve projecting into the LA.

Fig. 2-49. (cont'd)

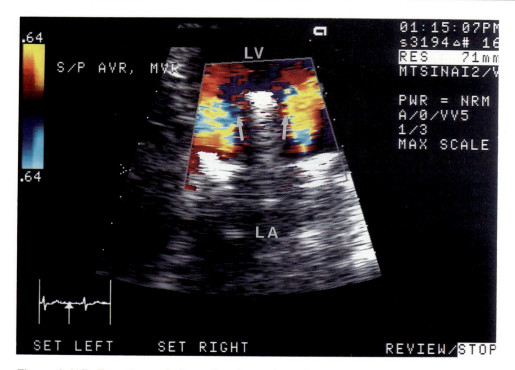

Figure 2-49B: Transthoracic four-chamber apical view. Two distinct jets (arrows) are seen going around the ball entering into the left ventricle (LV). Extra echoes shadowing into the left atrium (LA) would obscure detection of mitral regurgitation.

Fig. 2-50.

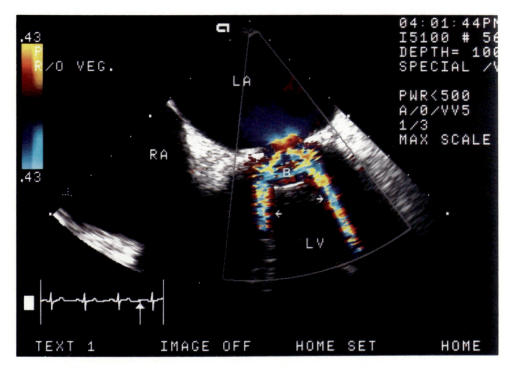

Figure 2-50: Transesophageal transverse four-chamber view. Two distinct jets of color flow are seen entering into the left ventricle (LV, arrows). The ball (B) is presented as the bluish oval in the middle of the flow velocity profile. With TEE, the ball valve projects shadows forward into the LV, while the left atrium (LA) is free of artifacts. RA = right atrium.

Fig. 2-51.

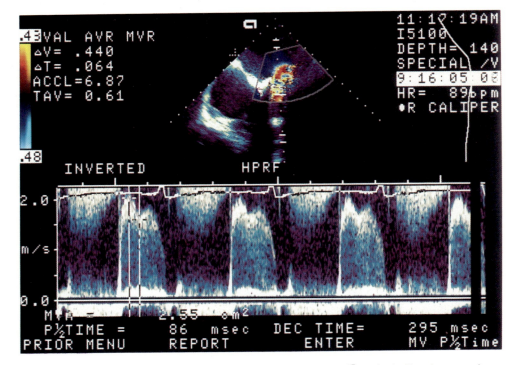

Figure 2-51: Doppler pressure half-time through Starr-Edwards ball valve requires placing the sample volume into one of the two parallel inflow jets. The valve area was 2.55 cm².

Fig. 2-52.

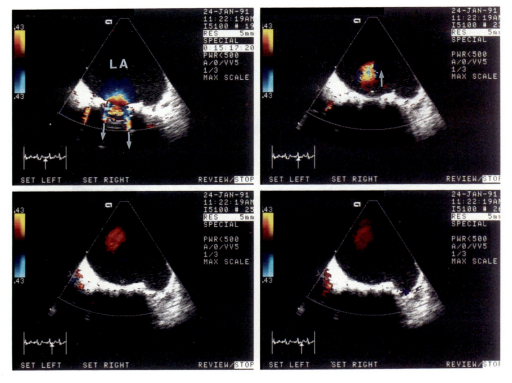

Figure 2-52: Sequence of flow dynamics of a ball valve. The upper left demonstrates two jets of mitral inflow during diastole around the ball valve. The upper right demonstrates mild mitral regurgitation, which is acceptable for a ball valve. The low velocity regurgitant jet dissipates in the left atrium in the two lower figures.

Fig. 2-53.

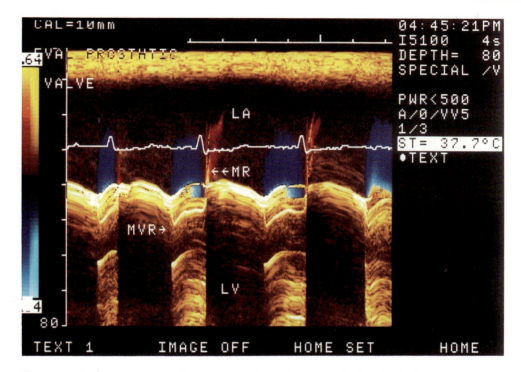

Figure 2-53: Color M-mode Starr-Edwards valve demonstrates diastolic heavy reverberation of echoes into the left ventricle (MVR). Systole is marked by minimal early mitral regurgitation (MR) in red.

Fig. 2-54.

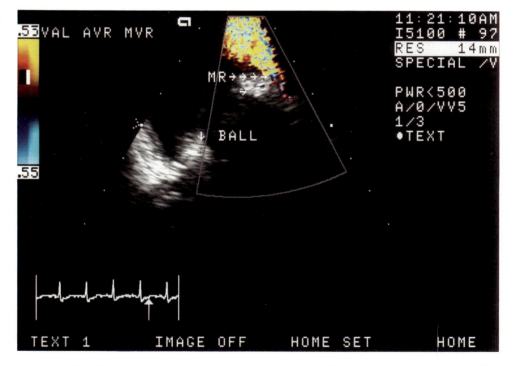

Figure 2-54: Mitral regurgitation paravalvular leak: systolic frame demonstrates the two struts (single arrows) with the ball seated within them. The mitral regurgitation jet (MR) is emanating from the lateral border of the sewing ring and is clearly a paravalvular jet of mitral regurgitation.

Fig. 2-55.

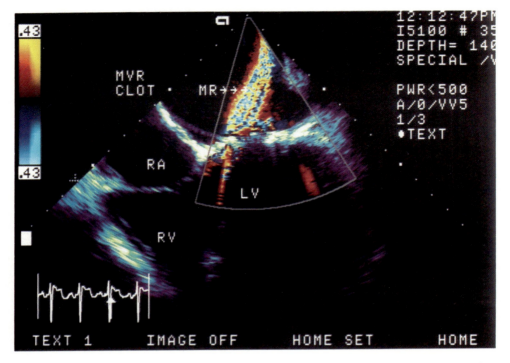

Figure 2-55A: Four-chamber transverse plane Starr-Edwards prosthesis. An excessive amount of mild-moderate mitral regurgitation (MR) originating from the medial border of the prosthesis. RA = right atrium; RV = right ventricle; LV = left ventricle.

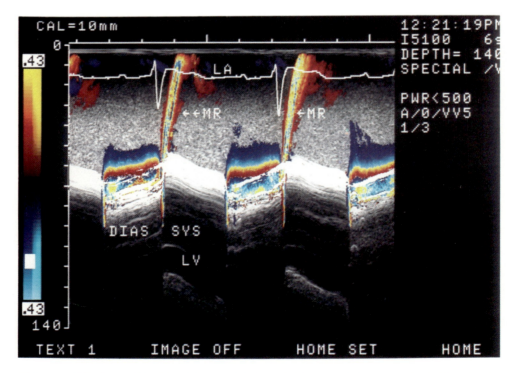

Figure 2-55B: Color flow M-mode demonstrated the high velocity jet of mitral regurgitation (MR) initiating immediately with onset of systole (SYS). Note the high velocity jet compared to the lower velocity normal regurgitation in Figure 2-53. LA = left atrium; LV = left ventricle; DIAS = diastole.

Fig. 2-55. (cont'd)

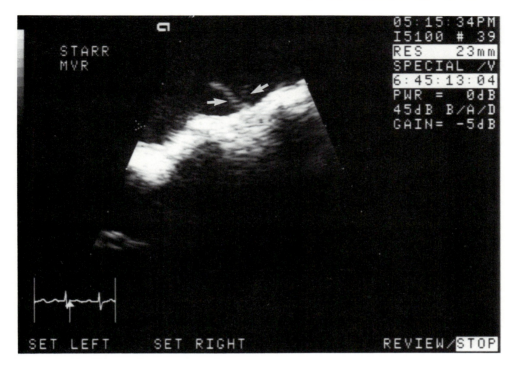

Figure 2-55C: Further investigation of the left atrial side of the ball valve demonstrated several mobile strands of fibrin (arrows).

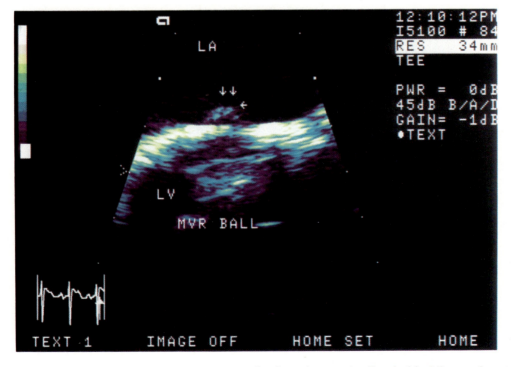

Figure 2-55D: Color B-mode demonstrated a thrombus protruding behind the sewing ring into the left atrium (arrows). LA = left atrium; LV = left ventricle.

Mitral Valve Replacement: Disc Valve Prosthesis

Disc valves may consist of two semilunar discs (St. Judes) or a single-hinged or free-floating disc valve (Medtronic-Hall, Omniscience).

Prosthetic valves may develop dysfunction secondary to endocarditis, thrombosis, paravalvular leak, dehiscence, or strut fracture. Because of the shadowing created by the metallic sewing ring, struts, and valve itself, TTE frequently cannot adequately evaluate the presence of prosthetic valve dysfunction even if there is extensive mitral regurgitation. TEE provides a total panoramic view of the left atrium. Therefore, the extent of mitral regurgitation is easily discerned. Also, with better resolution than TTE, TEE can visualize small fibrin strands or vegetations on the valve.

Fig. 2-56.

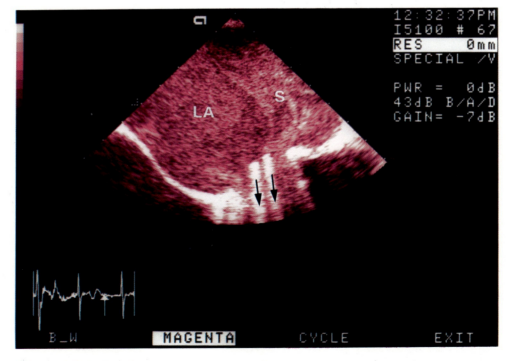

Figure 2-56A: The St. Judes prosthetic valve consists of two semilunar discs that ideally open parallel to flow (two arrows). This patient had echogenic smoke (S) in the left atrium (LA).

Fig. 2-56.
(cont'd)

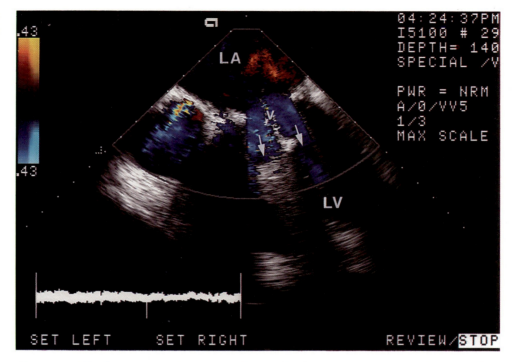

Figure 2-56B: Transverse plane: the mitral valve is seen as a central linear white density (V). There are two inflow jets seen with no turbulence by color Doppler.

Fig. 2-57.

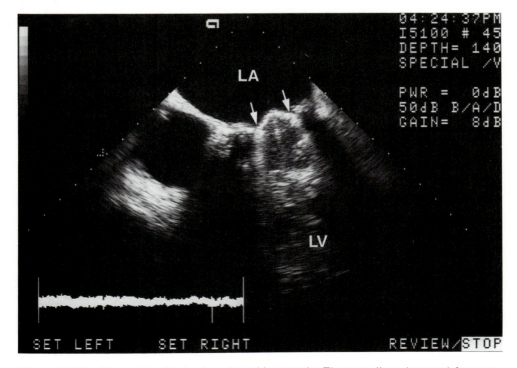

Figure 2-57A: St. Judes mitral valve closed in systole. The two discs (arrows) form an inverted "V." Note the shadowing in the left ventricle (LV). LA = left atrium.

80 • Clinical Atlas of Transesophageal Echocardiography

Fig. 2-57. (cont'd)

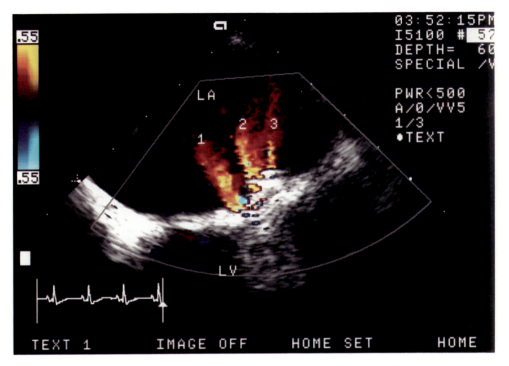

Figure 2-57B: St. Judes mitral valve in systole, with color Doppler. Three distinct jets of minimal regurgitation are normal for this valve. LA = left atrium; LV = left ventricle.

Fig. 2-58.

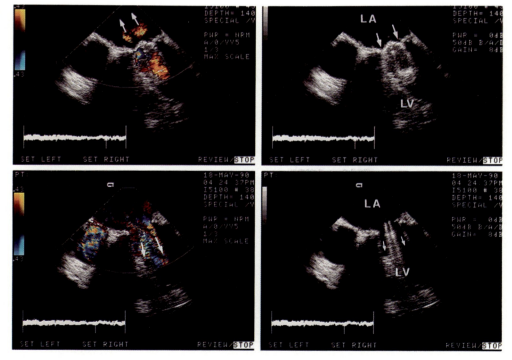

Figure 2-58: Multisequence of normal St. Judes valve. The upper right demonstrates systolic opening; the lower left depicts color Doppler in diastole; the upper left shows minimal systolic regurgitation. LA = left atrium; LV = left ventricle.

Fig. 2-59.

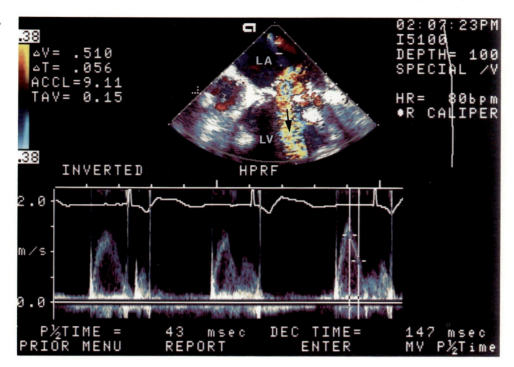

Figure 2-59A: Single disc mitral valve (Omniscience) in diastole. One major inflow jet is seen (arrow). Doppler pressure half-times can calculate valve area. LA = left atrium; LV = left ventricle.

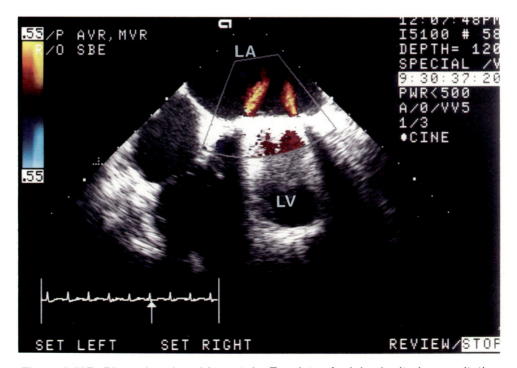

Figure 2-59B: Disc valve closed in systole. Two jets of minimal mitral regurgitation are normal for this valve. LA = left atrium; LV = left ventricle.

Fig. 2-60.

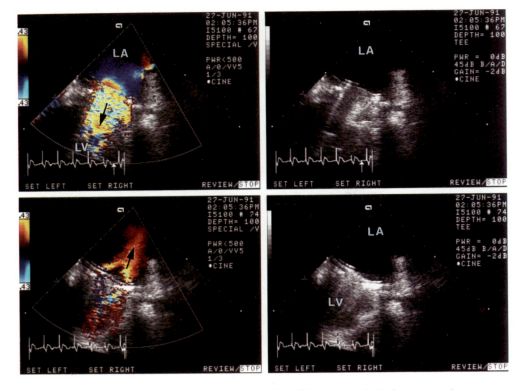

Figure 2-60: Multisequence of single disc valve. The upper right images valve open in diastole; in the lower right, the valve is closed; the upper left is color Doppler view of diastolic inflow; the lower right shows two jets of mitral regurgitation, which is acceptable for a large orifice disc valve. LA = left atrium; LV = left ventricle.

Fig. 2-61.

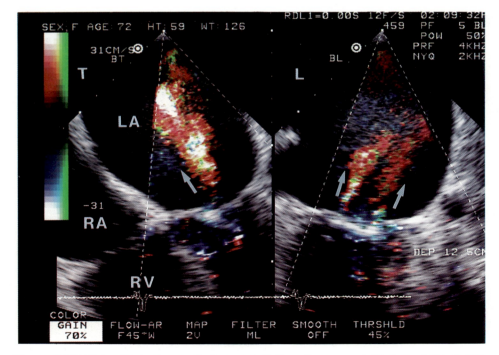

Figure 2-61: Disc mitral valve, systolic regurgitation. Transverse (T) plane (left) demonstrates a single jet, while the longitudinal (L) plane (right) images two distinct jets. LA = left atrium; RA = right atrium; RV = right ventricle.

Fig. 2-62.

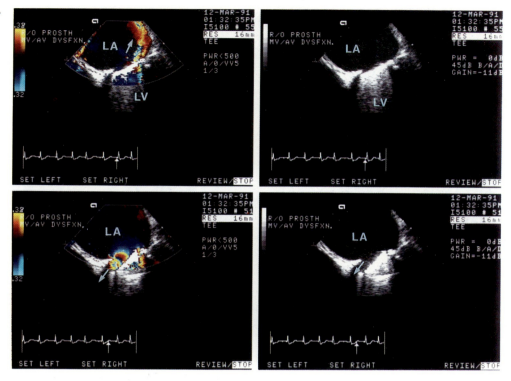

Figure 2-62: Multisequence of disc valve paravalvular leak. The upper right depicts valve systolic closure; in the lower right, the valve is tilted open; the lower left demonstrates mitral inflow; the upper left images a moderate paravalvular jet extending along the lateral atrial wall. LA = left atrium; LV = left ventricle.

Fig. 2-63.

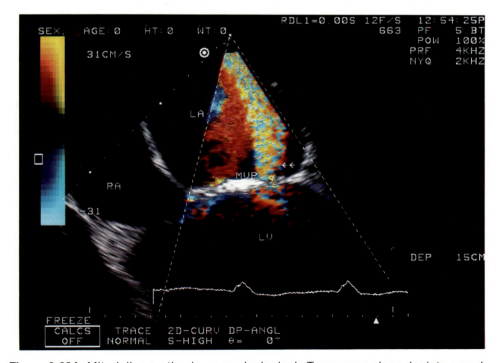

Figure 2-63A: Mitral disc prothesis, paravalvular leak. Transverse plane depicts a moderate regurgitant leak. LA = left atrium; LV = left ventricle; RA = right atrium; MVR = mitral valve replacement.

Fig. 2-63. (cont'd)

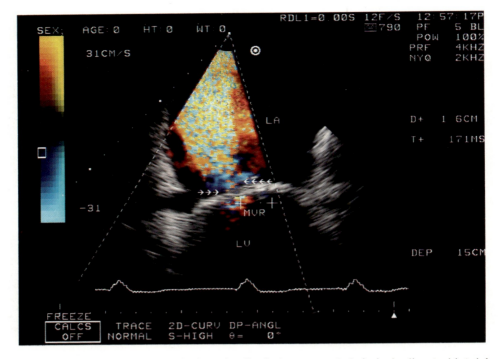

Figure 2-63B: Paravalvular leak. Longitudinal plane reveals inferiorly directed jet. LA = left atrium; LV = left ventricle; MVR = mitral valve replacement.

Fig. 2-64.

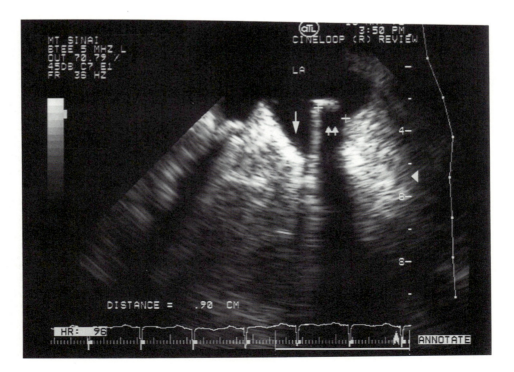

Figure 2-64A: Severe paravalvular leak, longitudinal plane. Diastolic frame images the valve open (single arrow) and the partial dehiscence (double arrow) measuring 0.9 cm. LA = left atrium.

Fig. 2-64. (cont'd)

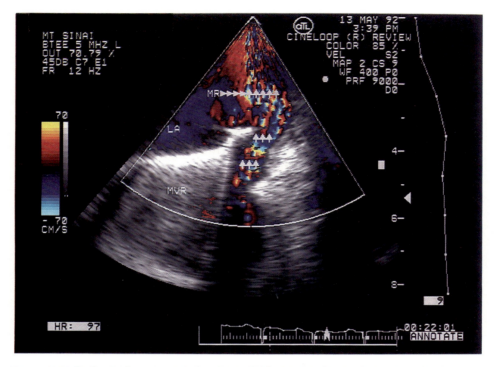

Figure 2-64B: Color Doppler confirms the dehiscence with a moderate systolic regurgitant jet (MR, arrows). LA = left atrium; MVR = mitral valve replacement.

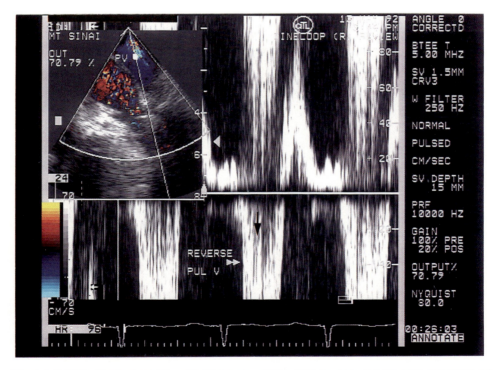

Figure 2-64C: Hemodynamic significance of the MR is documented by reversal of early systolic (see ECG) pulmonary vein (Pul V) inflow (arrow). Note sample volume in left upper pulmonary vein in upper left.

Fig. 2-65.

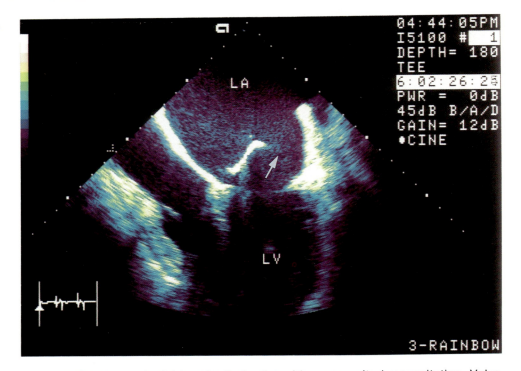

Figure 2-65A: Dramatic dehisced mitral valve with severe mitral regurgitation. Valve in systole clearly swings into the left atrium (LA, arrow). LV = left ventricle.

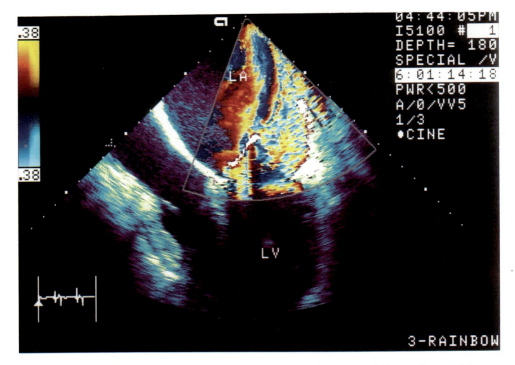

Figure 2-65B: Severe mitral regurgitation. LA = left atrium; LV = left ventricle.

Fig. 2-65.
(cont'd)

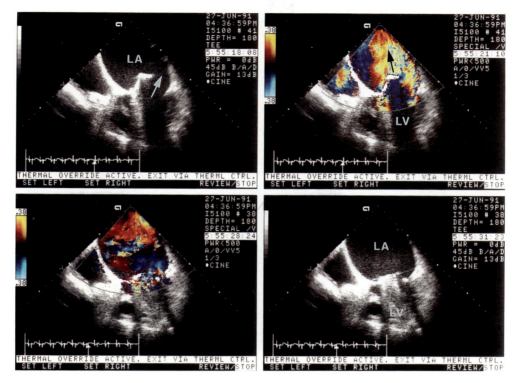

Figure 2-65C: Sequence of dehisced mitral disc valve. In the lower left and right, the valve is seated in very early systole before regurgitation occurs; the upper left reveals the detached lateral aspect of the prosthesis, confirmed by color Doppler, upper right. LA = left atrium; LV = left ventricle.

Fig. 2-66.

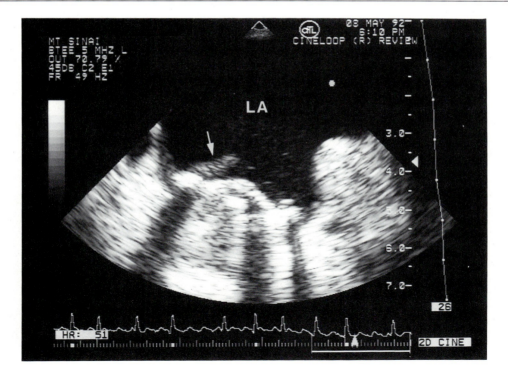

Figure 2-66A: Small vegetation on mitral double disc (St. Judes) disc valve, left atrial (LA) side (longitudinal plane).

Fig. 2-66. (cont'd)

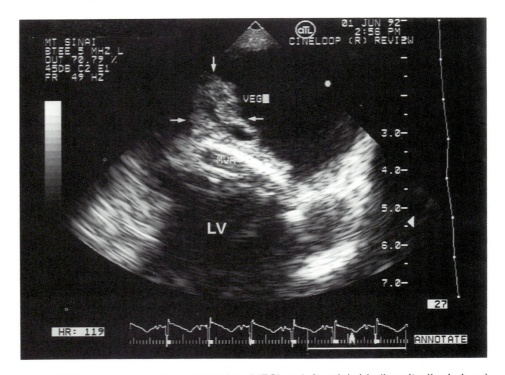

Figure 2-66B: Larger, complex vegetation (VEG) on left atrial side (longitudinal plane). Endocarditis is more prone to develop on the atrial side because of the turbulence created by the inherent regurgitation into the LA and more of the sewing ring is in the LA. LV = left ventricle; MVR = mitral valve replacement.

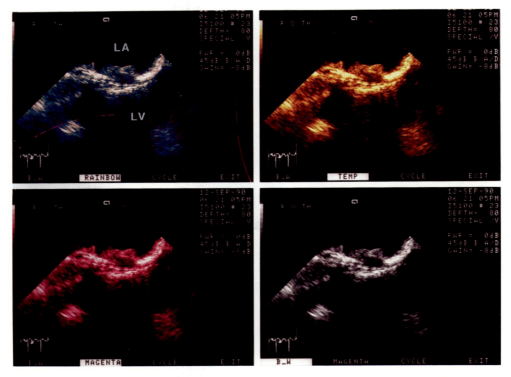

Figure 2-66C: Color B-mode may assist in detection of valve endocarditis or thrombosis. This thrombus in a patient with an embolic event was confirmed to be sterile at surgery. LA = left atrium; LV = left ventricle.

Mitral Valve Replacement: Heterografts

Heterografts are tissue valves—either a native porcine aortic valve or a reconstructed pericardial valve to conform to the mitral orifice. Tissue valves have distinct advantages over mechanical valves because they are less thrombogenic. Anticoagulation is usually indicated only for the first few months following surgical implantation. Subsequently, the patient does not require chronic anticoagulation (unless the patient is in atrial fibrillation). Also, because of their lower profile, heterografts may cause less left ventricular outflow tract obstruction and interfere less with normal ventricular contraction since the chordae tendineae can remain attached to at least the posterior annulus. Additionally, porcine heterografts have a lower incidence of endocarditis than mechanical valves possibly because of the decreased capacity for bacteria to adhere to the tissue surface compared to the mechanical valve surface.

Bibliography

1. Nellessen U, Schnittger I, Appleton CP, Masuyama T, Bolger A, Fishell TA, Tye T, Popp RL: Transesophageal two-dimensional echocardiography and color Doppler velocity mapping in the evaluation of cardiac valve prostheses. *Circulation* 78:848–855, 1988.
2. Taams MA, Gussenhover EJ, Cahalan MK, Roclandt TC Jr., Herwerden LA, The HE, Bom N, Jong N: Transesophageal Doppler color flow imaging in the detection of native and Bjork-Shiley mitral valve regurgitation. *J Am Coll Cardiol* 13:95–99, 1989.
3. Khanderia BK, Seward JB, Oh JK, et al: Value and limitation of transesophageal echocardiography in assessment of mitral valve prothesis. *Circulation* 83:956–968, 1991.
4. Scott PJ, Ettles DF, Wharton GA, Williams GJ: The value of transesophageal echocardiography in the investigation of acute prosthetic valve dysfunction. *Clin Cardiol* 13:541–544, 1990.
5. Ramirez ML, Wong M, Sadler N, Shah PM: Doppler evaluation of bioprosthetic and mechanical aortic valves: data from four models in 107 stable, ambulatory patients. *Am Heart J* 115:418–424, 1988.
6. Van den Brink RBA, Visser LA, Bassart DCG, et al: Comparison of transthoracic and transesophageal color Doppler imaging in patients with mechanical prostheses in the mitral position. *Am J Cardiol* 63:1471–1474, 1989.
7. Alam M, Serwin J, Rosman H, et al: Transesophageal echocardiography features of normal and dysfunctioning bioprosthetic valves. *Am Heart J* 121:1149–1155, 1991.
8. Daniel LB, Grigg LE, Weisel RD, et al: Comparison of transthoracic and transesophageal assessment of prosthetic valve dysfunction. *Echocardiography* 7:83–95, 1990.
9. Reisner SA, Meltzer RS: Normal valves of prosthetic valve Doppler echocardiographic parameters: a review. *J Am Soc Echocardiogr* 1:203–210, 1988.

Fig. 2-67.

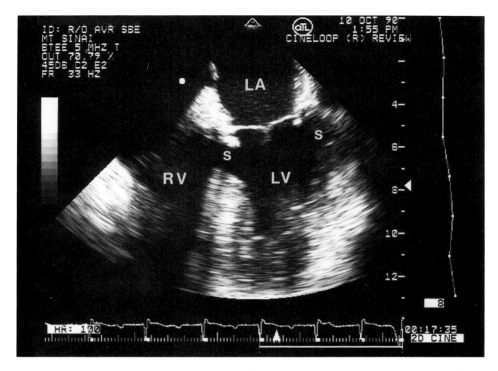

Figure 2-67A: Transverse four-chamber view, porcine mitral valve. The leaflets are coapted during systole. The valve struts project shadows (S) into the left ventricle (LV). LA = left atrium; RV = right ventricle.

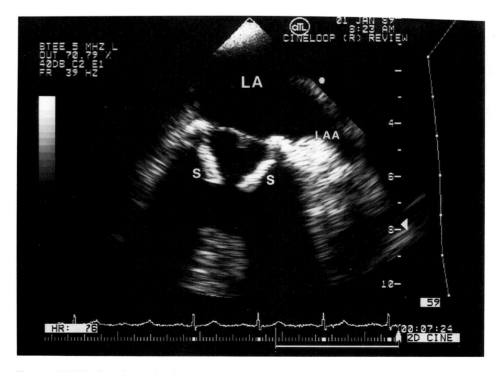

Figure 2-67B: Porcine mitral valve longitudinal plane, two-chamber view. The mitral valve (in systole) with the leaflets coapting well. The mitral valve struts (S) project further in the left ventricle in this plane. Additionally, note the shadow projected into the left ventricle by the dense prosthesis, thereby obviating adequate evaluation of the left ventricle and possible mitral regurgitation. LA = left atrium; LAA = left atrial appendage.

Fig. 2-68.

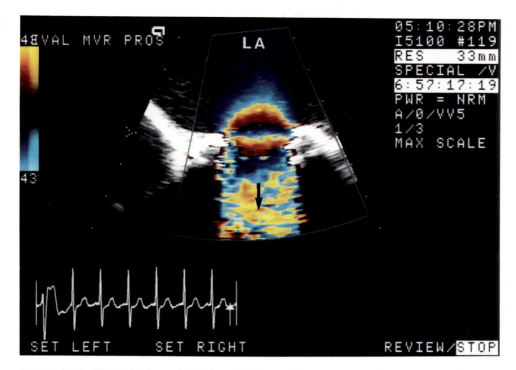

Figure 2-68: Diastolic flow through a porcine mitral valve. Note the proximal isovelocity concentric rings on the left atrial (LA) side of the prosthesis due to relative stenosis and the turbulent flow on the ventricular side of the prosthesis.

Fig. 2-69.

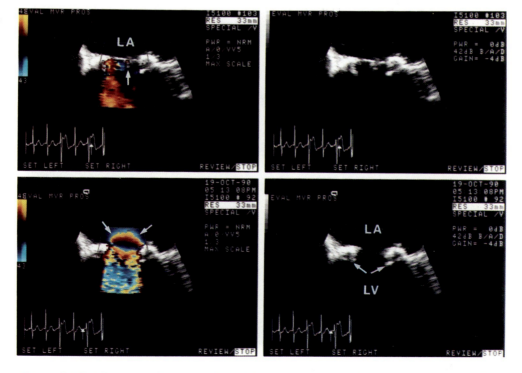

Figure 2-69: Mitral porcine valve closed in systole (upper right) with corresponding color flow Doppler (upper left) showing no mitral regurgitation. Diastolic flow through the opened mitral valve seen in color flow (bottom left). The leaflets are fully extended and opened (lower right). LA = left atrium; LV = left ventricle.

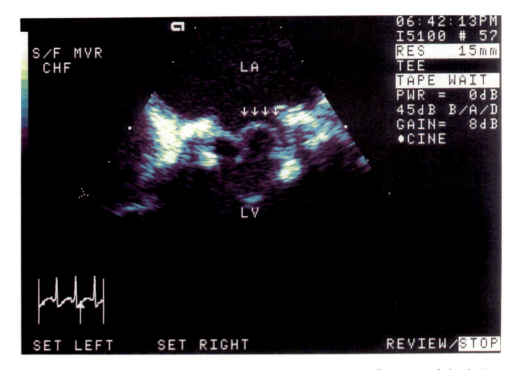

Figure 2-70: Porcine mitral valve prolapse, transverse plane. Because of the better resolution and closer proximity to the left atrium (LA) and mitral valve in the transesophageal approach, subtle details of valvular dysfunction such as prolapse of a porcine leaflet (arrows) can be detected. LV = left ventricle.

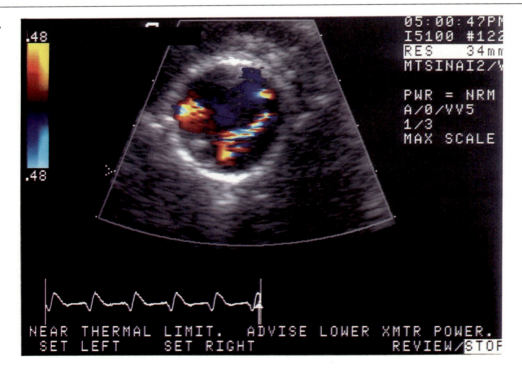

Figure 2-71: The short axis transgastric view. An important view in the evaluation of mitral prosthesis is the transverse transgastric or subxiphoid short axis plane just below the diaphragm. In this plane, the entire annular ring is seen, demonstrating mild mitral regurgitation originating between all the commissure lines of the older mildly fibrosed prosthesis.

Fig. 2-72.

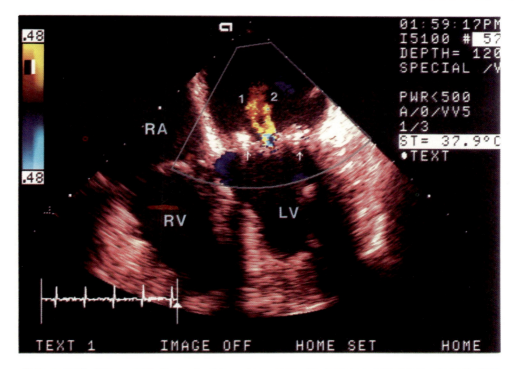

Figure 2-72: Transverse four-chamber view, stenotic porcine mitral heterograft. The struts are seen (two arrows) and the fibrosed mitral valve with poor coaptation has two small jets of mild mitral regurgitation. RA = right atrium; RV = right ventricle; LV = left ventricle.

Fig. 2-73.

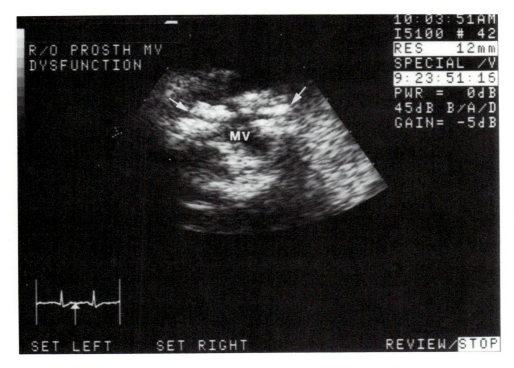

Figure 2-73A: Short axis transverse plane. This porcine heterograft has stippled calcification (arrows). MV = mitral valve.

Fig. 2-73. (cont'd)

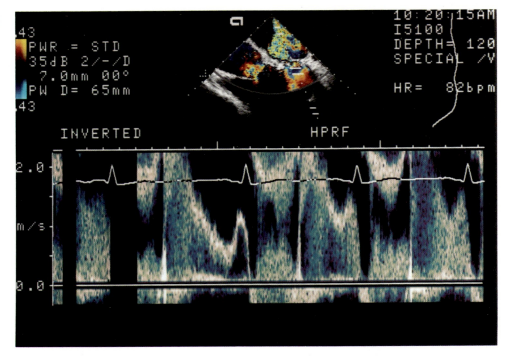

Figure 2-73B: Pressure half-time of the calcified mitral valve demonstrates moderate mitral stenosis.

Fig. 2-74.

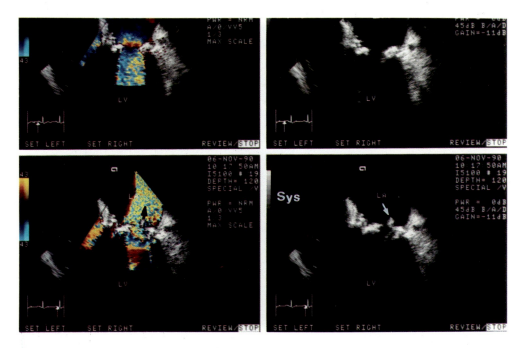

Figure 2-74: Severe MR due to flail posterior leaflet porcine valve due to endocarditis. Upper right: thickened valve open in diastole; upper left: diastolic color flow appears normal; lower right: thickened leaflets with flail posterior leaflet; lower left: moderate-severe MR.

Fig. 2-75.

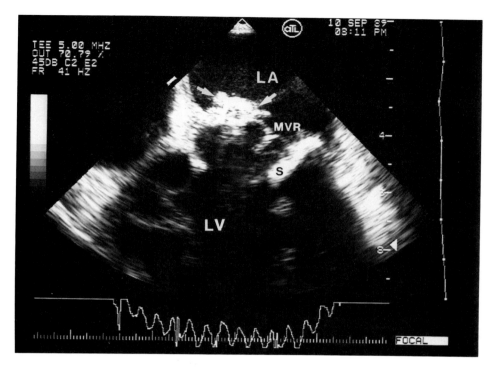

Figure 2-75A: Mitral valve heterograft endocarditis, transverse four-chamber plane. A white, dense, irregular vegetation (arrows) is seen at the junction of the prosthetic valve (MVR) to the septal annulus. LA = left atrium; LV = left ventricle; S = struts.

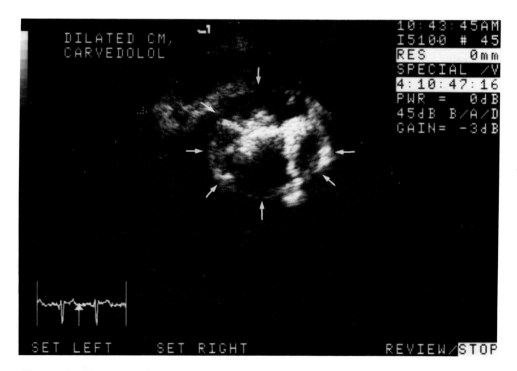

Figure 2-75B: Vegetations can also be seen in the transverse subxiphoid short axis plane. The infectious process involves all three leaflets. The porcine sewing ring (arrows) can be seen.

Fig. 2-75. (cont'd)

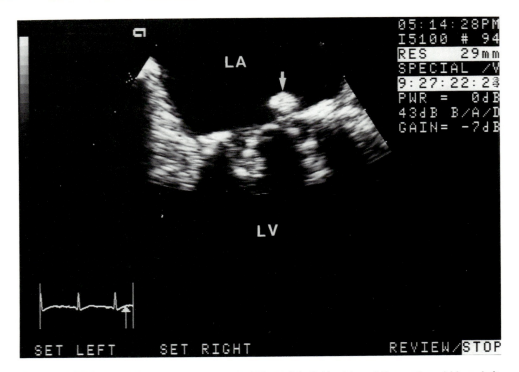

Figure 2-75C: Small vegetation on the left atrial (LA) side of the valve. LV = left ventricle.

Fig. 2-76.

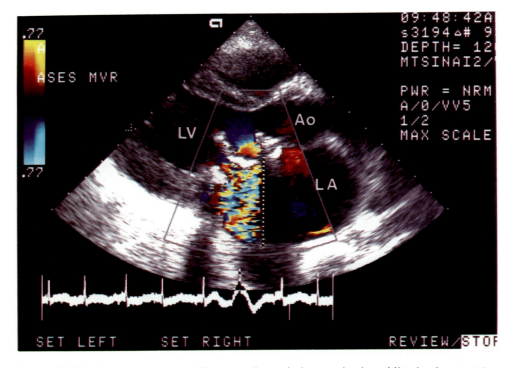

Figure 2-76A: Porcine endocarditis, transthoracic long axis view. Mitral valve vegetation causing mitral regurgitation. However, due to the shadowing behind the prosthesis (dotted line), the full extent of the regurgitation cannot be adequately accessed. LA = left atrium; LV = left ventricle; Ao = aorta.

Fig. 2-76. (cont'd)

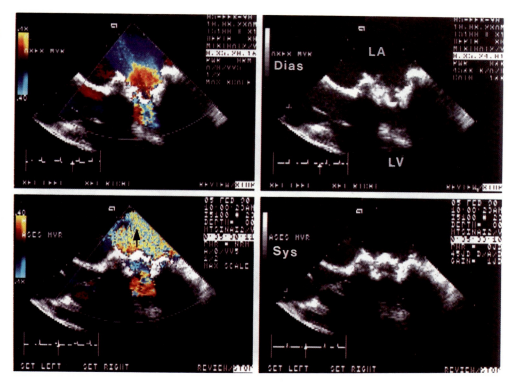

Figure 2-76B: Mitral endocarditis, transesophageal transverse four-chamber view from the same patient as in Figure 10A. The upper left and right views demonstrate the vegetation affecting the valve, in diastole (Dias). The lower right demonstrates the dense vegetation in systole (Sys), and the lower left depicts severe mitral regurgitation which fills most of the left atrium.

Fig. 2-77.

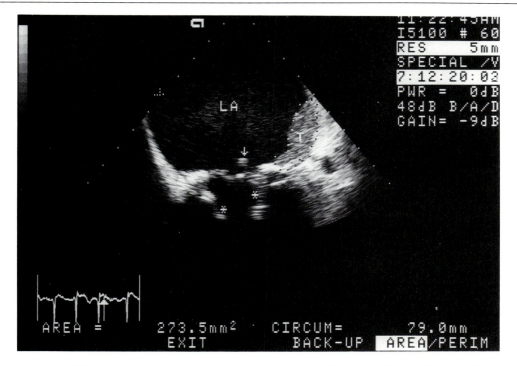

Figure 2-77A: A small pedunculated vegetation (arrow) is seen in the four-chamber view. The prosthetic struts are noted by asterisks. Additionally, this large left atrium (LA) was filled with "smoke" and a thrombus (T) behind the lateral aspect of the annulus measuring 2.7 cm^2.

Fig. 2-77. (cont'd)

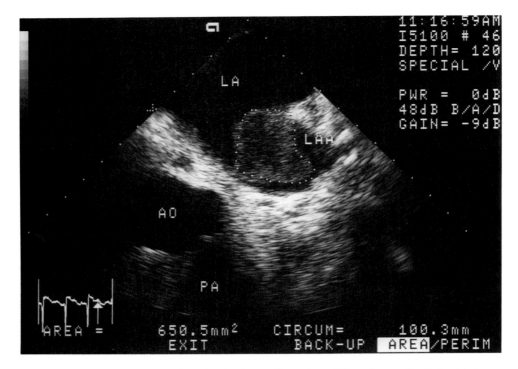

Figure 2-77B: The same patient had a large thrombus filling the entire left atrial appendage (LAA) measuring 6.5 cm². LA = left atrium; LV = left ventricle; PA = pulmonary artery; AO = aorta.

Fig. 2-78.

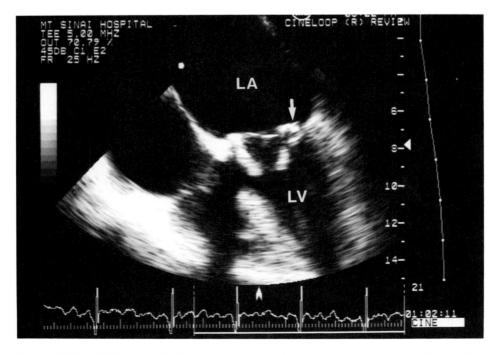

Figure 2-78A: Dehisced mitral valve: four-chamber view of porcine prosthesis. Note lateral separation of the valve from annulus (arrow) and moderately dilated left atrium (LA). LV = left ventricle.

Fig. 2-78. (cont'd)

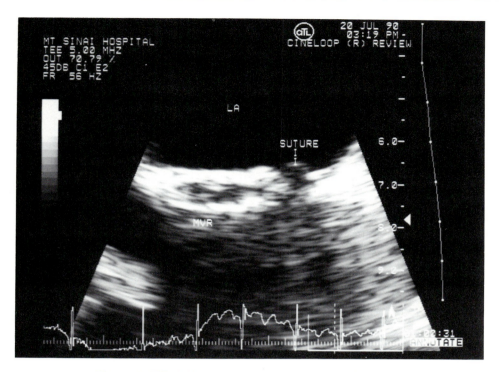

Figure 2-78B: A fluttering loose suture seen laterally.

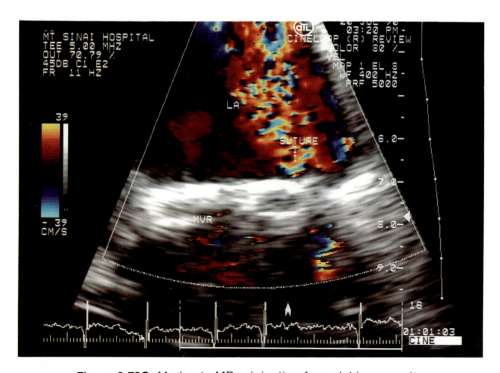

Figure 2-78C: Moderate MR originating from dehiscence site.

**Fig. 2-78.
(cont'd)**

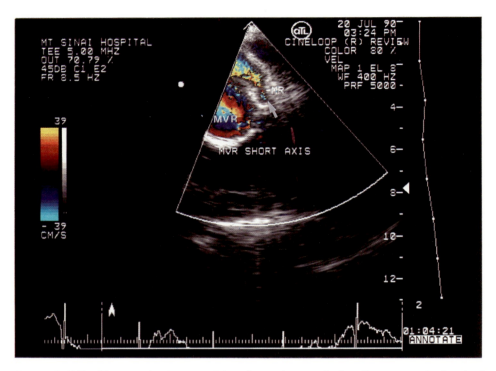

Figure 2-78D: Short axis transgastric plane demonstrates the paravalvular leak (arrow).

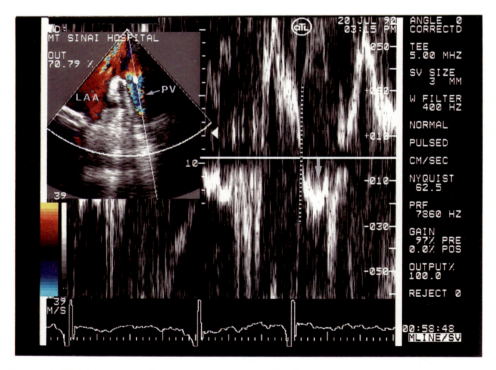

Figure 2-78E: Reversal of normal pulmonary vein (PV) flow due to markedly elevated early systolic LA pressures from the severe MR. Normal early pulmonary venous flow into the LA has positive forward flow. LAA = left atrial appendage.

Mitral Valve Repair

Over the last few years, the trend in mitral valve surgery for mitral regurgitation is to repair rather than to replace the valve whenever possible. The rationale behind mitral valve repair is that retention of the papillary muscles and chordae tendineae preserve ventricular function better than mitral prosthesis insertion with excision of the papillary muscles. The pathophysiological importance of the papillary muscles is to coordinate ventricular contraction from left ventricular apex to base. When the apical to basal connection provided by the papillary muscles is detached, ventricular dysfunction ensues. Additionally, the repair of the mitral valve negates the need for anticoagulation (if the patient is in sinus rhythm) and also has a lower incidence of mitral valve endocarditis. The mitral valve repair may sometimes appear echocardiographically as a porcine valve if there is a prominent mitral annulus inserted. The only contraindications to valve repair are calcification, fibrosis, and retraction of the leaflet and the subvalvular apparatus.

Bibliography

1. Daniel WG, Shroder RE, Nonnast-Daniel B, et al: Conventional and transesophageal echocardiography in the diagnosis of infective endocarditis. *Eur Heart J* 8(Suppl):278–293, 1987.
2. Erbel R, Rohmann S, Drexler M, et al: Improved diagnostic value of echocardiography in patients with infective endocarditis by transesophageal approach: a prospective study. *Eur Heart J* 9:43–53, 1988.
3. Mugge A, Daniel WG, Frank G, Lechtlen PR: Echocardiography in infective endocarditis: reassessment of prognostic implications of vegetation size determined by transthoracic and the transesophageal approach. *J Am Coll Cardiol* 14:631–638, 1988.
4. Shiveley BK, Gurule FT, Roldan CA, et al: Diagnostic value of transesophageal compared with transthoracic echocardiography in infective endocarditis. *J Am Coll Cardiol* 18:391–397, 1991.

Fig. 2-79.

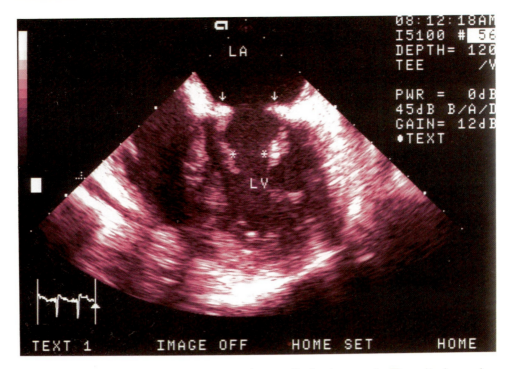

Figure 2-79A: Four-chamber transverse plane, mitral valve repair. The mitral annulus is almost a complete circular annulus which is seen into left atrial (LA) side of the mitral valve to strengthen the support of the mitral valve and to reduce the size of the mitral annulus. In this figure, the annular ring is seen by arrows and the elongated leaflets by asterisks. There are no struts in annular repair as seen in a porcine valve. LV = left ventricle.

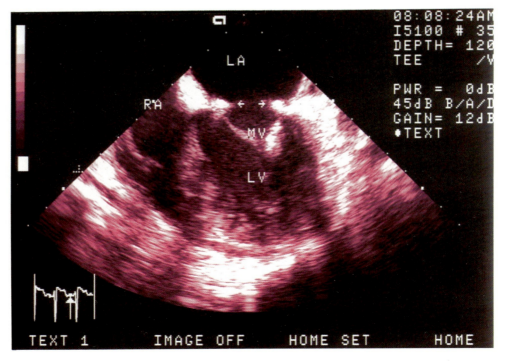

Figure 2-79B: The annulus as seen by arrows is very low profile, and in systole the mitral valve (MV) is seen to coapt well. LA = left atrium; LV = left ventricle; RA = right atrium.

Mitral Valve Disease • 103

Fig. 2-80.

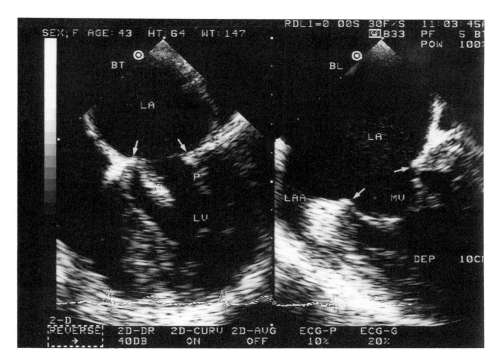

Figure 2-80: Transverse plane (left) and longitudinal plane (right) image the annulus prosthesis (arrows) and myxomatous valve. LA = left atrium; LV = left ventricle; LAA = left atrial appendage; MV = mitral valve.

Fig. 2-81.

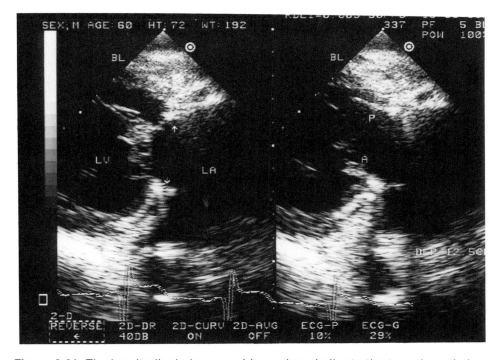

Figure 2-81: The longitudinal plane provides a view similar to the transthoracic long axis plane. The diastolic (right) and systolic (left) function of the annulus (arrow) and anterior (A) and posterior (P) leaflets can be assessed. LA = left atrium; LV = left ventricle.

Fig. 2-82.

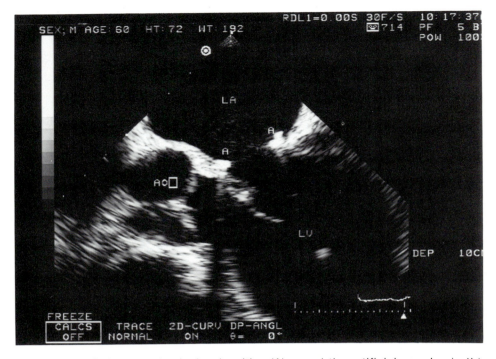

Figure 2-82A: Only two subvalvular densities (A) reveal the artificial annulus in this patient. LA = left atrium; LV = left ventricle; AO = aorta.

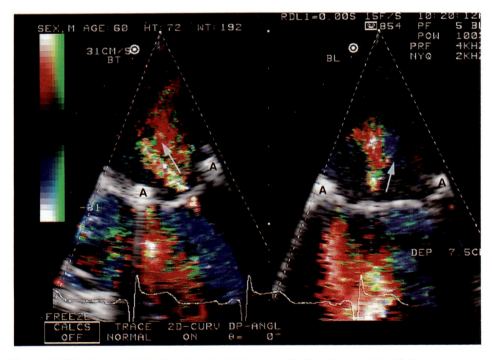

Figure 2-82B: A central jet of residual mitral regurgitation is seen in both the transverse (left) and the longitudinal (right) four-chamber views. A = annulus.

3

Aortic Valve Disease

Normal Variants and Aortic Valve Stenosis

The aortic valve is normally trileaflet with three distinct cusps: the left, the right, and the noncoronary, named for the origin of a coronary artery from the respective sinus.

The aortic valve can be evaluated in several different planes. It may be seen in the transgastric five-chamber view in the transverse plane as well as in the five-chamber view in a transverse plane above the diaphragm as the transducer is raised superiorly; it can also be seen in the transverse short axis at the level of the aorta and pulmonary artery (similar to the short axis transthoracic echo view), and in the longitudinal plane, the aortic valve can be seen in a three-chamber view as well as a modified long axis view.

Specific aortic pathology that can be evaluated includes the number of cusps, aortic valve prolapse, severity of aortic stenosis, endocarditis, perivalvular abscess, and severity of aortic regurgitation.

Bibliography

1. Mugge A, Daniel WG, Wolpers HG, Klopper JW, Lichtlen PR: Improved visualization of discrete subvalvular aortic stenosis by transesophageal color-coded Doppler echocardiography. *Am Heart J* 117:474–475, 1989.
2. Hofmann T, Kasper W, Meinertz T, Spillner G, Schlosser V, Just H: Determination of aortic valve orifice area in aortic valve stenosis by two-dimensional transesophageal echocardiography. *Am J Cardiol* 59:330–335, 1987.
3. Hoffman R, Flachskamf FA, Hanrath P: Planimetry of stenotic aortic valve area using multiplane transesophageal echocardiography. *Circulation* 84: II-129, 1991.

Fig. 3-1.

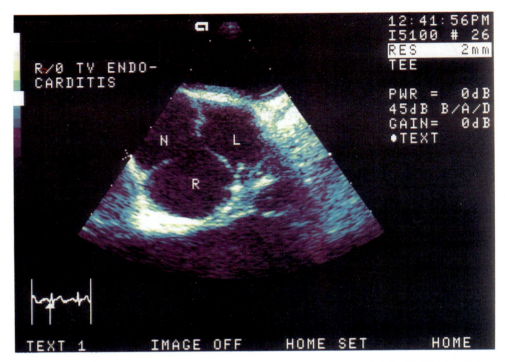

Figure 3-1A: The aortic valve in diastole in the transverse short axis plane; the three cusps of the aortic valve are labeled. L = left; N = noncoronary; R = right cusp.

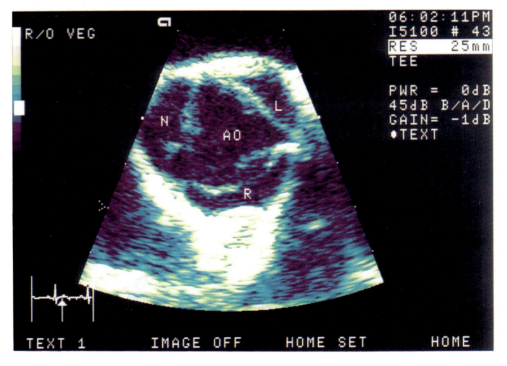

Figure 3-1B: In systole, the aortic leaflets retract into their respective sinuses, forming a round outflow orifice. In this transverse plane, the pulmonary artery is posterior to the aortic valve, because it is more distant from the TEE transducer imaging from a retrocardiac position. L = left; N = noncoronary; R = right cusp; AO = aorta.

Aortic Valve Disease • 107

Fig. 3-1. (cont'd)

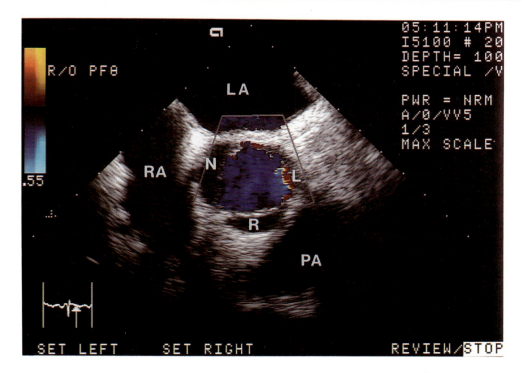

Figure 3-1C: Color flow outlines the systolic aortic valve orifice. L = left; N = noncoronary; R = right cusp; RA = right atrium; LA = left atrium; PA = pulmonary artery.

Fig. 3-2.

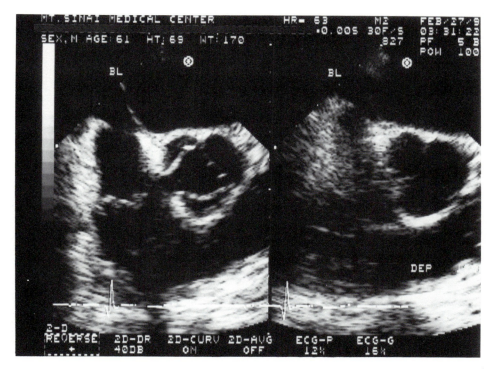

Figure 3-2: The longitudinal plane of the aortic valve in systole (left) and in diastole (right). L = left; N = noncoronary; R = right cusp; RA = right atrium; LA = left atrium.

Fig. 3-3.

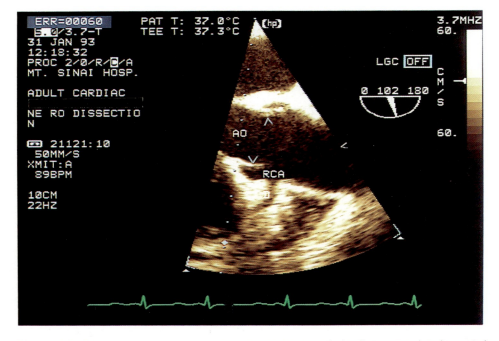

Figure 3-3: The longitudinal plane can also assess aortic leaflet excursion in systole (arrowheads). AO = aorta; RCA = origin of right coronary artery (multiplane probe at 102° axis, as seen in dial at the upper right of figure).

Fig. 3-4.

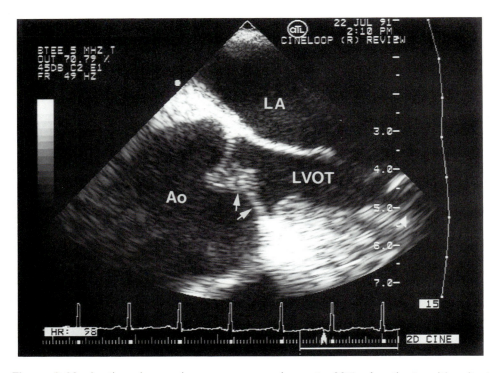

Figure 3-4A: Aortic valve *prolapse* may occur in up to 20% of patients with mitral valve prolapse and may be the source of aortic regurgitation. In this transverse plane, the right coronary cusp is seen to prolapse into the left ventricular outflow tract (LVOT) in diastole (arrows). LA = left atrium; Ao = aorta.

Aortic Valve Disease • 109

Fig. 3-4. (cont'd)

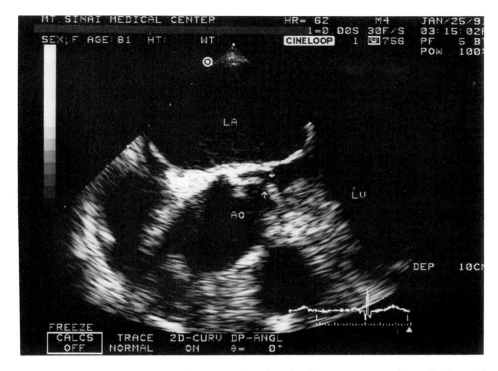

Figure 3-4B: In this modified five-chamber view in the transverse plane, both aortic leaflets (arrows) prolapse into the left ventricular outflow tract with poor coaptation. LA = left atrium; LV = left ventricle; AO = aorta.

Fig. 3-5.

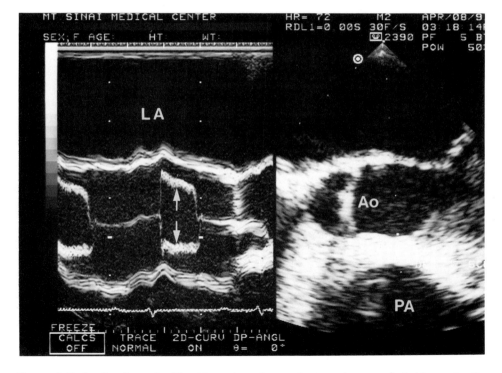

Figure 3-5: Aortic stenosis. The M-mode echocardiogram is very useful in evaluating leaflet mobility. The M-mode echocardiogram of the aortic valve demonstrates good excursion and only mild thickening of the leaflets also seen in the 2-D echo (right side). LA = left atrium; PA = pulmonary artery; Ao = aorta.

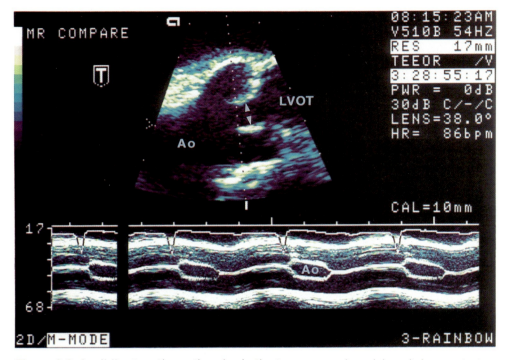

Figure 3-6: A mildly stenotic aortic valve in the transverse plane (above) demonstrates restricted M-mode excursion (below). Ao = aorta; LVOT = left ventricular outflow tract.

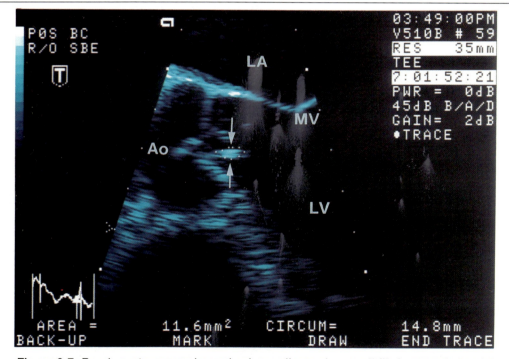

Figure 3-7: Rarely on transesophageal echocardiography, small fibrin strands can be seen on the left ventricular (LV) side of the aortic valve (Ao). These excrescences are probably related to mild degeneration of the valve with aging and denuding of the endothelial layer, with small fibrin strands developing on the exposed surfaces. These should not be confused with vegetations but may have embolic implications. They can be found in totally normal asymptomatic patients. Excrescenses may be recognized as short, thin, fluttering linear densities (arrows on left ventricular side of the valve). LA = left atrium; MV = mitral valve.

Fig. 3-8.

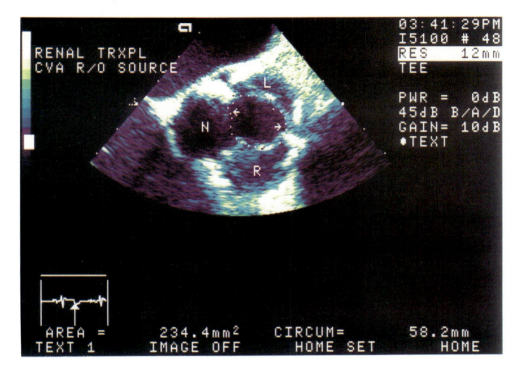

Figure 3-8A: Planimetry of the aortic orifice area can be performed to determine the severity of stenosis. Calcification of the posterior aortic root and leaflets themselves may distort the orifice, affecting the accuracy of this TEE method. The valve area of this patient was 2.3 cm² (see dotted circle outlining orifice). L = left; N = noncoronary; R = right cusp.

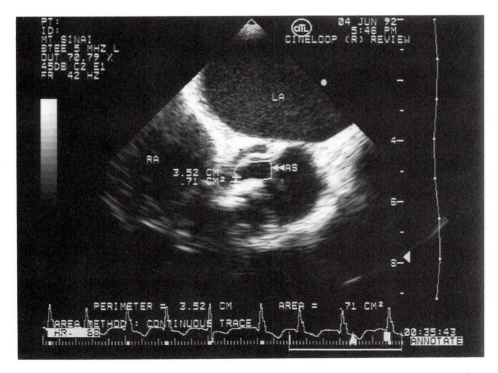

Figure 3-8B: More severe aortic stenosis (AS) planimetered in the transverse plane (valve area, 0.71 cm²). LA = left atrium; RA = right atrium.

Fig. 3-9.

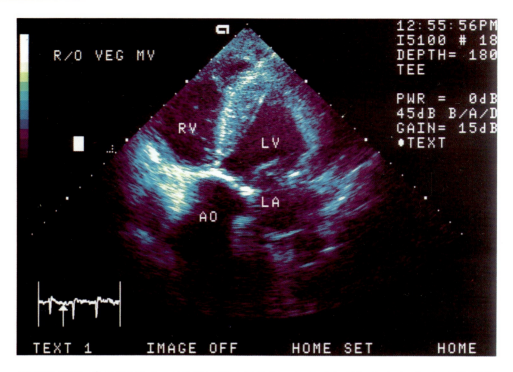

Figure 3-9A: Continuous wave Doppler can measure actual transvalvular gradient in the subxiphoid, gastric transverse five-chamber view. LA = left ventricle; RV = right ventricle; LA = left atrium; AO = aorta.

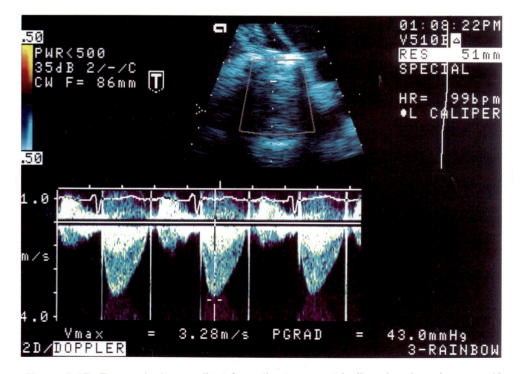

Figure 3-9B: Transvalvular gradient from the transgastric five-chamber view was 43 mm Hg.

Aortic Regurgitation

Aortic regurgitation may be due to primary disease of the aortic valve itself or of the aortic root and may be congenital or acquired. Minimal degrees of aortic regurgitation may be seen in normal patients, particularly in older patients with mild sclerosis of the valve. Other acquired etiologies of aortic regurgitation include rheumatic disease, endocarditis, calcific aortic stenosis, trauma, and hypertension. Congenital etiologies of valvular aortic regurgitation include bicuspid aortic valve, ventricular septal defect, subaortic membrane, and congenital valvular aortic stenosis. Dilatation of the aortic root and ascending aorta may cause poor coaptation of the aortic leaflets leading to varying degrees of aortic regurgitation. Diseases of the aorta causing regurgitation include aortic dissection, Marfan's disease, syphilis, ankylosing apondylitis, and cystic medial aortic necrosis. Aortic regurgitation produces a volume overload condition with the ventricular response of left ventricular eccentric hypertrophy and elongation. Echocardiography with Doppler can document the etiology of aortic regurgitation, measure ventricular size and function, and quantify severity of regurgitation, which are important considerations in determining an appropriate pharmacological or surgical response. Quantification of aortic regurgitation by transesophageal echo is similar to transthoracic echocardiography. The length and area of the aortic regurgitant jet by color Doppler is evaluated in the left ventricular outflow tract and compared to the length and area of the entire outflow tract. The ratio of color area divided by outflow tract area estimates severity of aortic regurgitation: <10% = mild; <25% = mild to moderate; >40% = moderate; >60% = severe.

Fig. 3-10.

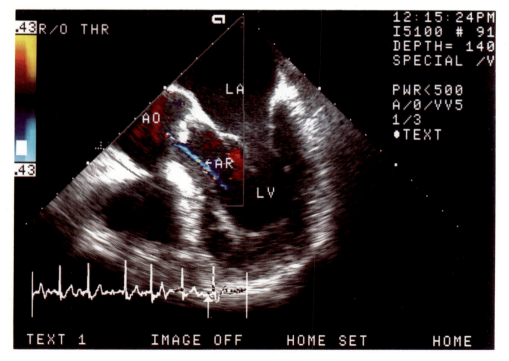

Figure 3-10: Aortic four-chamber transverse plane: minimal aortic regurgitation. A tiny jet of aortic regurgitation (AR) is seen to course along the interventricular septum (arrow). LA = left atrium; LV = left ventricle; AO = aorta.

Fig. 3-11.

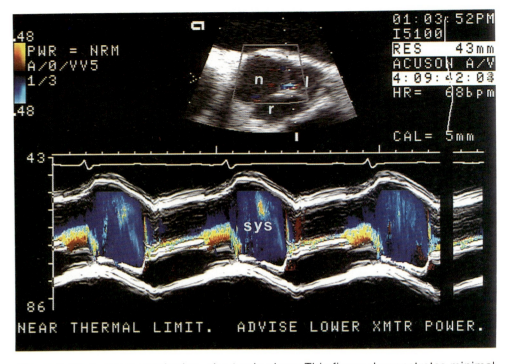

Figure 3-11: Aortic regurgitation, short axis plane. This figure demonstrates minimal aortic regurgitation seen in the short axis basal plane (above) and the corresponding M-mode echocardiogram (below). The tiny jet of aortic regurgitation is seen to be in the middle of the coaptation point between the three leaflets on both the 2-D and the M-mode color Dopplers. Though the jet is seen to be holodiastolic by color M-mode, it represents only minimal aortic regurgitation. Aortic valve cusps: l = left; r = right; n = noncoronary.

Fig. 3-12.

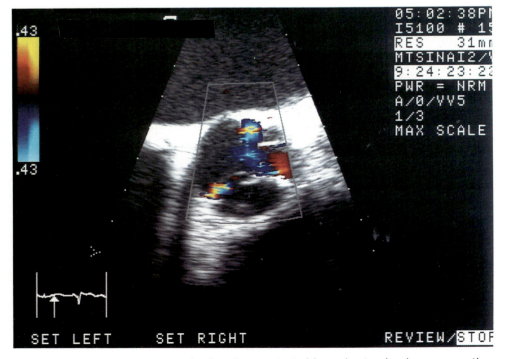

Figure 3-12: Mild aortic regurgitation demonstrated in a short axis plane emanating from the coaptation points of all three leaflets and a mildly rheumatic aortic valve.

Fig. 3-13.

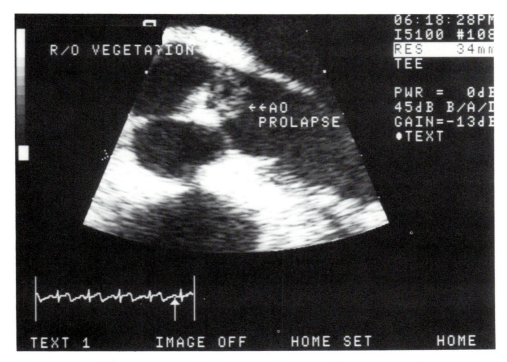

Figure 3-13A: Transverse plane, aortic valve prolapse. The aortic leaflet prolapses into the left ventricle, generating mild aortic regurgitation. AO = aorta.

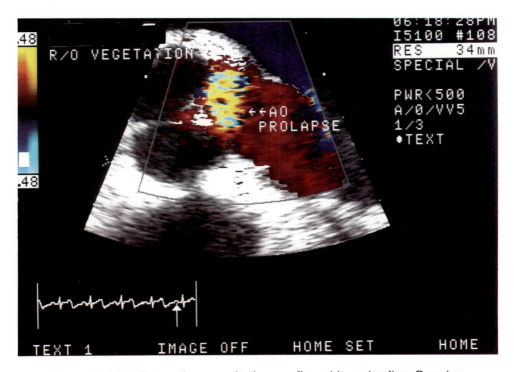

Figure 3-13B: Mild aortic regurgitation confirmed by color flow Doppler.

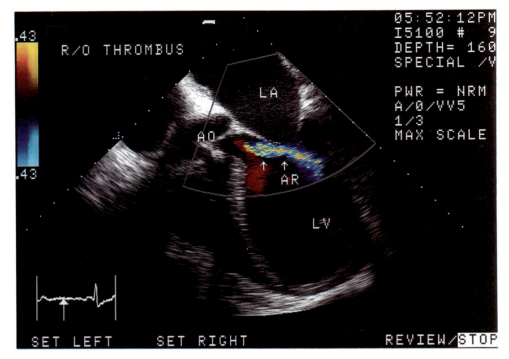

Figure 3-14: Mild aortic regurgitant jet (AR) directed over the anterior leaflet of the mitral valve. LA = left atrium; LV = left ventricle; AO = aorta.

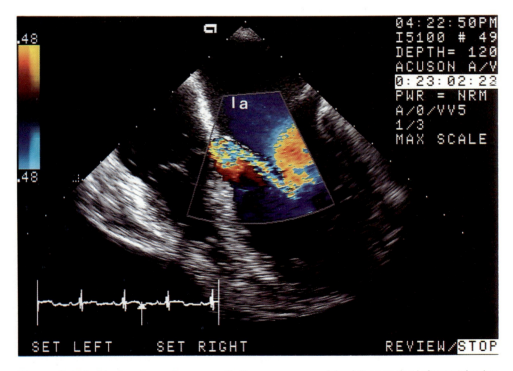

Figure 3-15A: Moderate aortic regurgitation seen as a wider jet near the left ventricular outflow jet and narrowing over the anterior leaflet of the mitral valve. The aortic regurgitant jet may be directed superiorly or inferiorly out of the plane of this view. The severity of aortic regurgitation in quantified in the outflow tract and not by its size or extent in the left ventricle. la = left atrium.

Fig. 3-15. (cont'd)

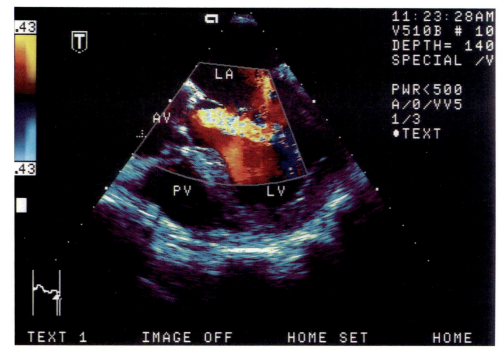

Figure 3-15B: A more uniform jet of moderate aortic regurgitation. LA = left atrium; LV = left ventricle; PV = pulmonary valve; AV = aortic valve.

Fig. 3-16.

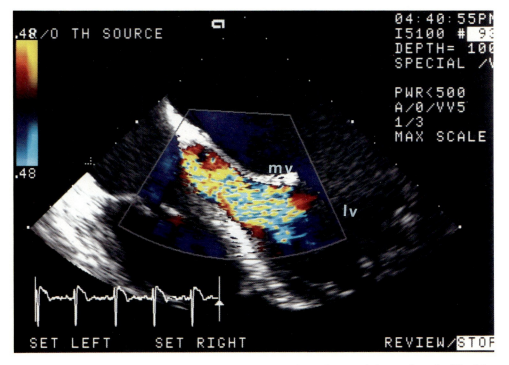

Figure 3-16: Severe aortic regurgitation. The entire left ventricle outflow is filled by a color regurgitant jet. mv = mitral valve; lv = left ventricle.

Fig. 3-17.

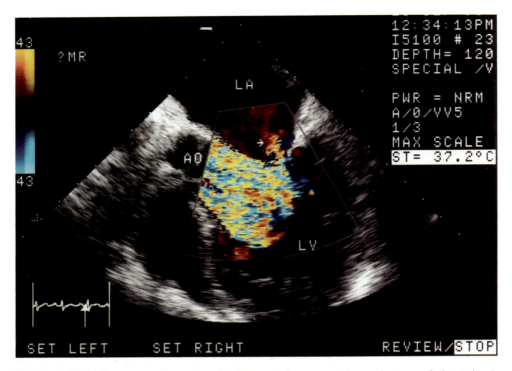

Figure 3-17A: Severe aortic regurgitation causing premature closure of the mitral valve with late diastolic mitral regurgitation (the arrow in the left atrium, LA). This is indicative of severe acute aortic regurgitation causing a significant rise in left ventricular diastolic pressure above the left atrial pressure causing premature closure of the mitral valve. This severity of aortic regurgitation is considered a medical emergency in which prompt pharmacological or surgical intervention is required. LA = left atrium; LV = left ventricle; AO = aorta.

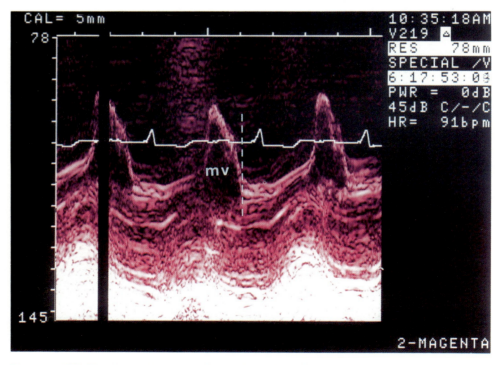

Figure 3-17B: The M-mode echo of the mitral valve (MV) can also document premature mitral valve closure (transthoracic view). Normally, the MV closes at the onset of the QRS. Premature closure indicates marked increase in left ventricular diastolic pressures.

Fig. 3-18.

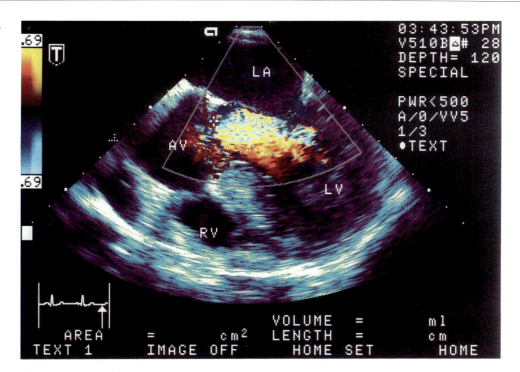

Figure 3-18A: A 60-year-old man with severe aortic regurgitation. The entire left ventricular outflow tract is outlined by the color aortic regurgitation jet. LA = left atrium; LV = left ventricle; RV = right ventricular; AV = aortic valve.

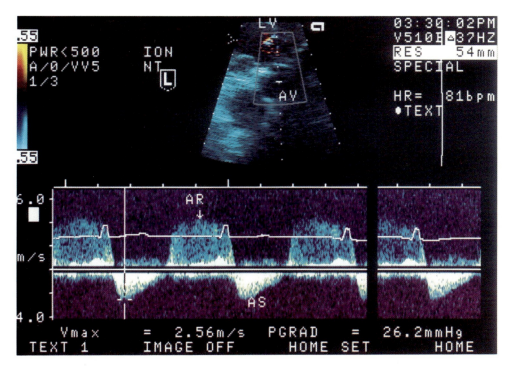

Figure 3-18B: Continuous wave Doppler through the aortic valve (transgastric longitudinal plane) demonstrates a peak gradient of 26 mm Hg, and a high velocity aortic regurgitant jet (arrow). The flat slope of the aortic regurgitation (AR) jet connotes that there is slow equilibration of diastolic aortic and left ventricular (LV) pressures, suggesting the lack of hemodynamic compromise. If the AR jet slope is rapid, the left ventricular diastolic pressure rises precipitously. AS = aortic stenosis; AV = aortic valve.

Fig. 3-18. (cont'd)

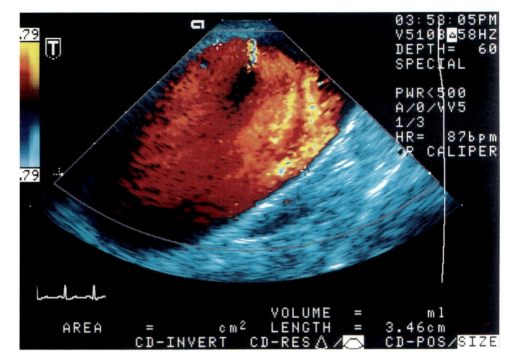

Figure 3-18C: This patient also had a mildly dilated ascending aorta (diameter, 3.46 cm).

Fig. 3-19.

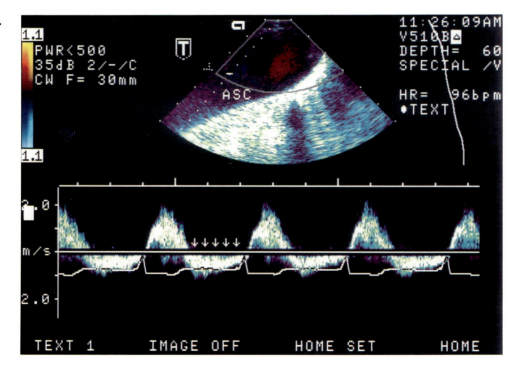

Figure 3-19: Severe aortic regurgitation causes diastolic reversal of flow in the ascending aorta (ASC, arrows, in pulsed Doppler tracing below).

Aortic Valve Endocarditis

Aortic endocarditis is usually related to an infection of a valve with underlying pathology such as rheumatic disease, degenerative aortic sclerosis, aortic stenosis, bicuspid aortic valve, or aortic insufficiency. Because of its high resolution, transesophageal echo is extremely valuable in differentiating the sclerotic or calcific aortic valve from an infected valve. By detecting smaller vegetations earlier in the course of the disease process, transesophageal echo may facilitate prompt therapy before extensive damage is done to the valve.

Fig. 3-20.

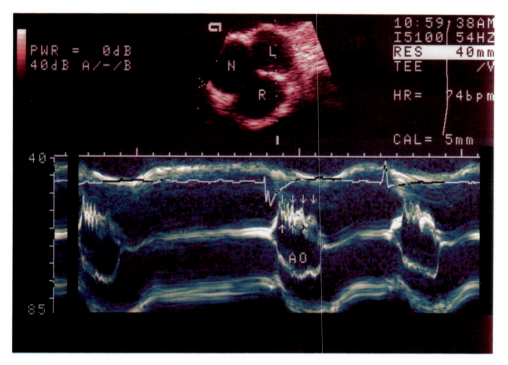

Figure 3-20: A trileaflet aortic valve echo was thickened between the left (L) and right (R) cusps seen by transthoracic echo, but endocarditis could not be confirmed. Transesophageal echo was performed and by color M-mode demonstrated that there was a high frequency fluttering irregularity on the valve consistent with a small vegetation on the left coronary cusp (arrows in figure below). N = noncoronary cusp; AO = aortic valve.

Fig. 3-21.

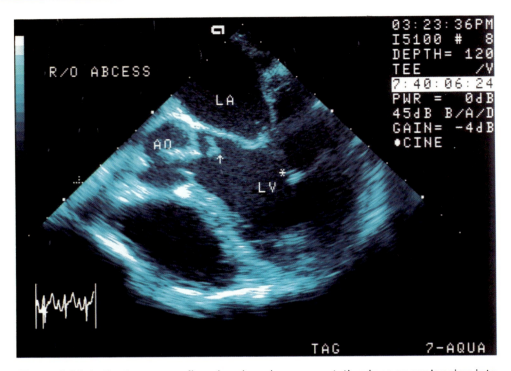

Figure 3-21: In the transverse five-chamber view, a vegetation is seen prolapsing into the left ventricular outflow tract off of the left coronary cusp of the aortic valve (arrow). The bulbous distal end of ruptured chordae is seen and marked by an asterisk in the left ventricle. LA = left atrium; LV = left ventricle; AO = aortic valve.

Fig. 3-22.

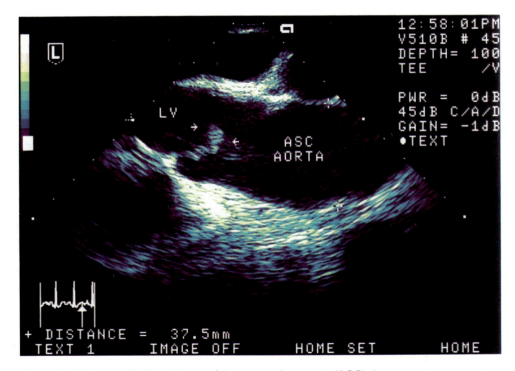

Figure 3-22A: Longitudinal plane of the ascending aorta (ASC) demonstrates a vegetation on the left cusp of a bicuspid aortic valve that extends into the aortic root during systole (arrows). The ascending aorta is dilated (3.75 cm). LV = left ventricle.

Fig. 3-22.
(cont'd)

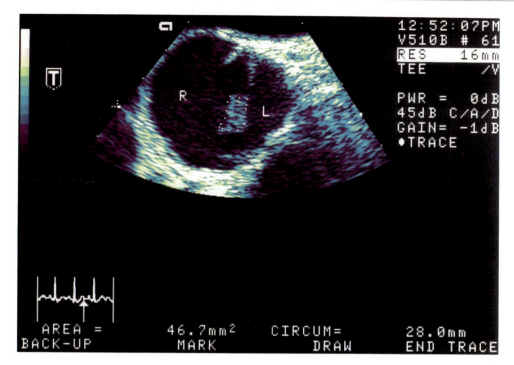

Figure 3-22B: The transverse plane confirms the irregular density on the bicuspid aortic valve. R = right cusp; L = left cusp.

Fig. 3-23.

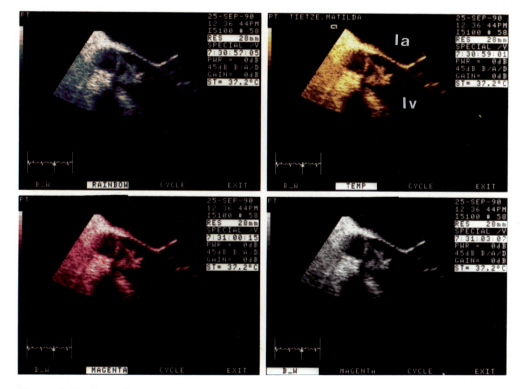

Figure 3-23: Color B-mode facilitates better differentiation of this irregular, heterogeneous mass prolapsing into the left ventricular outflow tract off of the aortic valve consistent with a vegetation. LA = left atrium; LV = left ventricle.

Fig. 3-24.

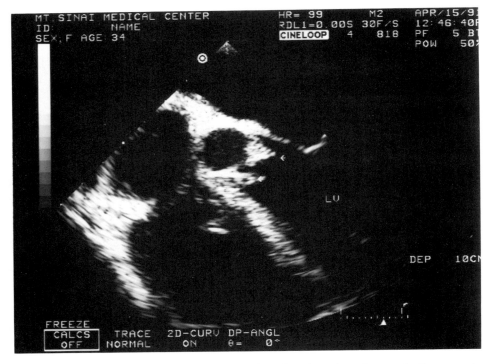

Figure 3-24A: Transverse transesophageal five-chamber view demonstrating vegetations on both the left and right coronary cusps prolapsing into the left ventricle (LV, small arrows).

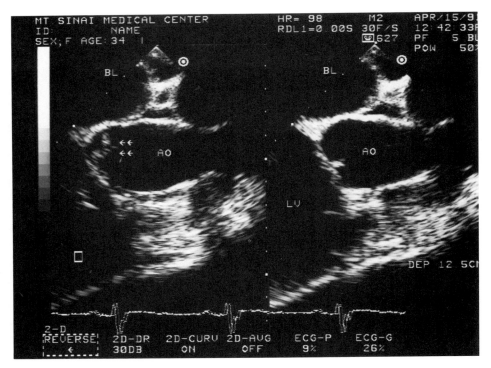

Figure 3-24B: The longitudinal plane (right side) shows a normal valve in diastole, but the valve during systole (left) demonstrates the irregular vegetation which was seen better in the transverse plane. LV = left ventricle; AO = aorta.

Fig. 3-24. (cont'd)

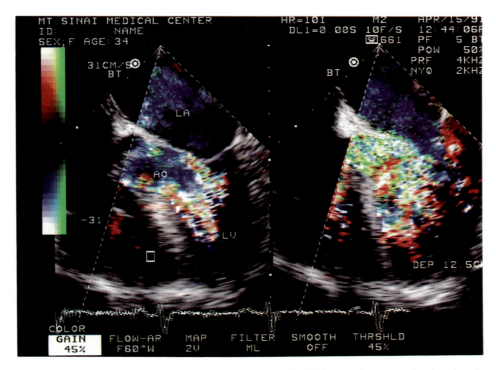

Figure 3-24C: With isovolumetric relaxation (left side), aortic regurgitation begins before the opening of the mitral valve and becomes severe regurgitation during mid-diastole (right side). LA = left atrium; LV = left ventricle; AO = aortic valve.

Fig. 3-25.

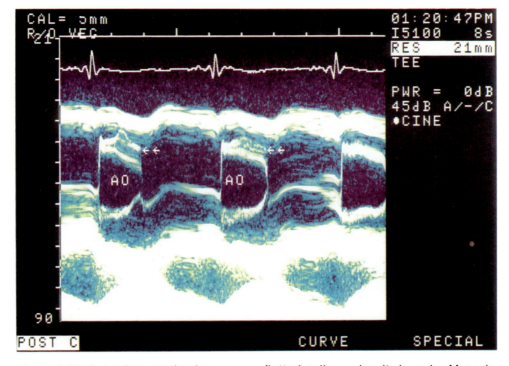

Figure 3-25: A small vegetation is seen as a fluttering linear density by color M-mode echocardiography. Because of its higher sampling rate, color M-mode facilitates resolution of very small abnormalities that are not easily perceivable by routine two-dimensional echocardiography. AO = aortic valve.

Fig. 3-26.

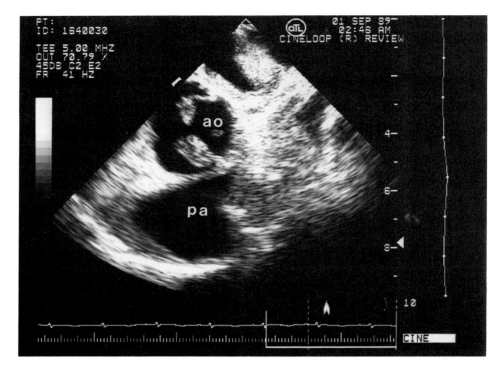

Figure 3-26: A bicuspid aortic valve with bulbous vegetations on both doming leaflets. Ao = aortic valve; PA = pulmonary artery.

Fig. 3-27.

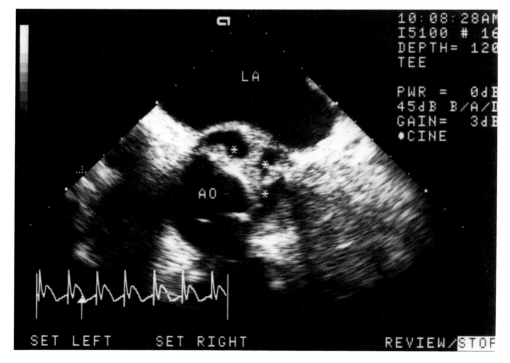

Figure 3-27A: A serious complication of endocarditis is abscess formation. In this figure, there are multiple small abscess cavities between the aortic root and the left atrium (LA, asterisks). AO = aortic valve.

Fig. 3-27. (cont'd)

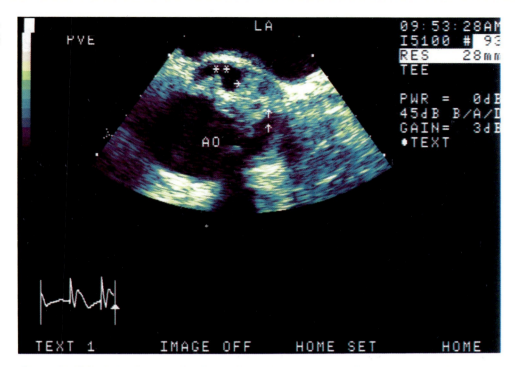

Figure 3-27B: Color B-mode further defines the abscess and the arrows point to communication between the aorta (AO) and the left ventricle generating aortic insufficiency.

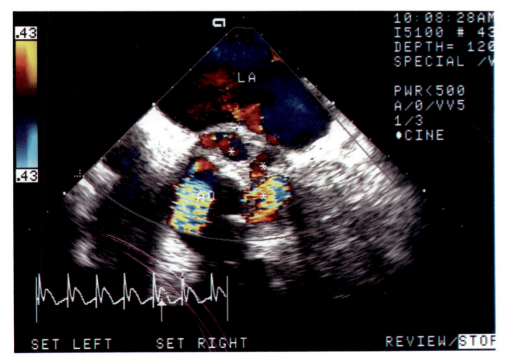

Figure 3-27C: Color Doppler demonstrates aortic insufficiency and small amounts of flow inside the multiloculated abscess cavity. Low velocity flow (red) confirmed communication the the left atrium. LA = left atrium; AO = aortic valve.

Aortic Valve Prostheses

Aortic valve prostheses are usually easily imaged by transthoracic echo (TTE). Since the TTE ultrasound beam originates from the left ventricular apex in the apical chamber view, the ventricular outflow tract is not obstructed by shadows generated by the prosthesis. Peak gradient and valve area can be calculated by CW Doppler measurement, and regurgitant jets detected by color Doppler.

However, with TEE imaging, the aortic prosthesis projects shadows into the LV outflow tract, thereby obscuring potential regurgitant flow. Therefore, the transgastric five-chamber TEE view (transverse or longitudinal) is invaluable since its perspective is similar to the apical transthoracic approach. An accurate CW Doppler peak transaortic gradient can be obtained from this plane.

Complications of aortic heterograft (tissue) prostheses include leaflet abnormalities (stenosis, prolapse, endocarditis) and paravalvular leak, dehiscence, and abscess formation. Leaflets and struts of either heterografts or mechanical valves must be interrogated very carefully for thrombus or fibrin strands in the patient being evaluated for a potential cardioembolic source.

Fig. 3-28.

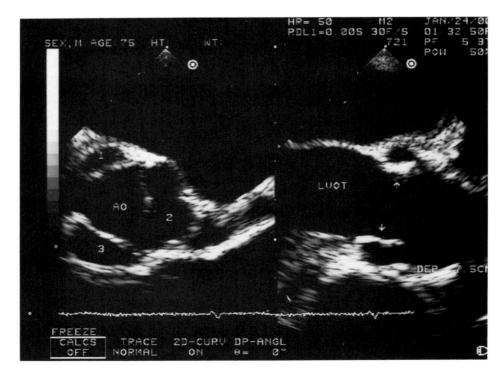

Figure 3-28: Normal aortic valve. The transverse plane (left side) images the three coronary cusps (1 = noncoronary, 2 = left coronary, 3 = right coronary cusp), open in systole. While the longitudinal plane (right side) visualizes the valve (arrow), left ventricular outflow tract (LVOT), and ascending aorta. AO = aortic valve.

Fig. 3-29.

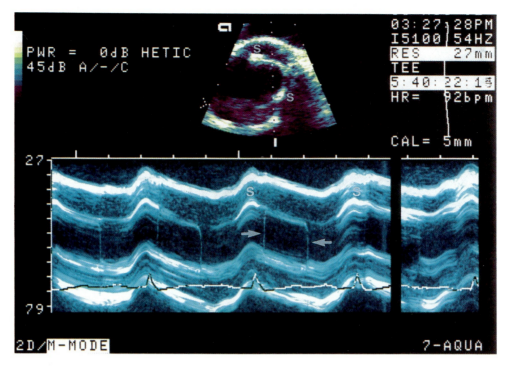

Figure 3-29A: Porcine aortic prosthesis. M-mode taken in the transverse basal plane demonstrates systolic excursion of the thin leaflets (arrows) between the dense struts (S).

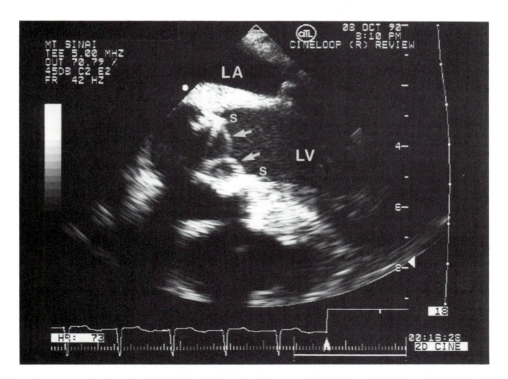

Figure 3-29B: Aortic heterograft prosthesis. The transverse five-chamber view, the thin tissue leaflets (arrows) are seen surrounded by the valve struts (S). LA = left atrium; LV = left ventricle.

Fig. 3-29.
(cont'd)

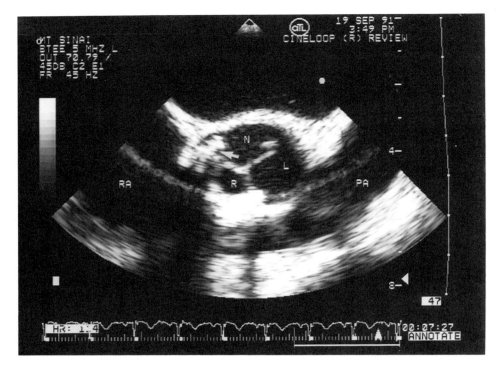

Figure 3-29C: Procine aortic prosthesis. In the longitudinal basal view, the three leaflets of the prosthesis are imaged (N = noncoronary, L = left, R = right coronary cusp). The density between the right and noncoronary cusp (arrow) was due to the strut and sutures. RA = right atrium; PA = pulmonary artery.

Fig. 3-30.

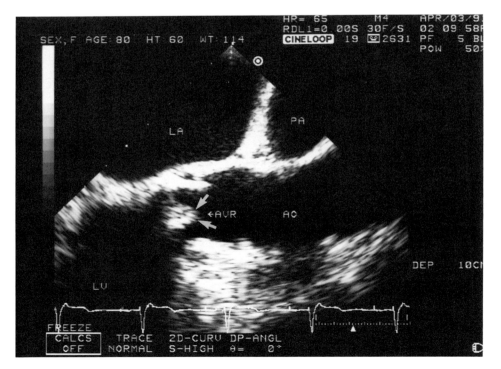

Figure 3-30: Heterograft aortic stenosis. In the longitudinal plane, the valve leaflets are thickened and calcified with decreased excursion arrows. LA = left atrium; LV = left ventricle; PA = pulmonary artery; AVR = aortic valve replacement.

Fig. 3-31.

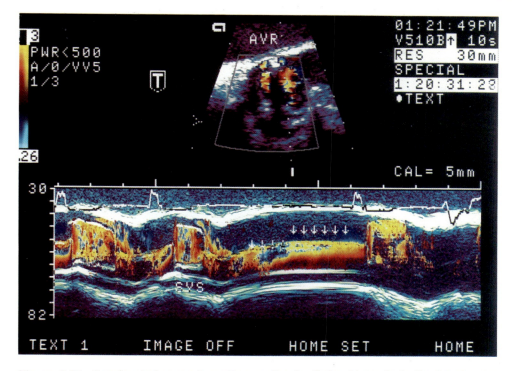

Figure 3-31: Porcine heterograft aortic prosthesis. Color M-mode in the transverse basal plane can depict the systolic (SYS) excursion of the open box as well as the diastolic regurgitant jet (arrows) which begins immediately with valve closure. AVR = aortic valve replacement.

Fig. 3-32.

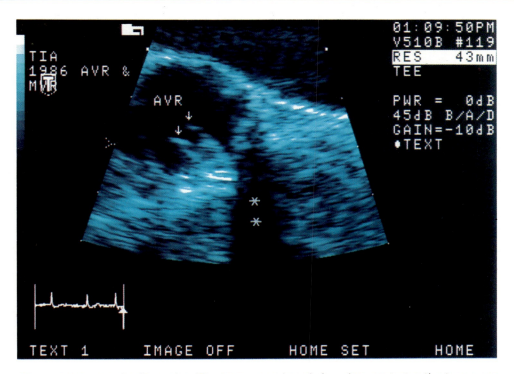

Figure 3-32A: Aortic disc valve. The transverse basal view demonstrates the two open discs of the St. Jude's prosthesis (arrows) in systole. Shadowing into the LVOT (asterisks) obscures full assessment of the valve in this plane. AVR = aortic valve replacement

**Fig. 3-32.
(cont'd)**

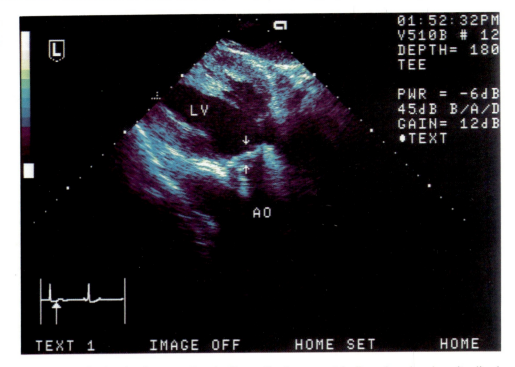

Figure 3-32B: Aortic disc prosthesis. From the transgastric five-chamber longitudinal plane, the aortic valve can be imaged (arrows) to assess excursion and to align the CW probe. LV = left ventricle; AO = aorta.

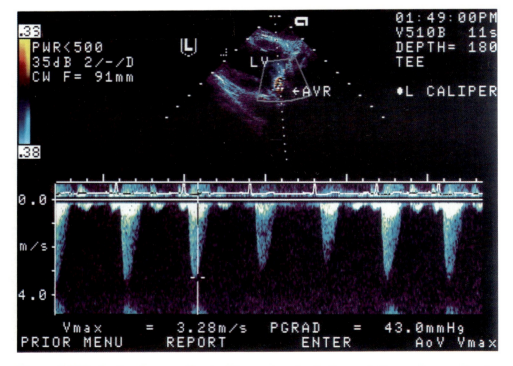

Figure 3-32C: Aortic disc prosthesis. The peak velocity through the aortic prosthesis can be measured in the transgastric view, in either the longitudinal (this figure) or the transverse planes. The peak gradient here was 43 mm Hg. LV = left ventricle; AVR = aortic valve replacement.

Fig. 3-33.

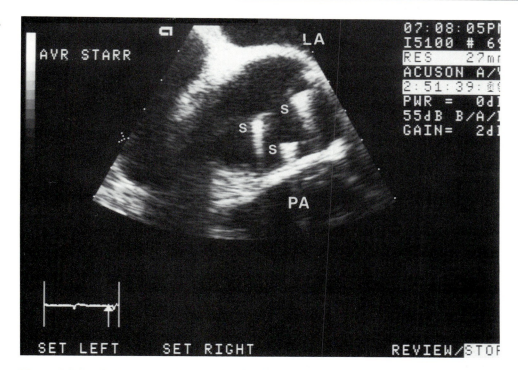

Figure 3-33A: Ball valve aortic prosthesis. Though not currently implanted, the Starr-Edwards ball valve prosthesis (ball in cage) was popular years ago. Thus, the distinctive appearance of the valve should be recognized. The three dense struts (S) are seen in the transverse basal view. LA = left atrium; PA = pulmonary artery.

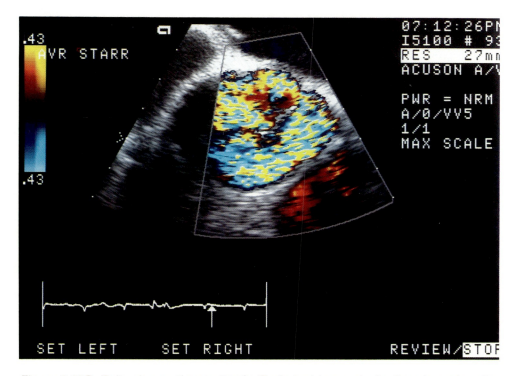

Figure 3-33B: Ball valve aortic prosthesis. Turbulent transvalvular flow (mosaic color jet) is due to blood flow circumnavigating around the ball.

Fig. 3-33. (cont'd)

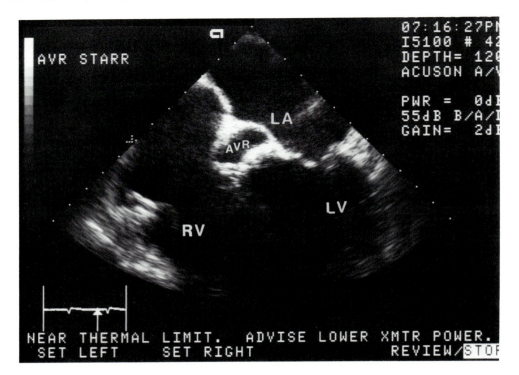

Figure 3-33C: Ball prosthesis. The transverse five-chamber view of the ball valve demonstrates extensive shadowing, virtually obscuring the septum. LA = left atrium; LV = left ventricle; RV = right ventricle; AVR = aortic valve replacement.

Fig. 3-34.

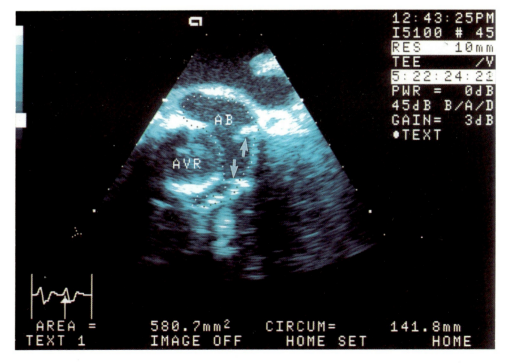

Figure 3-34A: Aortic abscess cavity (AB) measures 5.8 cm^2 in the transverse basal plane developed several months after implantation of a porcine valve (AVR). Two white strands (arrows) represent sutures breaching the abscess cavity.

Fig. 3-34. (cont'd)

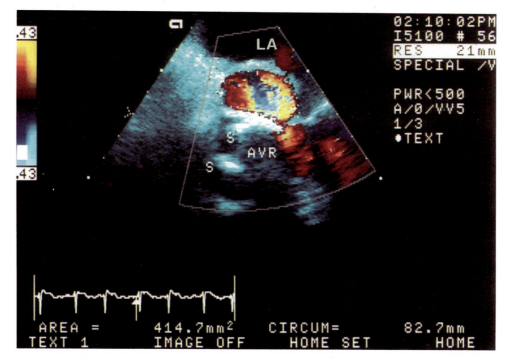

Figure 3-34B: Color flow Doppler demonstrates flow in the abscess cavity assisting in outlining its size. Aortic abscesses form most commonly between the left atrium (LA) and the aorta and they may bulge into the LA. S = prosthetic struts of the procine valve; AVR = aortic valve replacement.

Fig. 3-35.

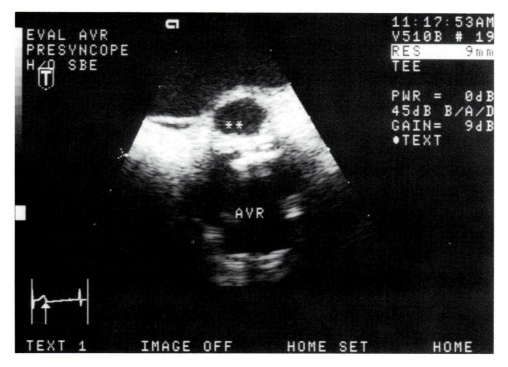

Figure 3-35A: Aortic abscess cavity in the transverse plane (asterisks). AVR = aortic valve replacement.

Fig. 3-35.
(cont'd)

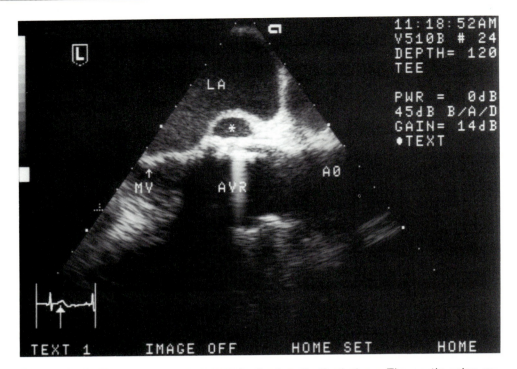

Figure 3-35B: The same abscess seen in the longitudinal plane. The aortic valve replacement (AVR) casts a reverberatory echo. LA = left atrium; AO = aorta; MV = mitral valve.

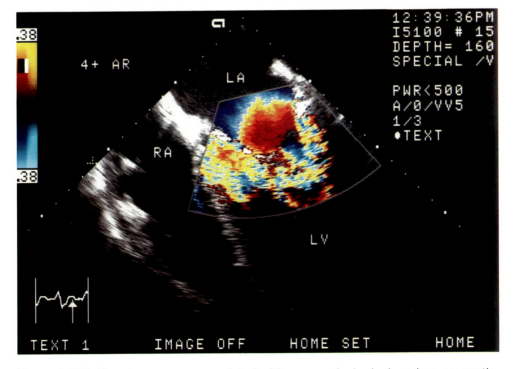

Figure 3-35C: The abscess was associated with a paravalvular leak and severe aortic regurgitation. LA = left atrium; RA = right atrium; LV = left ventricle.

Bicuspid Aortic Valve

Congenital aortic stenosis may occur in 3% to 6% of all patients with congenital cardiovascular defects and the most common anatomical abnormality is a bicuspid (two leaflets) instead of a tricuspid aortic valve. The two leaflets may be symmetrical with an anterior and posterior or right and left orientation or asymmetric in size. Usually, the left coronary artery originates from the left or the anterior cusp.

The bicuspid aortic valve may be recognized by the identification of only two leaflets, mild systolic doming, mild stenosis, and possible diastolic prolapse with aortic regurgitation. Because of the abnormal flow characteristics through the domed valve, gradually there may be progressive fibrosis and commissural fusion and the development of aortic stenosis by the fourth or fifth decade.

Fig. 3-36.

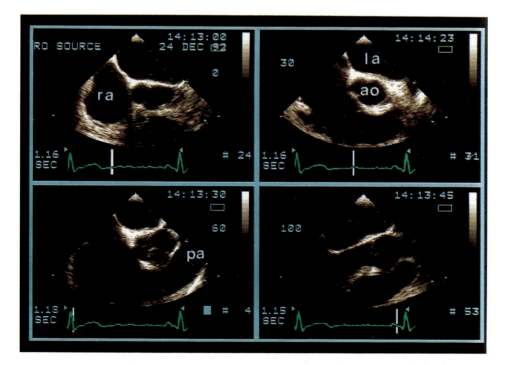

Figure 3-36: Complete interrogation of the aortic valve is possible with a multiplane probe. Starting at the upper left frame, the aortic valve is imaged at 0°, 30°, 60°, and 100° axes. ra = right atrium; la = left atrium; ao = aorta; pa = pulmonary artery.

138 • Clinical Atlas of Transesophageal Echocardiography

Fig. 3-37.

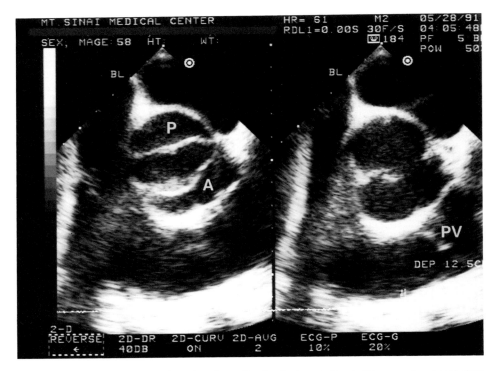

Figure 3-37A: Bicuspid aortic valve (longitudinal plane): the left image (systole) demonstrates a large anterior (A) and a large posterior (P) leaflet. The figure on the right demonstrates diastolic valve closure. PV = pulmonic valve).

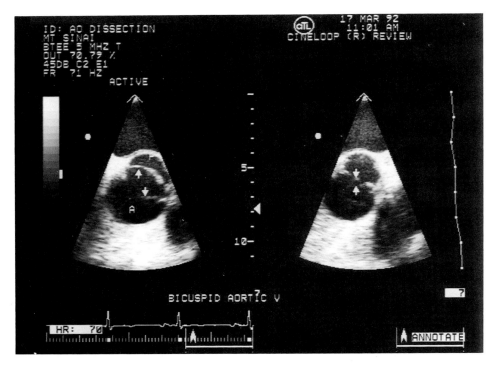

Figure 3-37B: Transverse plane of bicuspid aortic valve (left, during systole) with moderately stenotic valve. A = anterior.

Aortic Valve Disease • 139

Fig. 3-37. (cont'd)

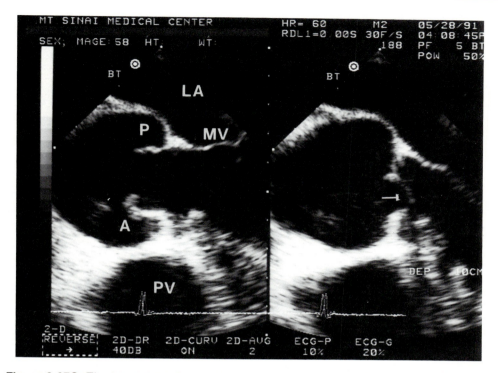

Figure 3-37C: The transverse plane demonstrates a bicuspid valve with mild doming of the lower cusp (A, anterior). The diastolic frame on the right demonstrates mild prolapse of that same leaflet. There is mild thickening of the leaflets. LA = left atrium; P = posterior; MV = mitral valve; PV = pulmonary valve.

Fig. 3-38.

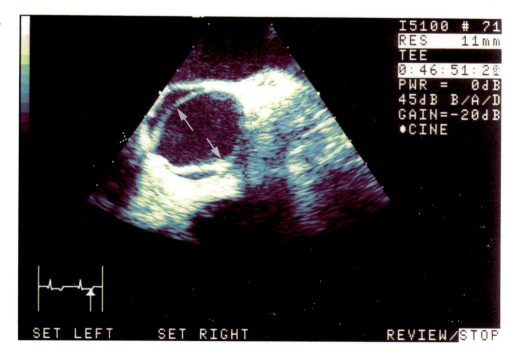

Figure 3-38A: B-color can highlight the valve leaflets demonstrating a symmetric large orifice of this bicuspid valve.

**Fig. 3-38.
(cont'd)**

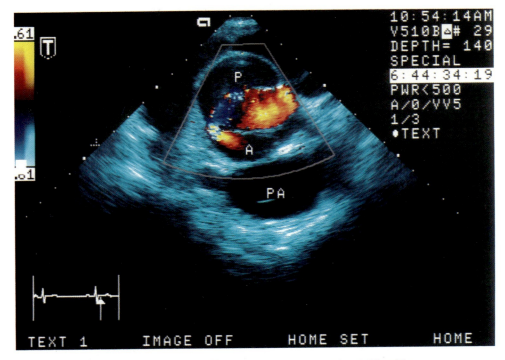

Figure 3-38B: Color Doppler outlines the bicuspid orifice.

Fig. 3-39.

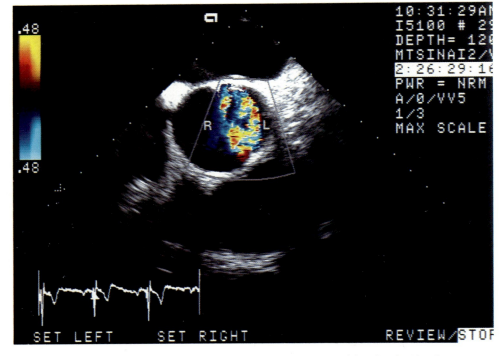

Figure 3-39A: Color Doppler clearly confirms this bicuspid valve in the transverse plane with asymmetric left (L) and right (R) coronary cusps.

Fig. 3-39.
(cont'd)

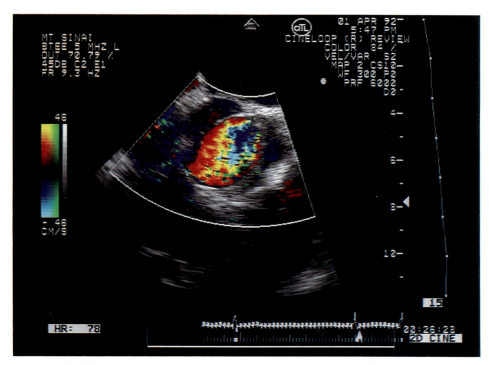

Figure 3-39B: The color Doppler accentuates a bicuspid valve in the longitudinal view. P = posterior; A = anterior; PA = pulmonary artery.

Fig. 3-40.

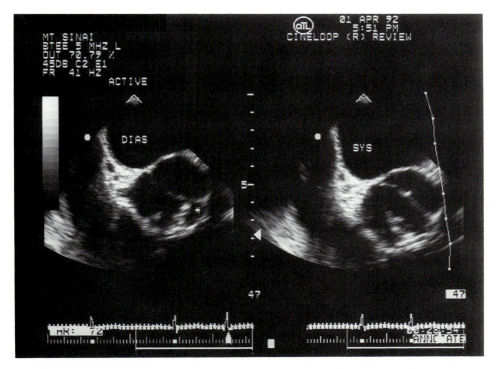

Figure 3-40: A thickened raphe of a bicuspid valve can mimic a tricuspid aortic valve. Careful interrogation in all views can define the bicuspid nature of the valve. The systolic (SYS) frame (right) has only two cusps, while the diastolic (DIAS) frame (left) has a dense raphe (asterisk) which can cause misdiagnosis as a tricuspid valve. A = anterior; P = posterior.

Fig. 3-41.

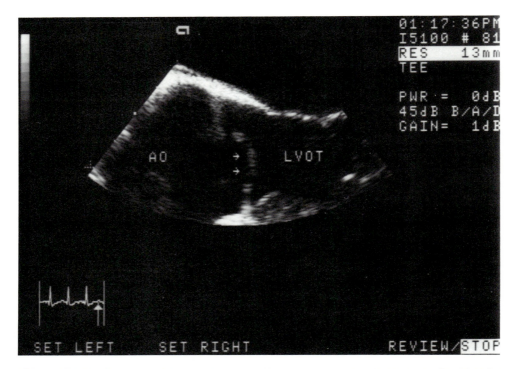

Figure 3-41A: Prolapse of the anterior leaflet (arrows) of a bicuspid aortic valve in the transverse plane. AO = aorta; LVOT = left ventricular outflow tract.

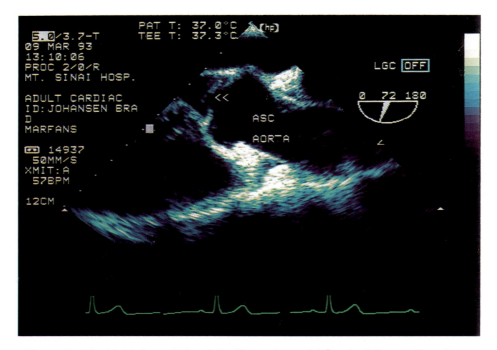

Figure 3-41B: Multiplane (72° axis) with prolapse (arrows) of the aortic valve.

Fig. 3-42.

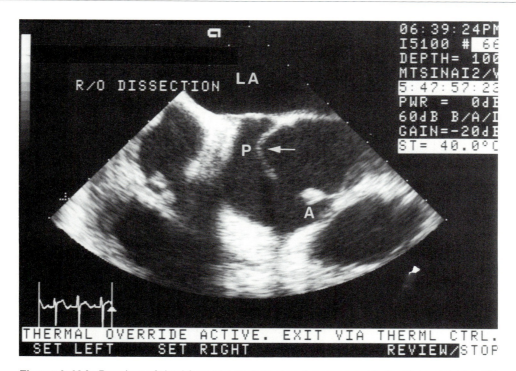

Figure 3-42A: Doming of the bicuspid aortic valve, transverse plane. The posterior (P) cusp is longer with more significant doming than the diminutive small and thickened anterior (A) leaflet. LA = left atrium.

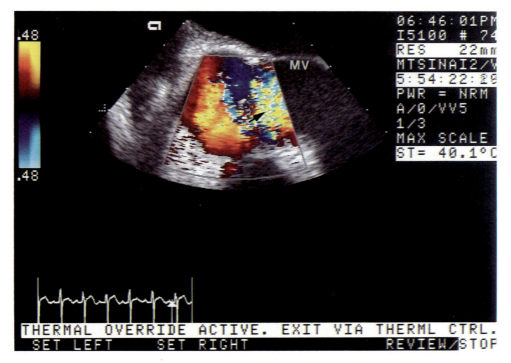

Figure 3-42B: Aortic insufficiency originating from the bicuspid aortic valve. The closure is asymmetric with an aortic regurgitation jet originating from the point of poor coaptation between the two leaflets (transverse plane). MV = mitral valve.

Fig. 3-42. (cont'd)

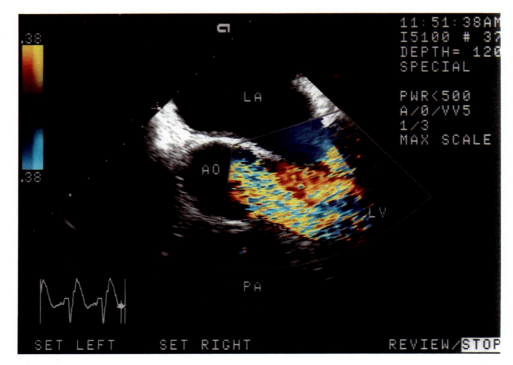

Figure 3-42C: Moderate aortic regurgitation. LA = left atrium; AO = aorta; PA = pumonary artery.

Fig. 3-43.

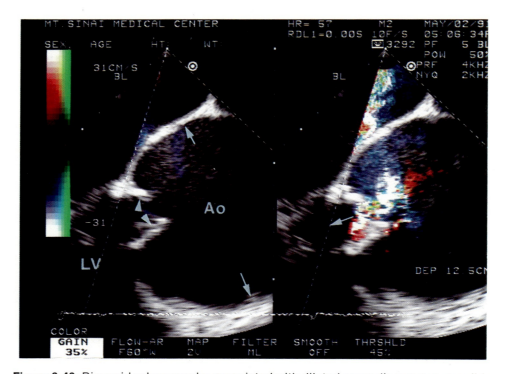

Figure 3-43: Bicuspid valves may be associated with dilated ascending aortas, possibly due to the turbulent systolic flow. The left frame demonstrates a doming aortic valve and aortic aneurysm (8 cm diameter) in the longitudinal plane. Aortic insufficiency is shown by color flow Doppler (right). LV = left ventricle; Ao = aorta.

Fig. 3-44.

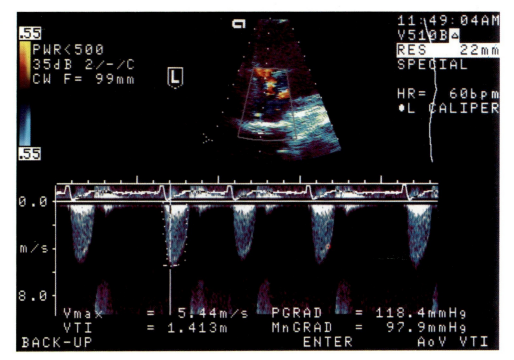

Figure 3-44: Late in the disease process, bicuspid aortic vaves may develop aortic stenosis. From the five-chamber transgastric view, continuous wave Doppler yielded a maximum transaortic gradient of 118.4 mm Hg and a mean gradient of 97.9 mm Hg, consistent with severe aortic stenosis.

4

Tricuspid Disease

Tricuspid Regurgitation

The most common etiology of tricuspid regurgitation is dilatation of the tricuspid annulus secondary to right ventricular dilatation due to pulmonary hypertension usually from left-sided heart disease. Transthoracic echocardiography can usually evaluate the severity of tricuspid regurgitation. However, since transesophageal echocardiography is frequently used to better evaluate mitral valve disease, the extent and severity of possible tricuspid regurgitation should also be determined because it may alter the clinical and surgical management of the patient. Mild tricuspid regurgitation is frequently seen in normal patients. The patients with pathological tricuspid regurgitation usually have more severe regurgitation manifested by a larger color flow area, greater systolic duration, more turbulent flow, and elevated calculated right ventricular systolic pressure. Continuous wave Doppler can be positioned to measure the transtricuspid regurgitant jet gradient from which right ventricular systolic pressure can be estimated by adding 5–12 mm Hg for right atrial pressures, 5 mm for normal right atrial pressure, 12 mm for elevated right atrial pressure, with dilated jugular neck veins (RV systolic pressure = (RV − RA gradient) + 5–12 mm Hg). See Figures 4-9A and 4-9B.

Fig. 4-1.

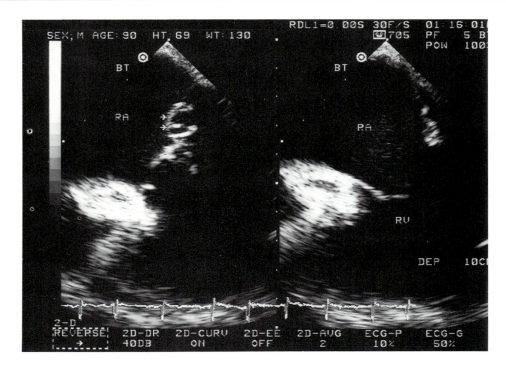

Figure 4-1: Right ventricular inflow view, transverse plane. The right side demonstrates diastolic opening of the tricuspid valve with mild thickening and doming. The left frame demonstrates prolapse of the septal leaflet (arrows). RA = right atrium; RV = right ventricle.

Fig. 4-2.

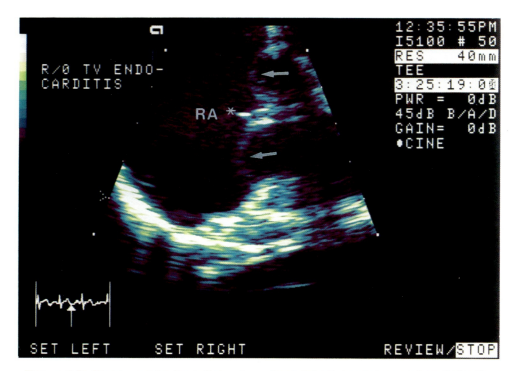

Figure 4-2: Right ventricular inflow view, demonstrating prolapse of both leaflets. Both the anterior and the septal leaflets have tiny fibrous strands or vegetations seen at their coaptation point (white densities, asterisks). RA = right atrium.

Fig. 4-3.

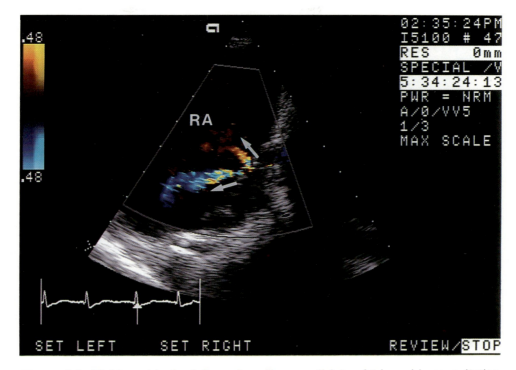

Figure 4-3: Right ventricular inflow view. Two small jets of tricuspid regurgitation (arrows) consistent with mild disease. This degree of tricuspid regurgitation is essentially a normal finding.

Fig. 4-4.

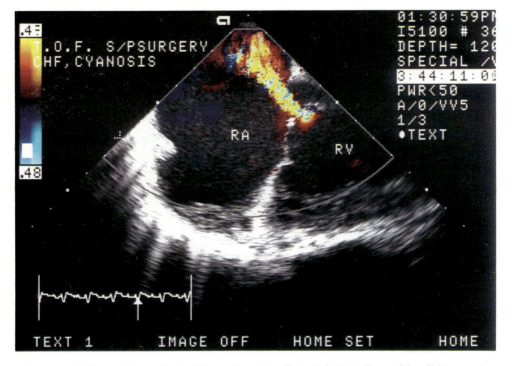

Figure 4-4: Shown is a patient with moderately dilated right atrium with mild to moderate tricuspid regurgitation. RA = right atrium; RV = right ventricle.

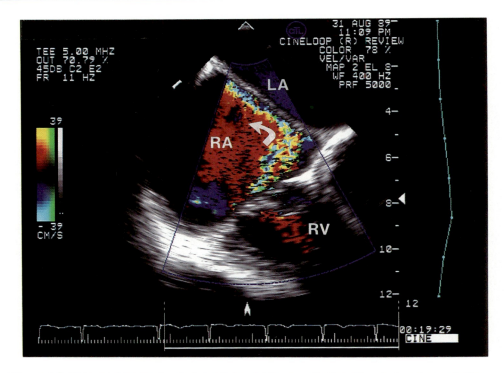

Figure 4-5: This mild to moderate jet of tricuspid regurgitation directed up towards the interatrial septum. Careful interrogation of the right atrium in all planes is important to quantify severity of tricuspid regurgitation. RA = right atrium; RV = right ventricle; LA = left atrium.

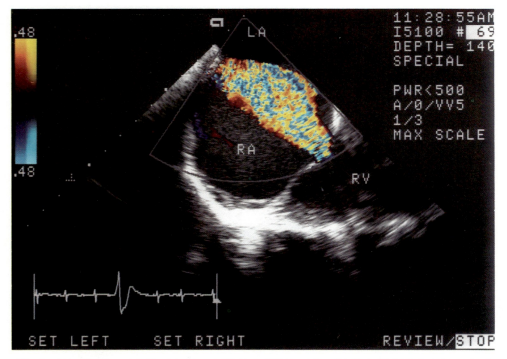

Figure 4-6: Moderate tricuspid regurgitation filling at least one-half of the right atrium. RA = right atrium; RV = right ventricle; LA = left atrium.

Fig. 4-7.

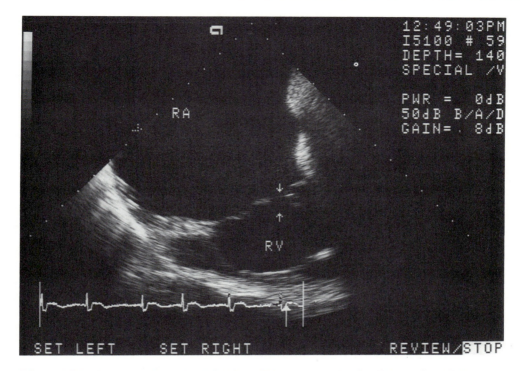

Figure 4-7A: Massively dilated right atrium (RA) and a markedly dilated tricuspid annulus causing poor coaptation of the leaflets (arrows). LV = left ventricle.

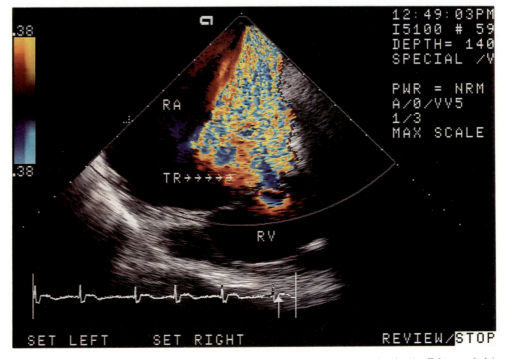

Figure 4-7B: Severe tricuspid regurgitation (tricuspid regurgitation). RA = right atrium; RV = right ventricle.

Fig. 4-8.

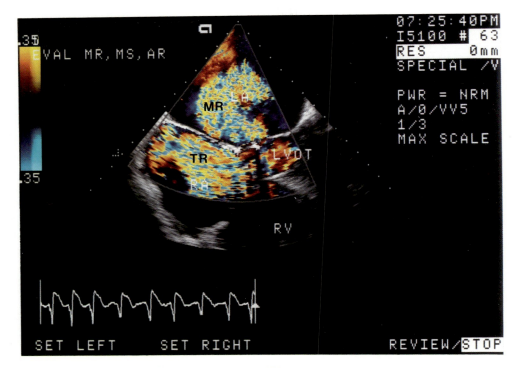

Figure 4-8: Transverse five-chamber view. Etiology of severe tricuspid regurgitation (tricuspid regurgitation) is due to moderate dilatation of the left atrium secondary to moderate mitral regurgitation. This patient required mitral valve repair (MR) as well as tricuspid valve repair. LVOT = left ventricular outflow tract; RV = right ventricle.

Fig. 4-9.

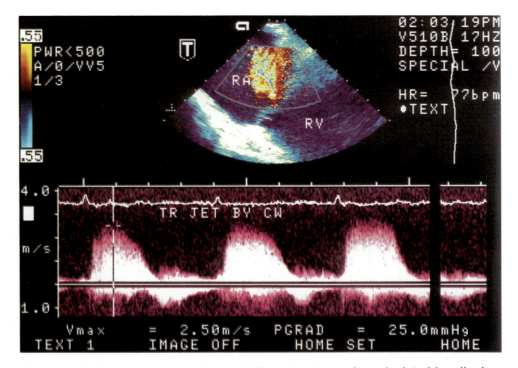

Figure 4-9A: Right ventricular (RV) systolic pressure can be calculated by aligning the CW Doppler beam parallel to the tricuspid regurgitation (TR) jet. This patient had moderate TR with a peak systolic gradient of only 25 mm Hg. Adding 5 mm Hg as the estimated right atrial (RA) pressure yields an estimated right ventricular systolic pressure of 30 mm Hg.

Fig. 4-9. (cont'd)

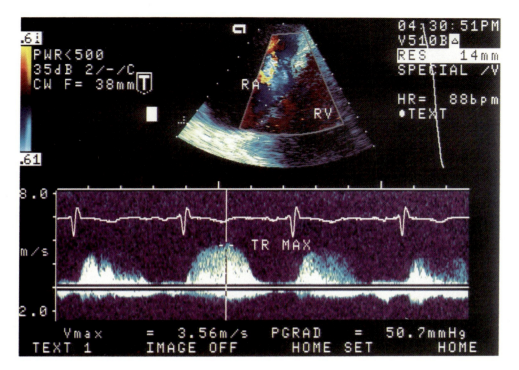

Figure 4-9B: A patient with moderate pulmonary hypertension due to mitral regurgitation had a transtricuspid valve gradient of 50 mm Hg. Because the jugular venous pressure was elevated, right atrial (RA) pressure was estimated to be 10 mm Hg. Therefore, right ventricular (RV) systolic pressure was estimated to be 60 mm Hg.

Fig. 4-10.

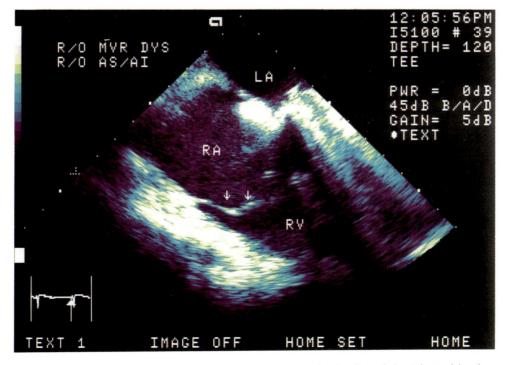

Figure 4-10A: Hockey stick configuration of the anterior leaflet of the tricuspid valve (arrows) consistent with mild to moderate tricuspid stenosis. Rheumatic involvement of the tricuspid valve may be seen in 15% of pathological studies of rheumatic heart disease. RA = right atrium; RV = right ventricle; LA = left atrium.

Fig. 4-10. (cont'd)

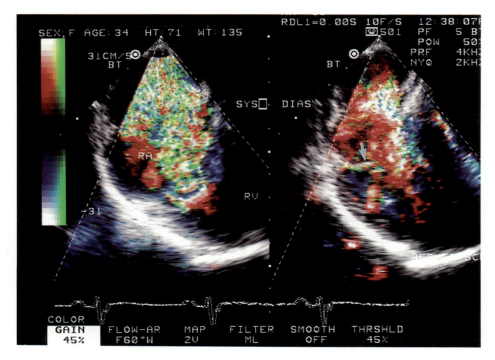

Figure 4-10B: Mild diastolic doming (arrow) of a mildly stenotic tricuspid valve (right frame) and severe systolic tricuspid regurgitation (left frame). RA = right atrium; RV = right ventricle. This patient had tricuspid stenosis and regurgitation and pulmonic stenosis due to carcinoid disease.

Tricuspid Valve Endocarditis

Endocarditis usually develops on a valve that is regurgitant or stenotic, generating a turbulent jet lesion that serves as a nidus for vegetation development. There may be tricuspid valve prolapse or rheumatic involvement predisposing to endocarditis. Importantly, intravenous drug abusers are particularly at risk for right-sided endocarditis because of the large dose of bacteria and irritant materials injected intravenously that is presented to the right side of the heart before it is filtered in the lungs. Drug abusers who develop tricuspid endocarditis may have had underlying mild tricuspid prolapse or regurgitation. Tricuspid endocarditis may present initially as fever, chills, or as a pulmonary embolus with marked dyspnea and chest pain.

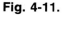
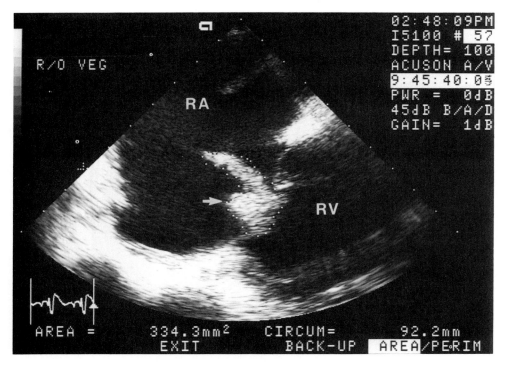

Figure 4-11A-C: A large vegetation (3.3 cm^2) (arrow) prolapses into the right atrium (RA) during systole and swings into the left ventricle (LV) during diastole (Fig. 4-11B) causing severe tricuspid regurgitation (TR) (Fig. 4-11C).

Fig. 4-11. (cont'd)

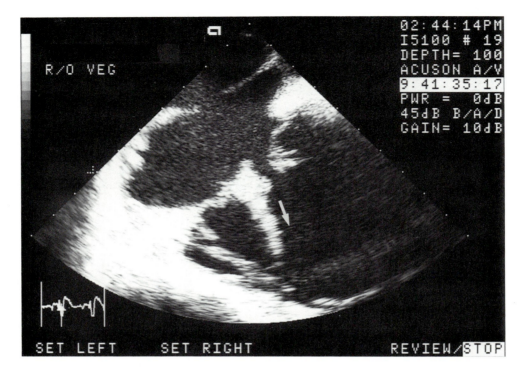

Figure 4-11B.

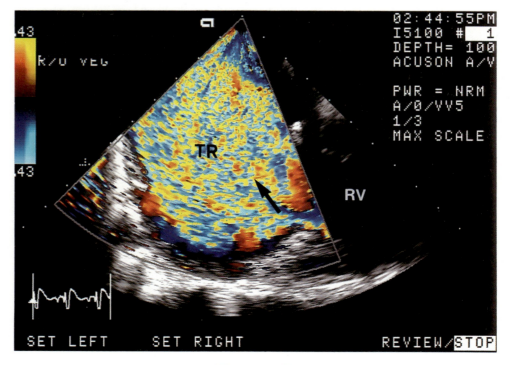

Figure 4-11C.

Fig. 4-12.

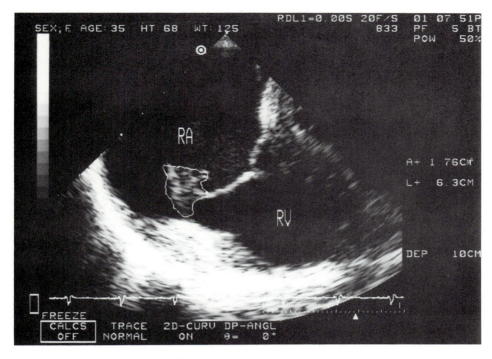

Figure 4-12A: A sessile vegetation is seen on the base of the anterior leaflet (1.76 cm² area). RA = right atrium; RV = right ventricle.

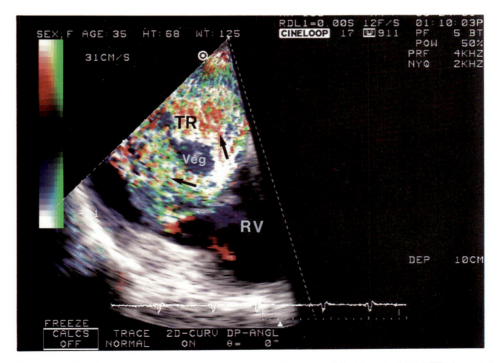

Figure 4-12B: Severe tricuspid regurgitation (TR) caused by the endocarditis is seen to envelop around the vegetation (Veg) in the middle of the tricuspid jet. RV = right ventricle.

Fig. 4-13.

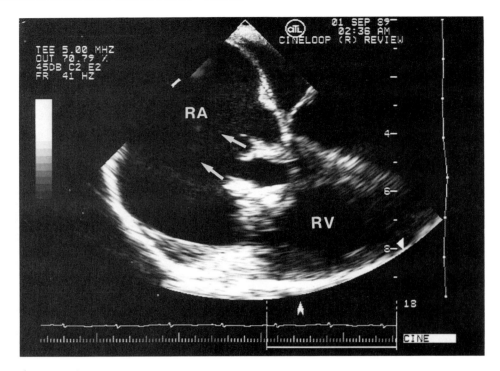

Figure 4-13: Two pedunculated vegetations are seen prolapsed into the right atrium (RA) during systole (arrows). RV = right ventricle.

5

Aortic Dissection

Aortic dissection is a potential medical emergency that requires immediate and accurate diagnosis and may necessitate urgent surgigal intervention. Aortic dissection is precipitated by a sudden tear of the aortic intima facilitating a column of blood to drive into the wall of the aorta. The primary pathophysiological event is a hemorrhage within the media that ruptures through the intima or primary tear of the intima leading to the dissection.

There are three types of aortic dissection (see Fig. 1):

Type I: originates in the ascending aorta within several centimeters of the aortic valve and continues to dissect antegrade up the anterior ascending aorta, arch, and down the descending.

Type II: begins in the ascending aorta near the aortic valve but does not continue to dissect antegrade to the arch.

Type III: occurs in distal or descending aorta just beyond the origin of the left subclavian artery at the side of the ligamentum arteriosum.

For practical purposes, thoracic aortic dissections can be categorized into either type A (for ascending dissections limited to the ascending aorta or which dissect into the descending aorta types I and II) and type B (dissections originating in the descending aorta, type III).

The most common presenting symptom of aortic dissection is chest pain, which initially can be severe and may radiate to the back and shoulders as the dissecting hematoma begins to extend the tear. Other symptoms may include neurological manifestations such as stroke or syncope, and nausea and vomiting, or heart failure. On physical exam, the patient may initially be hypertensive but may develop hypotension if significant dissection leads to cardiac tamponade, rupture, or if there is occlusion of the brachial arteries. With an ascending aortic dissection, there may be a pulse deficit in the left subclavian and the femoral artery. Aortic regurgitation occurs in 50% of proximal type dissections.

Appropriate management requires initial suspicion of aortic dissection. Once the diagnosis is considered, the fastest and most accurate method for diagnosing an aortic dissection is transesophageal echocardiography (TEE). Studies have reported specificity and sensitivity of over 95% for TEE for the diagnosis of aortic dissection. Importantly, there is a small TEE blind spot (<1 cm in length) where the trachea crosses the aorta, but an isolated dissection to just this region would be extremely rare. Though CT scan, MRI, and angiography have also been advocated as diagnostic methods for aortic dissection, they require more time, which may not be feasible if the patient is hemodynamically unstable. CT scan without contrast may not differentiate between thrombus or calcification in the lumen of the aorta from dissection. Though MRI may image the ascending aorta more accurately than TEE, a thorough transthoracic and biplane TEE should be able to exclude any type of dissection.

Transesophageal echocardiogram can be performed in the emergency room, providing prompt diagnostic accuracy which determines whether or not the patient is a surgical candidate. During the transesophageal echocardiogram, several features of the dissection need to be defined:

1. The type of dissection—type A or B: Type A requires emergency surgery, while type B can be treated medially if it is not expanding.

2. The site of the original tear and communication site between true and false lumens: Though the tear may occur high in the ascending aorta, because of retrograde flow of blood, a false lumen may be seen near the aortic valve. This may create the impression that the dissection tear began at that level. The actual tear site is important in determining the type of surgical intervention that is necessary. An intimal flap may be seen undulating between the true and false lumens.

3. The extent of the dissection: The entire thoracic aorta should be carefully interrogated as far as possible down the descending aorta.

4. The extent of aortic insufficiency and involvement of aortic valve: Dilation of the annulus caused by the dissection may cause aortic insufficiency, which may necessitate aortic valve replacement if there is severe aortic regurgitation. A Bental procedure entails replacement of the aortic valve as well as a graft placement in the ascending aorta. Occasionally, the surgeon can repair the aortic root adequately so that the native valve can be salvaged.

5. The presence of pericardial effusion: Patients may present with pericardial tamponade because of retrograde dissection involving the rupture of the aorta into the pericardium. These patients must be handled very carefully because removal of the pericardial effusion may cause exsanguination and death of the patient. The presence of effusion should mandate rapid surgical intervention.

6. Involvement of the ostia of the coronary arteries may mandate coronary bypass surgery.

Bibliography

1. Thorsen MK, San Dretto MA, Lawson TL, et al: Detection of aortic dissection by transesophageal echocardiography. *Br Heart J* 58:45–51, 1987.
2. Erbel R, Rennollet H, Engberding R, Visser C, Daniel W, Roelandt J (European Cooperative Study Group): Complementary role of echocardiography in the diagnosis of aortic dissection including transesophageal echocardiography. *Lancet* 1:457–461, 1989.
3. Mohr-Kahaly S, Erbel R, Rennollet H, Wittlich N, Drexler M, Oelert H, Meyer J: Ambulatory follow-up of aortic dissection by transesophageal two dimensional and color-coded Doppler echocardiography. *Circulation* 80:24–33, 1989.
4. Simon P, Owen AN, Havel M, Moidl R, Hiesmayr M, Wolner E, Mohl W: Transesophageal echocardiography in the emergency surgical management of patients with aortic dissection. *J Thorac CardioVasc Surgery* 103: 1113–1118, 1992.

5. Kronzon I, Demopoulos L, Schrem SS, Pasternack P, McCauley D, Freedberg RS: Pitfalls in the diagnosis of thoracic aortic aneurysm by transesophageal echocardiography. *J Am Soc Echocardiogr* 3:145–148, 1990.
6. Silvey SV, Stoughton TL, Pearl W, Collazo WA, Belbel RJ: Rupture of the outer partition of aortic dissection during transesophageal echocardiography. *Am J Cardiol* 68:286–287, 1991.
7. Adachi H, Kyo S, Takamoto S, Kirmura S, Yokote Y, Omoto R: Early diagnosis and surgical intervention of acute aortic dissection by transesophageal color flow mapping. *Circulation* 82:19–23, 1990.
8. Chan KL: Usefulness of transesophageal echocardiography in the diagnosis of conditions mimicking aortic dissection. *Am Heart J* 122:495–504, 1991.
9. Nienaber CA, Spielmann RP, Von Kodolitsch Y, Siglow V, Piepho H, Jaup T, et al: Diagnosis of thoracic aortic dissection: Magnetic resonance imaging versus transesophageal echocardiography. *Circulation* 85:434–447, 1992.
10. Ballal RS, Nanda NC, Gatewood R, Darcy B, et al: Usefulness of transesophageal echocardiography in assessment of aortic dissection. *Circulation* 84:1903–1914, 1991.
11. Mienaber CA, Von Kodolitsch Y, Nicholas V, et al: The diagnosis of thoracic aortic dissection by noninvasive imaging procedure. *N Engl J Med* 38:35–43, 1993.
12. Cigarroa JE, Isselbacher EM, DeSanctis RW, Eagle KA: Diagnostic imaging in the evaluation of suspected aortic dissection. *N Engl J Med* 328:35–43, 1993.

Fig. 5-1.

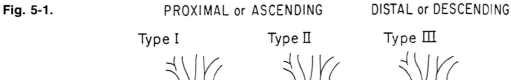

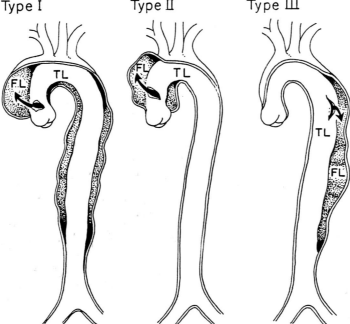

Figure 5-1: See text for discussion of three types of aortic dissection. TL = true lumen; FL = false lumen.

Fig. 5-2.

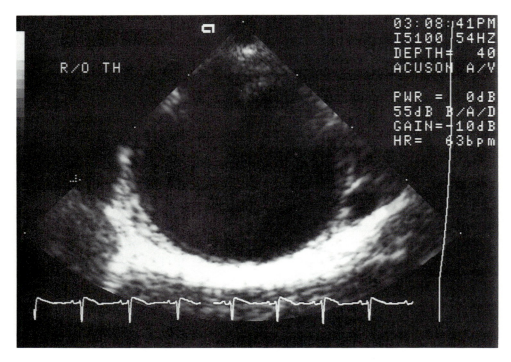

Figure 5-2: Normal descending aorta (transverse plane), with a round uniform lumen, usually with less than a 3 cm diameter.

Fig. 5-3.

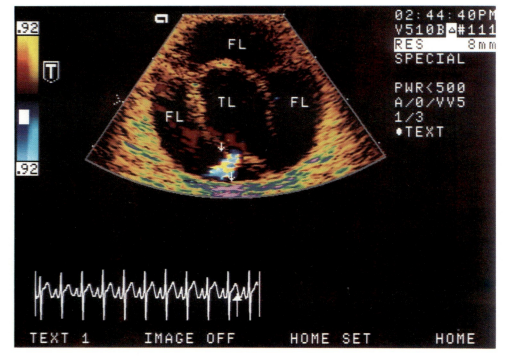

Figure 5-3A: Descending aortic dissection, transverse plane, demonstrates the true lumen (TL) surrounded circumferentially by the false lumen (FL) with communication between them (arrow, color Doppler jet) at the origin of a spinal artery.

Fig. 5-3. (cont'd)

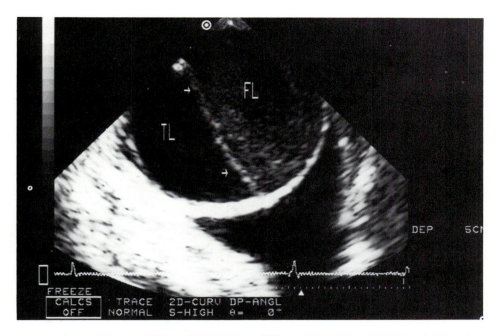

Figure 5-3B: True lumen (TL) and false lumen (FL) are demonstrated in the descending aorta separated by an intimal flap (arrows). A haze of echogenic "smoke" (seen in the FL because of the low flow state) may distinguish between the TL and FL when present. The clear space inferiorly is a pleural effusion.

Fig. 5-4.

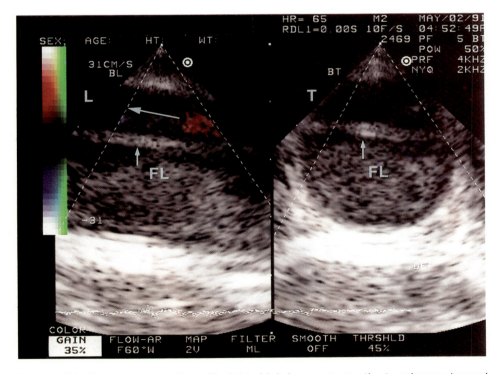

Figure 5-4A: The transverse plane (T, right side) demonstrates the true lumen (superiorly) and the false lumen (FL, below) with "smoke." The intimal flap (small arrow) separates the two chambers. The longitudinal plane (L, left side) demonstrates the two lumina with flow documented by color Doppler in the true lumen.

Fig. 5-4. (cont'd)

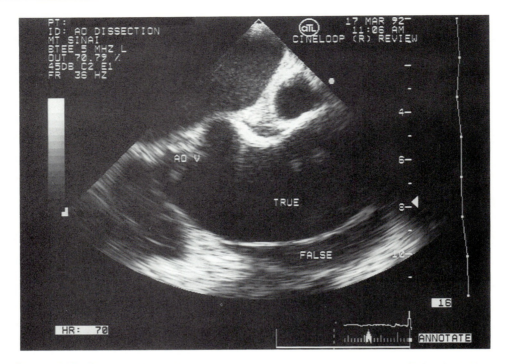

Figure 5-4B: The longitudinal plane can visualize the proximal aorta. This dissection extended to 4 cm above the aortic valve (AoV). An intimal flap separates the true lumen from the false.

Fig. 5-5.

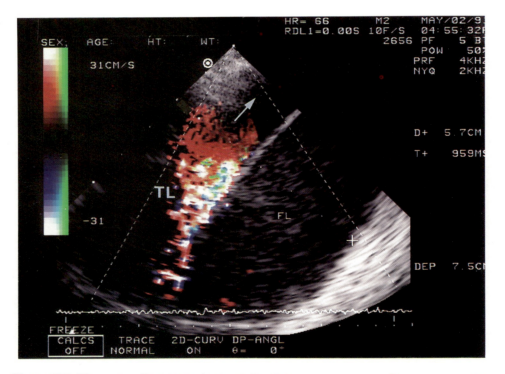

Figure 5-5: The ascending aorta (transverse plane) with the true (TL) and false (FL) lumina separated by the intimal flap. While there is flow in the true lumen, the false lumen is hazy due to echogenic smoke. The diameter of the aorta at this level was 5.7 cm (normal <3 cm) with the false lumen being twice as wide as the true lumen.

Fig. 5-6.

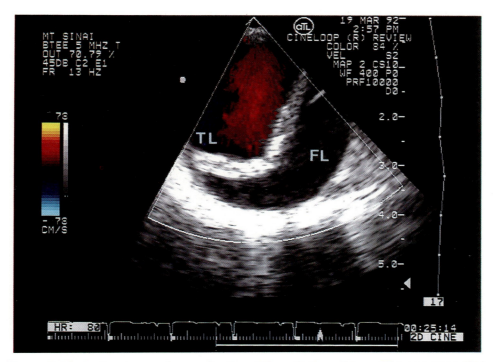

Figure 5-6A: In the descending aorta, the differentiation of true (TL) and false (FL) lumens can also be made by the presence of flow in the true lumen and the presence of smoke in the false lumen. The intimal flap is whiter, thicker, and denser, which may connote involvement of part of the media, a more atherosclerotic intima or a more chronic dissection. This intimal flap was fixed and did not undulate due to its rigidity.

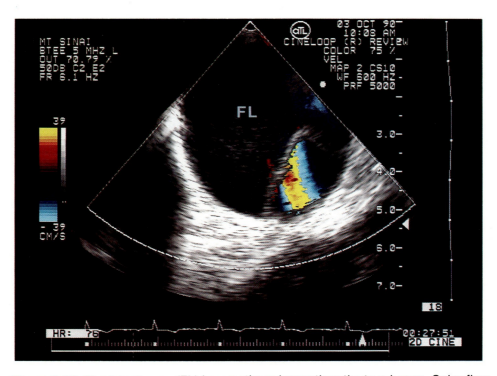

Figure 5-6B: The false lumen (FL) is sometimes larger than the true lumen. Color flow demonstrates predominant flow in the true lumen. Rarely, the false lumen may have the greater flow (aortic arch, longitudinal plane).

Fig. 5-7.

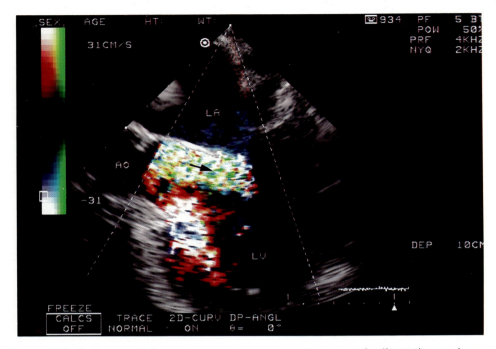

Figure 5-7: Aortic insufficiency frequently accompanies an aortic dissection and may predate the dissection because of underlying aortic dilatation or an aneurysm that may predispose to dissection. This transverse five-chamber view demonstrates aortic insufficiency (arrow) as the multicolor mosaic jet in the left ventricular outflow tract. LA = left atrium; LV = left ventricle; AO = aorta.

Fig. 5-8.

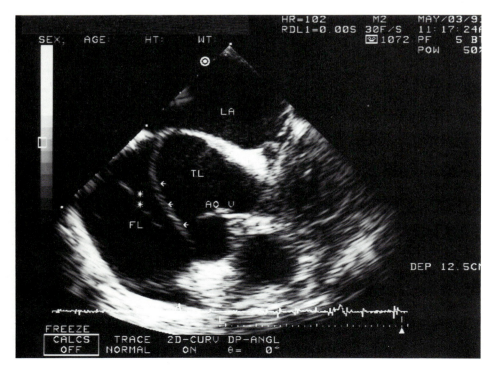

Figure 5-8A: In the transverse plane, an intimal flap (arrows), which separates the true lumen (TL) and false lumen (FL), begins approximately 2 cm anterior to the aortic valve (Ao V). There is a fibrous strand (asterisks) in the false lumen.

Fig. 5-8.
(cont'd)

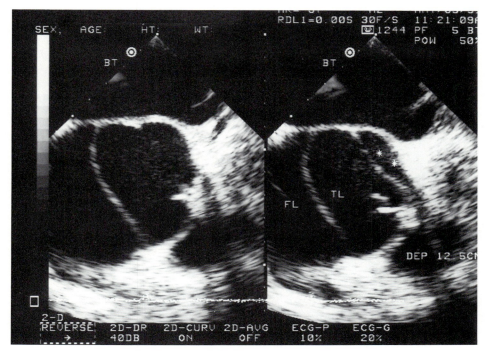

Figure 5-8B: The spiraling false lumen (FL and asterisks) surrounds the true lumen (TL) on both sides (right). The left frame demonstrates that the spiral effect of the false lumen was seen in only certain levels (transverse plane, proximal ascending aorta).

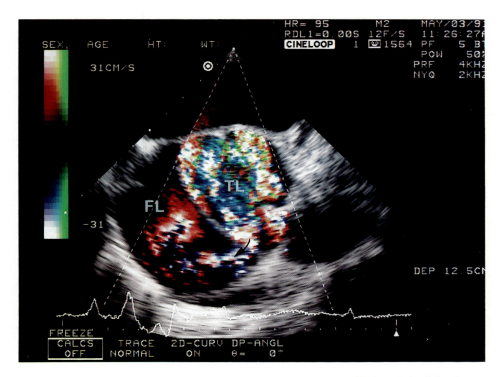

Figure 5-8C: A communication exists between the true lumen (TL) and the false lumen (FL) (mosiac flow), both in the more proximal segment to the right and anteriorly in the largest false lumen to the left (arrow), confirming this as a type A dissection.

Fig. 5-9.

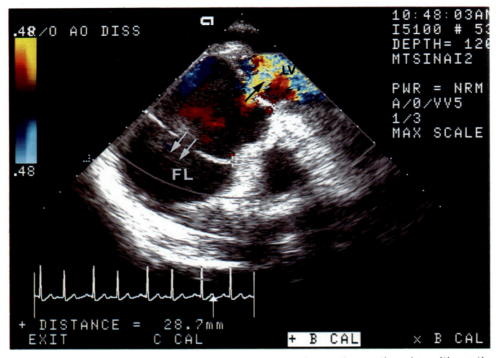

Figure 5-9A: An intimal flap is seen just 3 cm superior to the aortic valve with aortic insufficiency (single arrow) demonstrated by the mosaic jet refluxing the left ventricle (LV). There is flow in the true lumen and communication with the false lumen (FL, double arrows).

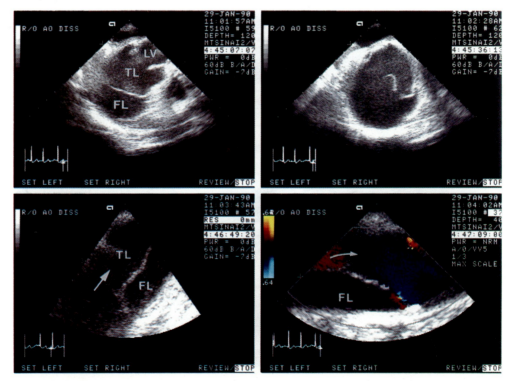

Figure 5-9B: The upper left frame demonstrates a proximal intimal flap with aortic valve open (systole). The lower left depicts the ascending aorta with intimal flap separating the true (TL) and false (FL) lumen. The lower right demonstrates the aortic arch with flow in the superior true lumen and the upper right images the intimal flap as an undulating membrane separating the true and false lumen. It appears that there is discontinuity of the intimal flap at that level (transverse plane). LV = left ventricle.

Fig. 5-9. (cont'd)

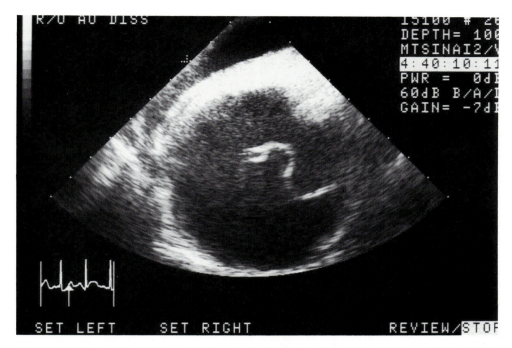

Figure 5-9C: Detail of the undulating intimal flap in the descending aorta in which there was communication between the true and false lumens (transverse plane).

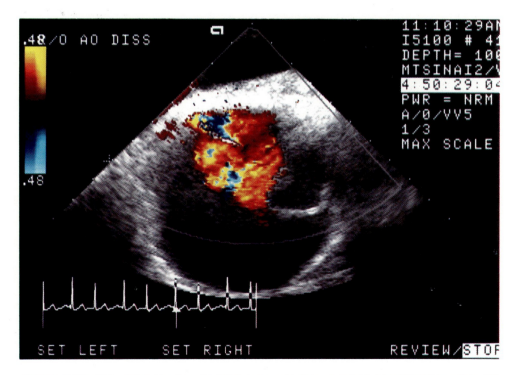

Figure 5-9D: Flow from the true to false lumen is documented. Identification of multiple entry sites is extremely important for determining the surgical approach.

Fig. 5-10.

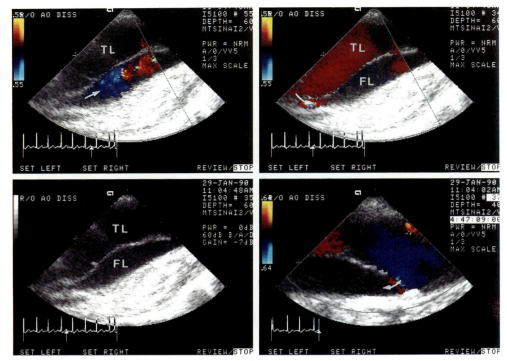

Figure 5-10A: An ascending aortic dissection is seen in the transverse plane. The two right frames demonstrate flow in the true lumen (TL) around the arch separated from the false lumen (F) by an undulating intimal flap. Communication between the two lumina is suspected by small color jets (curved arrows) and is confirmed by color flow Doppler in the FL (upper left).

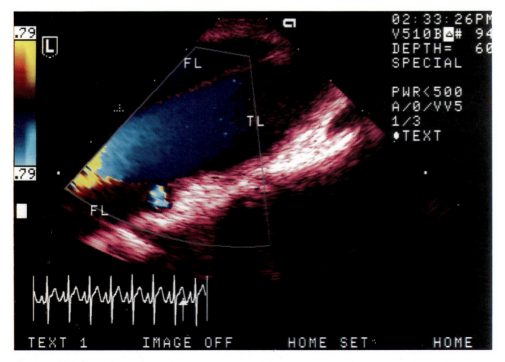

Figure 5-10B: The longitudinal plane can detect communication between the two lumina not visualized by the transverse plane alone. This proximal dissection demonstrated a small tear communication between the true lumen (TL) and the false lumen (FL) below. Very faint flow (low velocity blue color Doppler) is seen in the upper false lumen.

**Fig. 5-10.
(cont'd)**

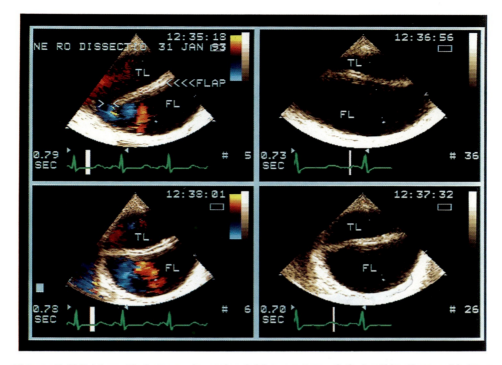

Figure 5-10C: A multiplane probe may yield even more information than a biplane probe in which the imaging axes are fixed at 0° and 90°. The upper left frame demonstrates a communication site (facing arrows) between the true lumen (TL) and the false (FL) obtained at a 75° axis. The standard longitudinal plane (upper right) or transverse planes (lower frames) did not detect the site of the tear.

Fig. 5-11.

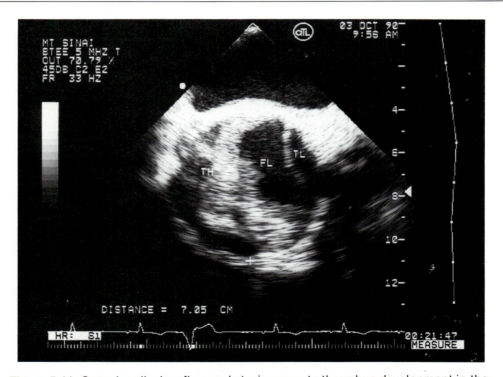

Figure 5-11: Occasionally, low flow and stasis promote thrombus development in the false lumen (FL) as seen in this proximal aortic dissection. The true lumen (TL) is separated from the FL by an intimal flap and the false lumen is almost completely filled by echodense thrombus (TH). The width of the ascending aorta at this level was 7 cm (transverse plane).

Fig. 5-12.

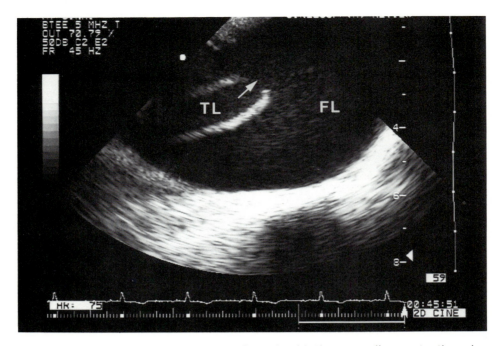

Figure 5-12A: At the junction of the aortic arch with the ascending aorta, there is a small lumen surrounded by a wider lumen with echo dropout at the apex of the smaller lumen (transverse plane). TL = true lumen; FL = false lumen.

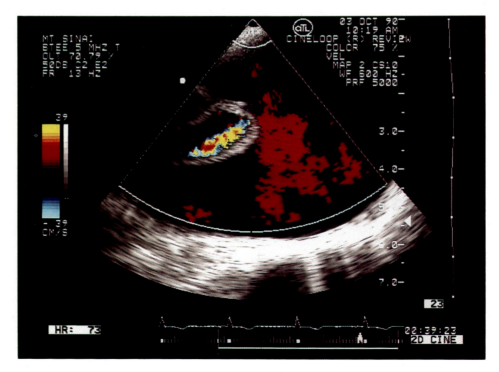

Figure 5-12B: Color flow Doppler demonstrates flow within both lumina; higher velocity (yellow) flow in the smaller true lumen and low velocity (red) in the larger false lumen. The arch diameter at this level is 6 cm.

Fig. 5-12. (cont'd)

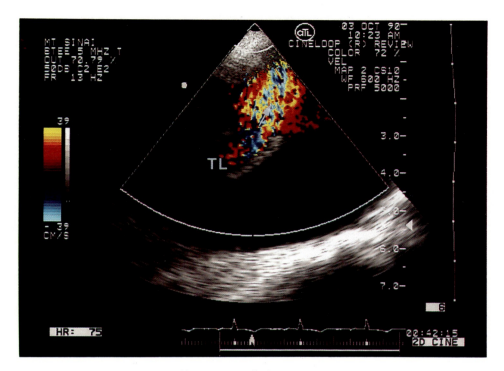

Figure 5-12C: Color flow Doppler documents systolic communication between the small true lumen (TL) and larger false lumen at this level.

Fig. 5-13.

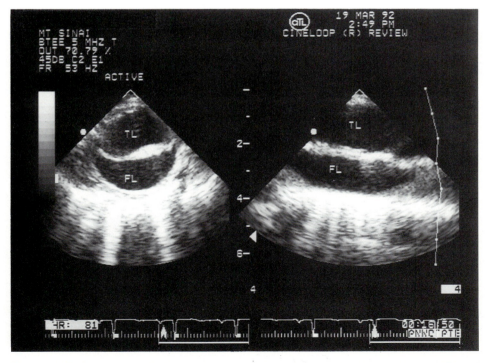

Figure 5-13: A patient with hypertension and mild upper back pain had a CT scan because of an enlarged aorta on chest X-ray, which could not differentiate calcium in the wall of the aorta from a dissection. A two-dimensional transesophageal echo in the transverse plane (left) demonstrated a false lumen (FL) separated from the true lumen (TL) by a calcified intimal flap in the descending aorta. The longitudinal plane (right) demonstrates the dense intimal flap.

Fig. 5-14.

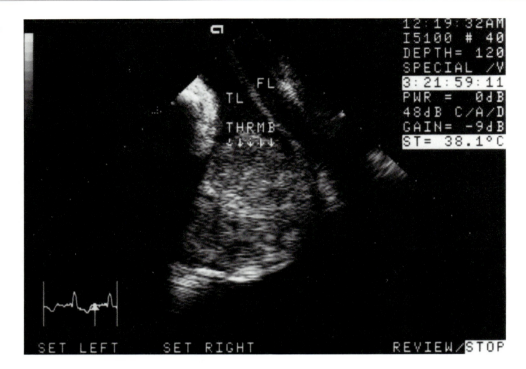

Figure 5-14A: A large thrombus (THRMB, arrows) is seen in the true lumen (TL) of this descending thoracic aneurysm (transverse with dissection plane). This patient probably had a prior aortic aneurysm with a preexisting thrombus that subsequently dissected creating a false lumen (FL).

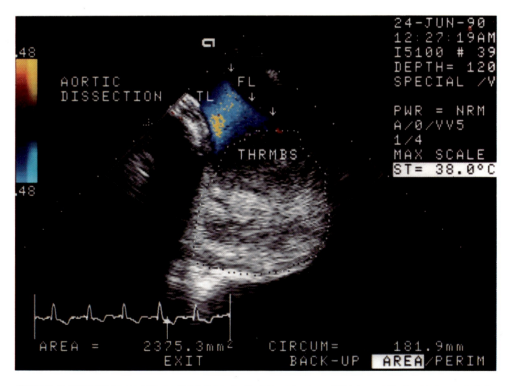

Figure 5-14B: This confirms that flow in the true lumen (TL) is partially obstructed by the thrombus (THRMBS). Occasionally, the false lumen (FL) may have more flow than the true lumen and may reenter more distally.

Fig. 5-15.

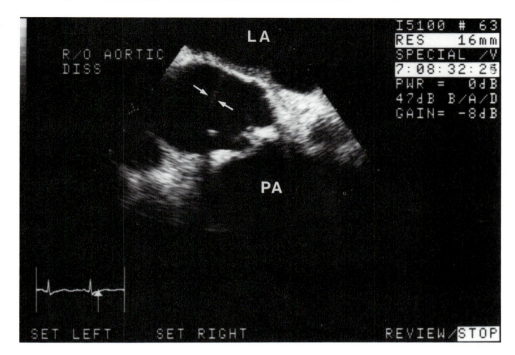

Figure 5-15A: Occasionally, artifacts can appear in the aorta due to calcium on the annulus, which may cause shadows that may appear to be an intimal flap. This transverse plane demonstrates the ascending aorta near the aortic valve with a hazy linear structure in the middle (arrows). LA = left atrium; PA = pulmonary artery.

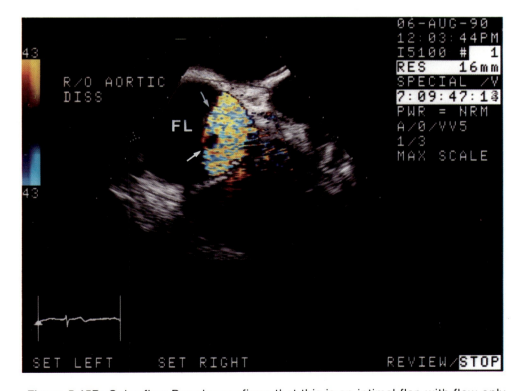

Figure 5-15B: Color flow Doppler confirms that this is an intimal flap with flow only in the true lumen. Color flow Doppler may differentiate the true from false lumen (FL) and confirm the presence of the intimal flap when imaging alone may be nondiagnostic.

Fig. 5-15. (cont'd)

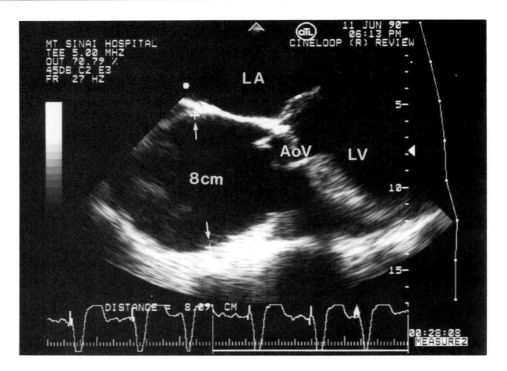

Figure 5-15C: Shadowing in this proximal aortic aneurysm (8 cm diameter) was artifactual and there was no dissection. LA = left atrium; LV = left ventricle; AoV = aortic valve.

Fig. 5-16.

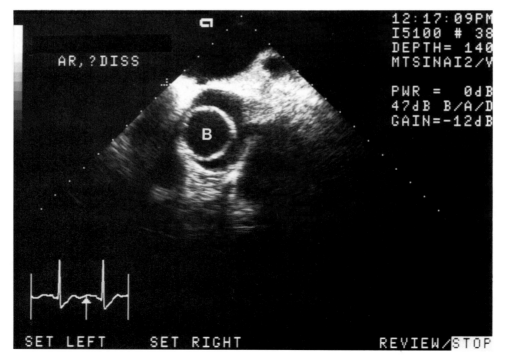

Figure 5-16A: Transesophageal echo following a Bental procedure demonstrates the inner lumen of the vascular prosthesis (B) surrounded by the lumen of the patient's native proximal ascending aorta.

Fig. 5-16. (cont'd)

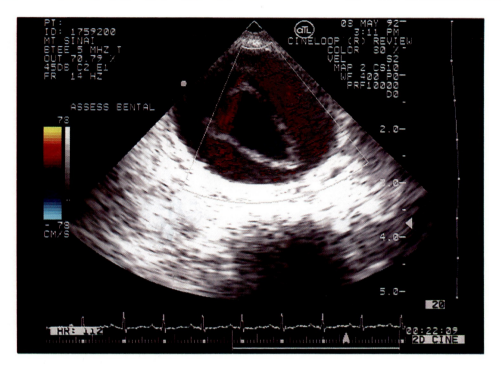

Figure 5-16B: Following a successful Bental procedure for an ascending aortic dissection, flow can still be seen in the false lumen (red) surrounding the true lumen (blue). The remaining descending aortic dissection was not repaired because it involves a much more complex operation. As long as the descending dissection does not expand, the patient will be treated medically.

Figure 5-17A–C: Case history: aortic dissection. A 42-year-old patient presented with back pain. He was seen by an orthopedist who suggested several days of bed rest and that he take muscle relaxants. He was still having discomfort. When he began having low-grade fever, he was seen by his local doctor who told him to take aspirin. However, he then began to develop a cough and was seen by a pulmonary specialist who did a chest X-ray and said that he had pulmonary infiltrates suggestive of "walking pneumonia" and treated him with erythromycin. His cough persisted and his chest pain grew worse. He presented to the emergency room and was admitted with a diagnosis of pneumonia. He was referred for an echocardiogram to evaluate the source of a heart murmur. The transthoracic echo was suspicious for an aortic dissection and the transesophageal echo was then performed.

See Figures 17A–C, pp. 178–179.

See Case History, p. 177.

Fig. 5-17.

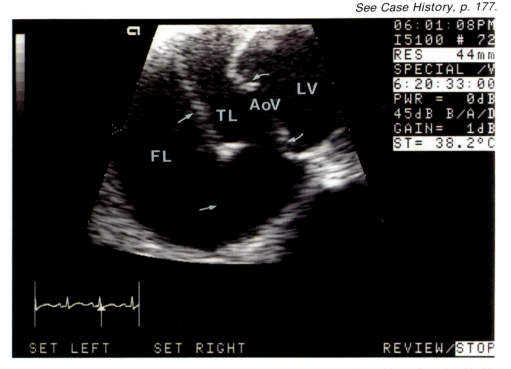

Figure 5-17A: The proximal ascending aorta with a doming bicuspid aortic valve (AoV, curved arrows) and an intimal flap (straight arrows) just 1 cm superiorly. FL = false lumen; TL = true lumen; LV = left ventricle.

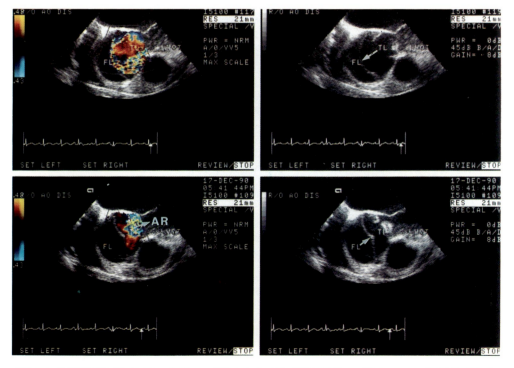

Figure 5-17B: Multiple sequences of the dynamic intimal flap. The upper right demonstrates the proximal aorta with a true lumen (TL) with systolic bowing of the intimal flap (arrow); the upper left demonstrates systolic color flow Doppler with blood flow in the true lumen separated from the false lumen (FL) by an intimal flap. During diastole (lower frames), the intimal flap swings closer towards the aortic valve because the systolic pressure jet has receded. The lower left demonstrates diastolic aortic insufficiency. AR = aortic regurgitation.

Fig. 5-17. (cont'd)

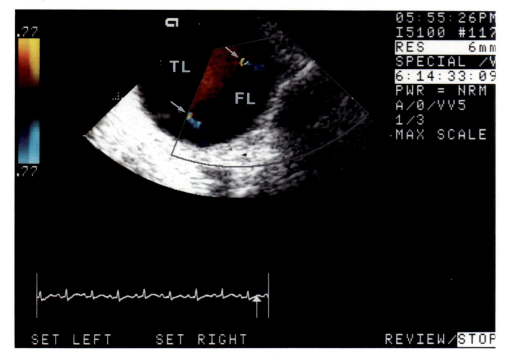

Figure 5-17C: Two more areas of communication between the true (TL) and false (FL) lumen are demonstrated, which may represent spinal arteries, explaining the cause of the patient's back pain. This patient was taken to surgery the same day and had successful repair of the ascending aorta with a Dacron graft placed inside of the patient's own aorta. The patient's aortic valve was salvaged by the surgeon, by narrowing the aortic annulus. This patient has had persistent low back pain and claudication which have been due to the dissection tearing several of those smaller spinal arteries.

Fig. 5-18.

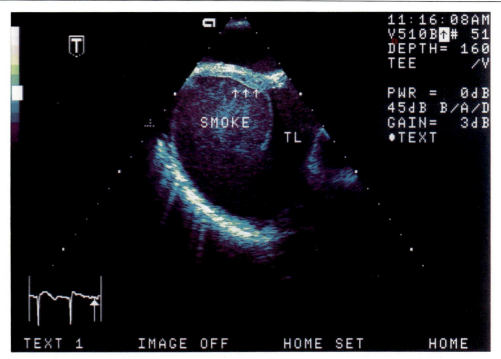

Figure 5-18A: Case history: aortic dissection. An elderly woman was admitted because of atypical chest pain and a wide mediastinum. TEE revealed a chronic proximal dissection in which a "pseudoaneurysm" developed in the false lumen. There was "smoke" and a layered thrombus (arrows) in the false lumen (transverse plane). TL = true lumen.

**Fig. 5-18.
(cont'd)**

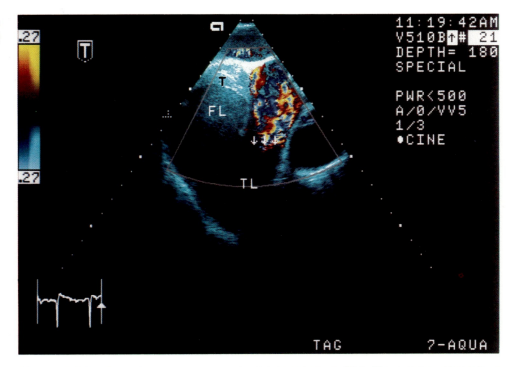

Figure 5-18B: Color flow defines flow in the true lumen (TL). The laminar thrombus (T) is seen in the false lumen (FL).

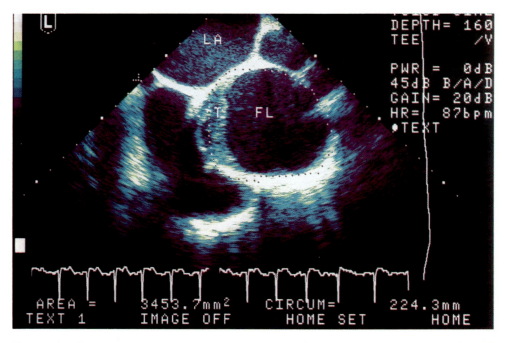

Figure 5-18C: In the longitudinal plane, the "pseudoaneurysm" had an area of 34.5 cm². LA = left atrium; FL = false lumen.

Fig. 5-19.

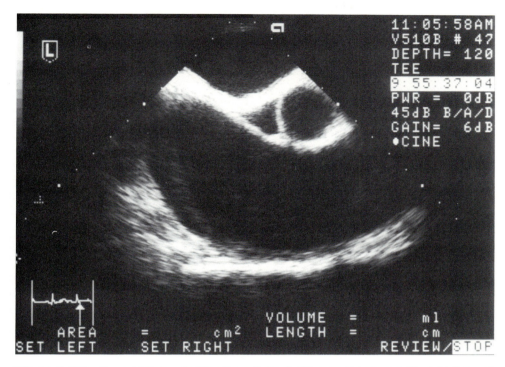

Figure 5-19A: Case history: aortic dissection. A 64-year-old man with a history of chronic back pain and hypertension. An MRI was read as "probable" type A dissection, while a CT scan was read as "aneurysm with thrombus." Longitudinal plane of the ascending aorta revealed a faint immobile line suspicious for an intimal flap.

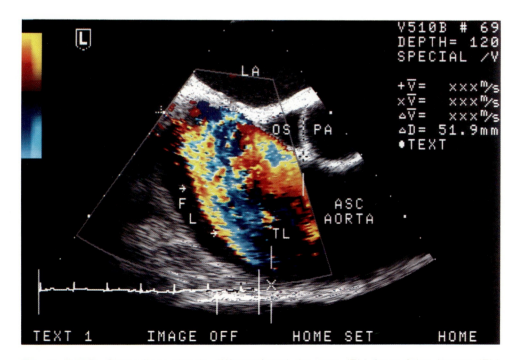

Figure 5-19B: Color flow clearly differentiated the true (TL) from false lumen (FL) separated by an intimal flap (arrows) that did not undulate due to lack of flow in the false lumen. The oblique sinus (OS) is a potential space in this plane. PA = pumonary artery. Asc = ascending aorta; LA = left atrium.

Fig. 5-19. (cont'd)

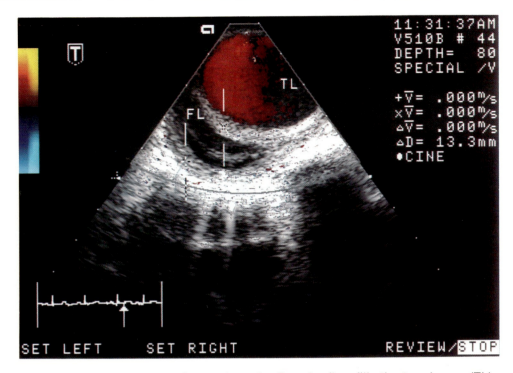

Figure 5-19C: In the descending aorta, color Doppler flow fills the true lumen (TL), with no flow in the false lumen (FL). The intimal flap is dense and thick. The false lumen contains layered thrombus and smoke. The patient underwent successful surgical repair.

6

Aortic Plaque

The examination of the aorta can be performed with transthoracic echocardiography by several planes. From the parasternal long and short axes, the proximal aortic root and its sinuses can be studied. From the right parasternal view, the ascending aorta is seen; and from the supersternal notch, the aortic arch can be seen. The descending aorta can be seen in the parasternal long axis view behind the left atrium. The transthoracic approach to the aorta is technically limited in many patients. However, the esophagus is posterior to the ascending aorta and directly anterior to the descending aorta. Therefore, pathology of the thoracic aorta such as dissections, plaque, and aneurysms can be studied very thoroughly with transesophageal echo.

More recently, studies have demonstrated the importance of plaque in the aorta as a potential source of cerebrovascular embolic events. The mechanism of the plaque formation may be similar to arteriosclerotic changes that occur in other arteries. The plaque may be sessile or nodular and rarely may have a pedunculated portion that is floating within the aortic lumen (a potential embolic source).

Careful examination of the aorta may be warranted in patients with suspected cardioembolic stroke or a transient ischemic event in whom there are no intracardiac or carotid sources for embolization.

The examination of the thoracic aorta with transesophageal echo can be divided into the ascending aorta, transverse arch, and descending aorta. Even with biplane imaging, there may be a "blind spot" near the trachea. Combining a thorough transthoracic exam with the transesophageal study facilitates complete interrogation of the aorta. The aortic sinus and proximal ascending aorta are well seen in both the transverse and longitudinal planes. Up to 8 cm of the ascending aorta can be imaged in the longitudinal slice. However, since the aorta is more distant from the transducer in this view, the resolution may not be adequate to detect endothelial irregularities.

The aortic arch is well seen in both the transverse and longitudinal views. The takeoff of the great vessels and fine intraluminal detail is possible.

The thoracic descending aorta is imaged by both planes. Circumferential detail of abnormalities is provided by the transverse plane and "length" of pathology is given by the longitudinal plane.

Bibliography

1. Karalis DG, Chandrasekaran K, Victor MF, Ross, JJ, Mintz GS: Recognition and embolic potential of intraaortic atherosclerotic debris. *J Am Coll Cardiol* 17:73–78, 1991.
2. Tunick PA, Kronzon I: Protruding atherosclerotic plaque in the aortic arch of patients with systemic embolization: a new finding seen by transesophageal echocardiography. *Am Heart J* 120:658–660, 1990.
3. Tunick PA, Culliford AT, Lamparello PJ, et al: Atheromatosis of the aortic arch as an occult source of multiple systemic emboli. *Am Intern Med* 11E: 391–392, 1991.
4. Mitchell M, Frankville D, Weinger M, et al: Detection of thoracic aortic atheroma with transesophageal echocardiography in patients without symptoms of embolism. *Am Heart J* 122:1768–1771, 1991.

Fig. 6-1.

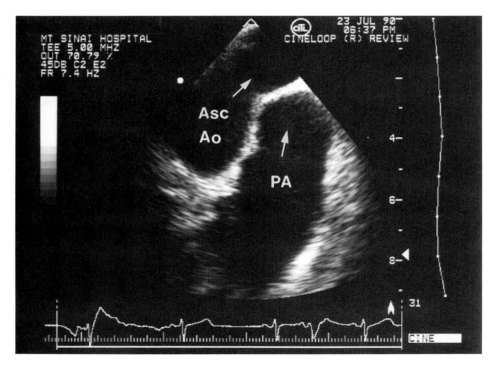

Figure 6-1A: After the aortic root is evaluated, the ascending aorta (Asc) can be appreciated in the transverse plane as the transducer is raised and slightly anteflexed. Ao = aorta; PA = pulmonary artery; arrows = flow direction.

Fig. 6-1.
(cont'd)

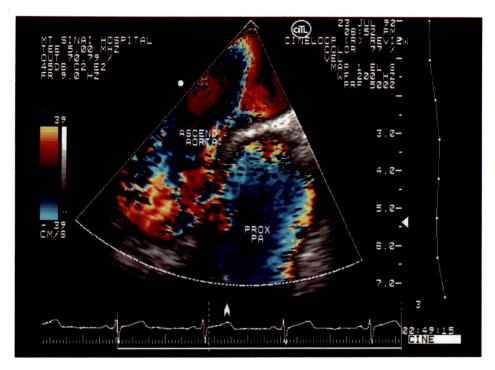

Figure 6-1B: Color flow Doppler in this transverse plane demonstrates flow in both the ascending aorta and proximal pulmonary artery.

Fig. 6-2.

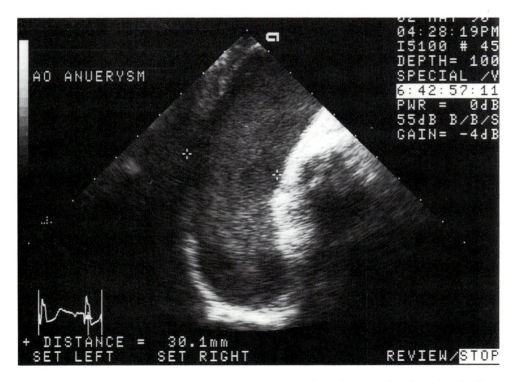

Figure 6-2: The ascending aorta is normally approximately 3 cm in diameter. In this particular patient, there is a gray "haze" or "smoke" in the aorta due to blood stasis.

186 • Clinical Atlas of Transesophageal Echocardiography

Fig. 6-3.

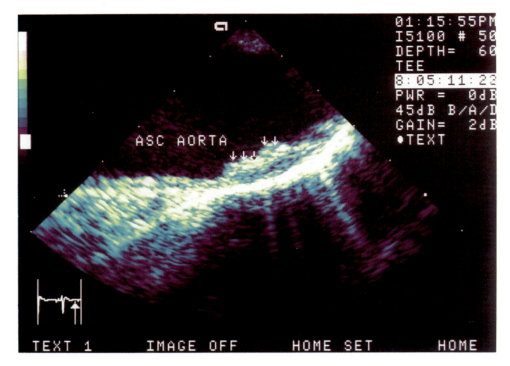

Figure 6-3: As the transducer is raised, the junction at the aortic arch is seen. In this patient, there is laminar plaque (arrows) (seen in the B-color mode) clearly distinct from the underlying media. The plaque is raised above the normal flat lumen contour in this transverse plane. Asc = ascending.

Fig. 6-4.

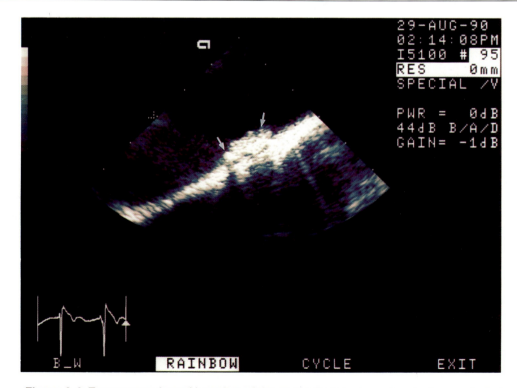

Figure 6-4: Transverse view of junction of the ascending aorta and arch demonstrated by B-color, a small area of isolated plaque raised and fairly dense, generating a shadow behind it, consistent with fibrosis or calcium in the plaque.

Fig. 6-5.

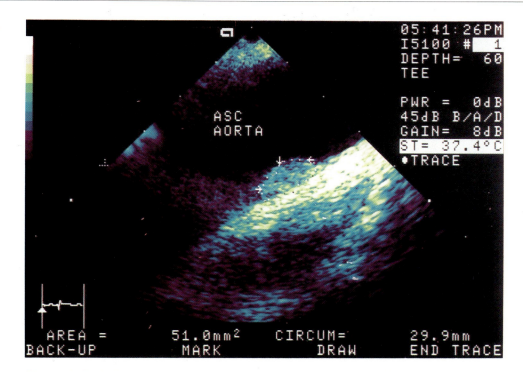

Figure 6-5A: In the transverse plane, softer plaque (arrows), less dense than the underlying lumen wall, may represent a fresh thrombus formed in an area of plaque rupture.

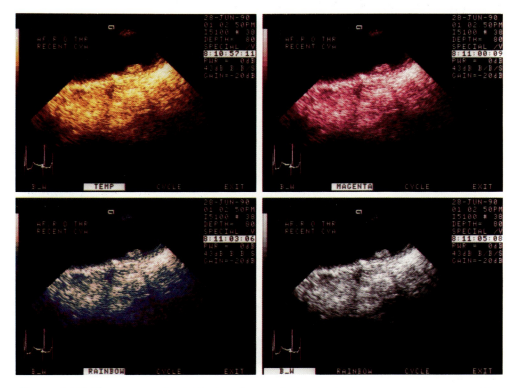

Figure 6-5B: B-color can be utilized to demonstrate the heterogeneous nature of this isolated plaque.

Fig. 6-6.

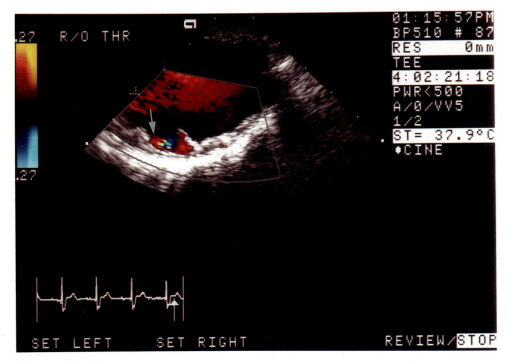

Figure 6-6A: The mechanism of these raised plaques may be related to hemorrhage in a sessile plaque. In this figure, there is Doppler flow seen between two edges of a probable ruptured plaque. This may be the nidus for thrombus formation even in a large grade vessel such as the aorta.

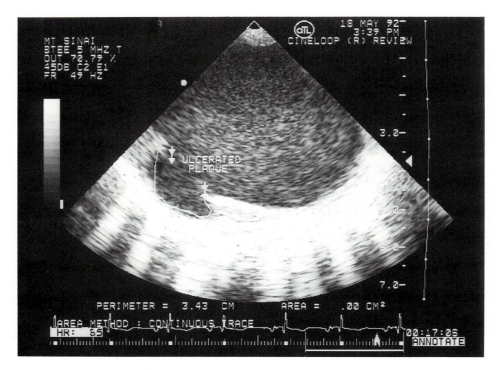

Figure 6-6B: Large ulcerated plaque in the descending aorta.

Fig. 6-7.

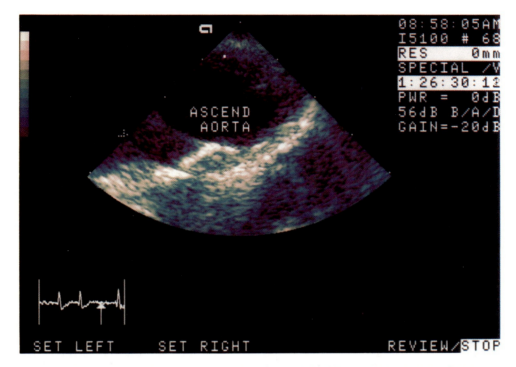

Figure 6-7: Another nodular plaque with a dense "shell" and softer lumen. This may represent hemorrhage under a plaque.

Fig. 6-8.

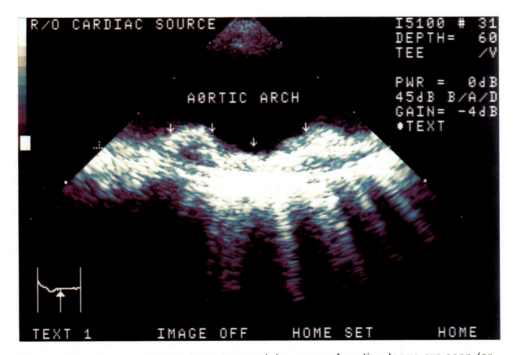

Figure 6-8: In the transverse plane, two nodular areas of aortic plaque are seen (arrows) in the arch. The one to the left has a more echolucent base than the one to the right, which may represent hemorrhage under this plaque.

Fig. 6-9.

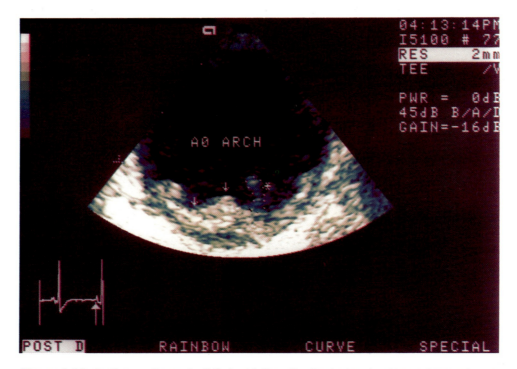

Figure 6-9A: In the aortic arch (AO Arch) (longitudinal plane), plaque (arrows) was seen protruding into the middle of the lumen with a fingerlike projection (asterisk) that was pedunculated and highly mobile. This particular patient had presented with a transient ischemic attack following a myocardial infarction.

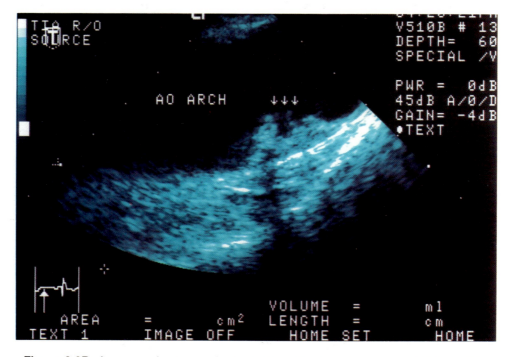

Figure 6-9B: Arrows point to mobile thrombi in the aortic arch, transverse plane.

Fig. 6-10.

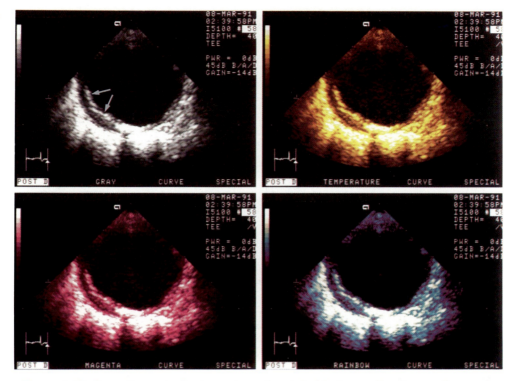

Figure 6-10: From the arch, the transducer is rotated to image the descending aorta. Eccentric raised laminar plaque is seen in these B-color images extending into approximately one-third of the entire left side of the lumen circumference. A softer plaque (arrows) is contrast with the denser, white, calcified plaque.

Fig. 6-11.

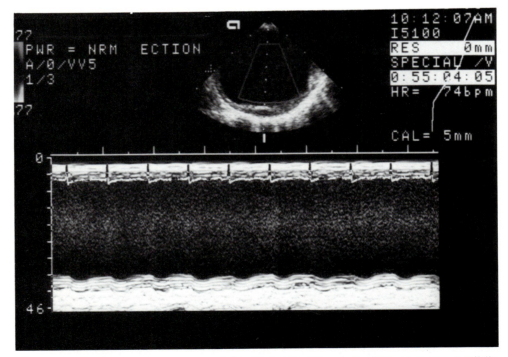

Figure 6-11A: The descending aorta in the transverse plane demonstrates a mildly dilated descending aorta (3.5 cm with normal being <3 cm). The wall appeared mildly thickened. There is a haze seen in the M-mode (below) consistent with "smoke" or low flow in the descending aorta.

Fig. 6-11. (cont'd)

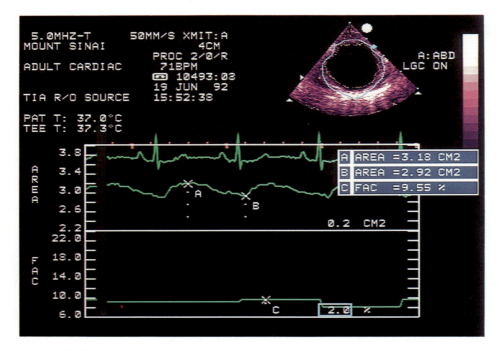

Figure 6-11B: Automated edge detection tracks the change in the aortic area with each systolic expansion in real time. This patient's aorta had a 9.55% change in area. The aorta becomes stiffer and less compliant with aging, hypertension, and atherosclerosis.

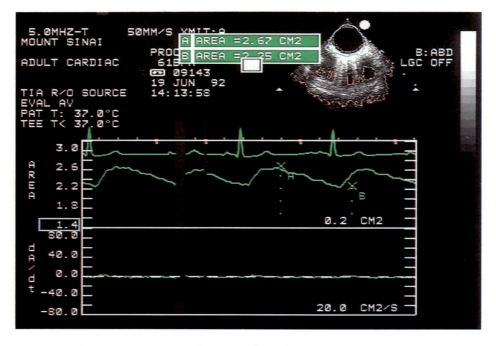

Figure 6-11C: Tracking of systolic expansion of the aorta revealed an end-systolic area of 2.67 cm² (point A on graph) and 2.25 cm² at end-diastole (point B) for an area change of 16%.

Aortic Plaque • 193

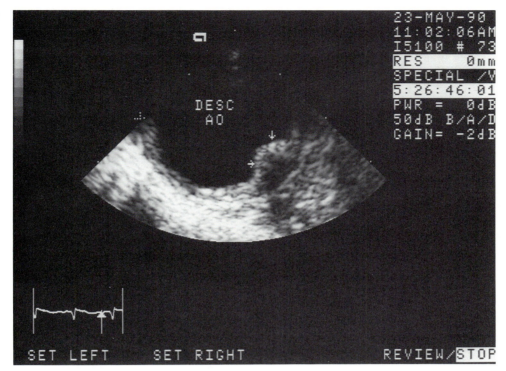

Figure 6-12: Raised plaque with underlying hemorrhage can also be seen in the descending aorta (DESC AO, arrows).

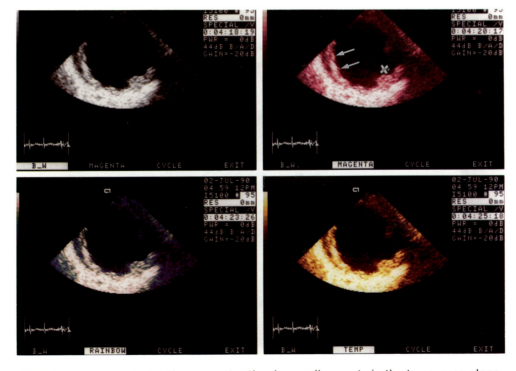

Figure 6-13: B-color echo demonstrates the descending aorta in the transverse plane with both laminar raised plaque (arrows to the left) and nodular plaque (asterisk to the right) with the same patient.

Fig. 6-14.

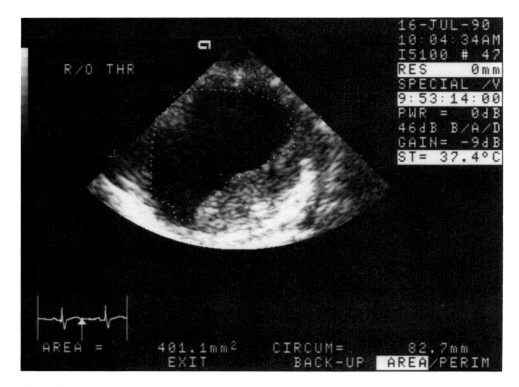

Figure 6-14A: Transverse plane of the descending aorta demonstrates extensive encroachment on the aortic lumen by the extensive thrombus.

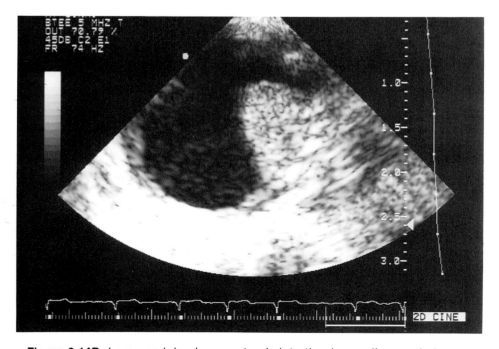

Figure 6-14B: Large nodule plaque extends into the descending aortic lumen.

Fig. 6-15.

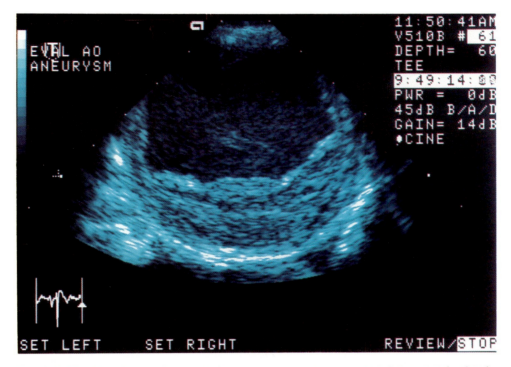

Figure 6-15A: The descending aorta (transverse plane), demonstrating extensive laminar thrombus. There is also "smoke" swirling in the lumen. Low flow states may predispose to this extensive thrombus formation.

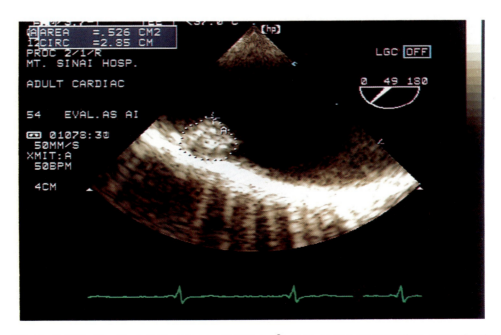

Figure 6-15B: Focal nodular plaque (0.586 cm^2) seen in the descending aorta (multiplane probe axis = 49°).

Fig. 6-16.

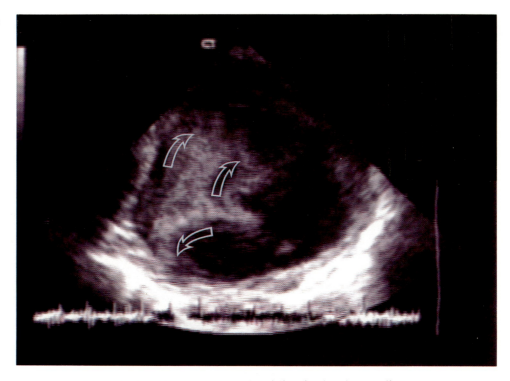

Figure 6-16: Hazelike "smoke" swirling in the descending aorta.

Fig. 6-17.

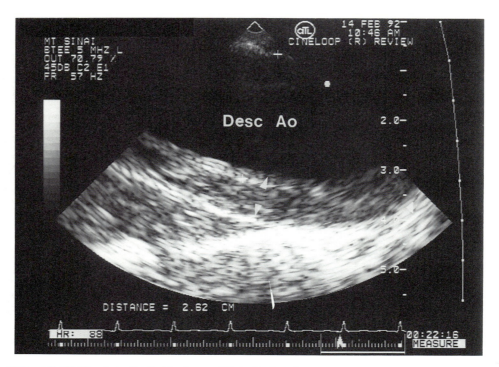

Figure 6-17: The longitudinal plane of the descending aorta (Desc Ao) demonstrates laminar plaque almost 1 cm thick (arrowheads).

Fig. 6-18.

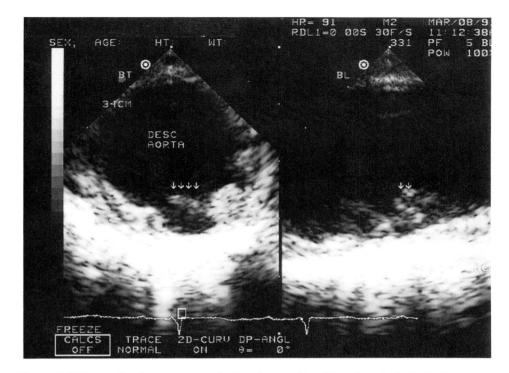

Figure 6-18A: Aortic plaque is seen in the descending (Desc) aorta in both the transverse (left) and longitudinal (right) planes. The transverse view on the left highlights a very mobile portion of plaque (arrows). The nodularity of the plaque (arrows) is well seen in the longitudinal plane (right side).

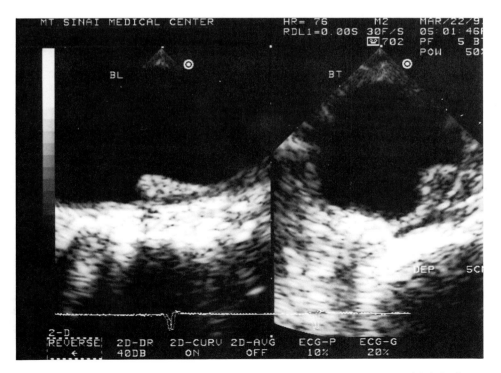

Figure 6-18B: Nodular plaque in the longitudinal (left) and transverse (right) planes.

Fig. 6-19.

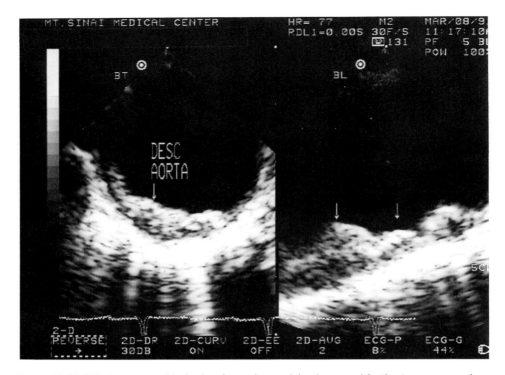

Figure 6-19: What appeared to be laminar plaque (single arrow) in the transverse plane (left) was actually nodular (possibly ulcerated) plaque, (arrows) better appreciated in the longitudinal plane (right).

Fig. 6-20.

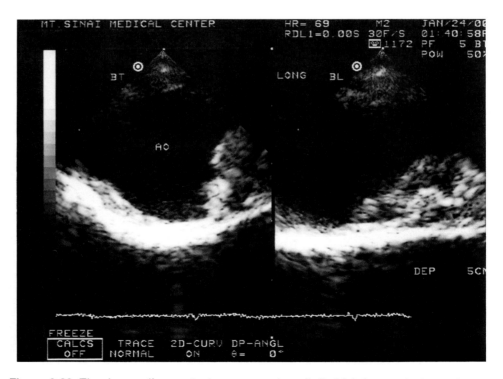

Figure 6-20: The descending aorta, transverse plane (left side) demonstrates a plaque that extends into the lumen. The degree of lumen compromise is better appreciated in the longitudinal plane (right side).

Fig. 6-21.

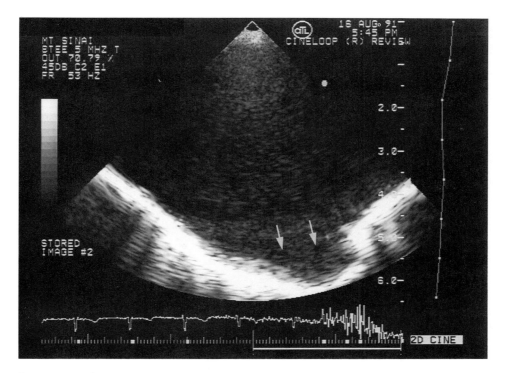

Figure 6-21: Occasionally the aorta is coiled and buckled, particularly at the junction of the descending aorta and aortic arch. This patient had a mildly dilated aorta (4 cm) with a sharp buckle at the junction of the arch and descending aorta. By transesophageal echo, it is represented by the evagination (arrows).

Fig. 6-22.

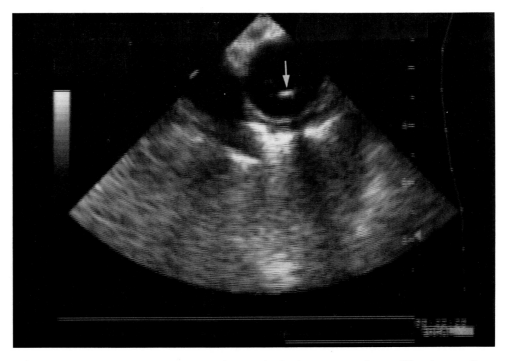

Figure 6-22: Intraaortic balloon pump is seen in the transverse plane of the descending aorta just distal to left subclavian artery. Transesophageal echo can be utilized to help guide or confirm proper placement of the intraballoon pump.

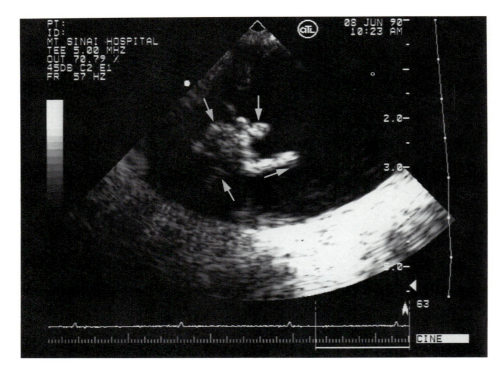

Figure 6-23A: Large pedunculated, mobile, fingerlike thrombus projecting into the aortic arch lumen. This patient had multiple cerebral emboli.

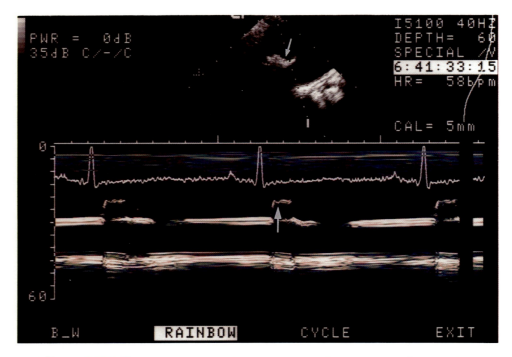

Figure 6-23B: The M-mode through the mass confirms its systolic mobility.

Fig. 6-23. (cont'd)

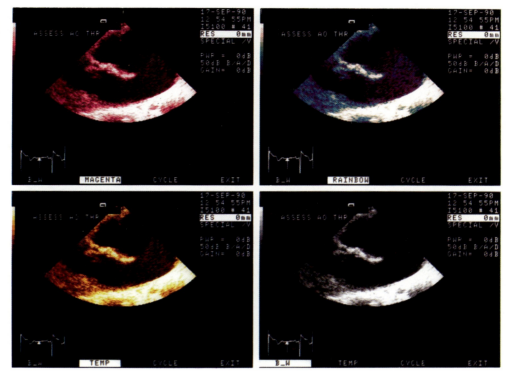

Figure 6-23C: B-color can emphasize a fingerlike thrombus at the junction of the ascending aorta and arch.

7

Left Ventricular Outflow Obstruction (Nonvalvular)

The distinguishing feature of hypertrophic cardiomyopathy (HCOM or idiopathic hypertrophic subaortic stenosis, IHSS) is idiopathic hypertrophy of the left ventricle in varying patterns: asymmetric basal septal hypertrophy; hypertrophy of the entire septum; apical hypertrophy or concentric hypertrophy. Transthoracic echocardiography is usually adequate to detect the major features of this disease. Importantly, there are several distinctive echocardiographic features that correlate with left ventricular outflow obstruction, including more severe septal hypertrophy, prolonged systolic anterior motion of the anterior leaflet of the mitral valve opposing the septum, and mid-systolic notching of the aortic valve. Pulsed and continuous wave Doppler can detect and quantify the left ventricular outflow tract gradient. The left ventricular septal to posterior wall thickness ratio should be greater than 1.3 to 1. However, because some patients with aortic stenosis or hypertension may have asymmetric hypertrophy, a ratio of 1.5 to 1 or more has the highest sensitivity for diagnosing HCOM. Color flow Doppler will demonstrate the development of the left ventricular outflow tract gradient with turbulent flow and varying degrees of mitral regurgitation. Because of the myocardial disarray and disorganization of the myofibrils and myofilaments, there may a ground-glass appearance of the involved muscle. Transesophageal echo will facilitate imaging of the left ventricular outflow tract both in the longitudinal and transverse planes, quantify the severity of mitral regurgitation, and determine the outflow gradient by continuous wave Doppler.

Fig. 7-1.

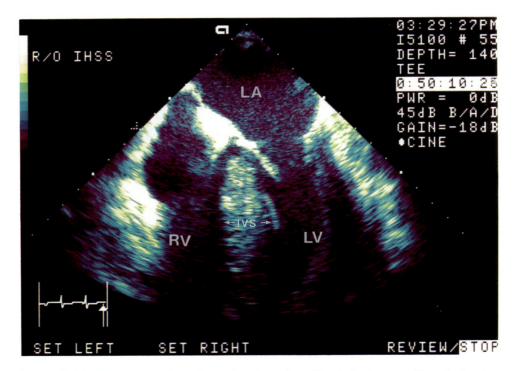

Figure 7-1A: Transverse plane four-chamber view. Diastolic frame with mitral valve open and a thickened intraventricular septum (IVS). LA = left atrium; RV = right ventricle; LV = left ventricle.

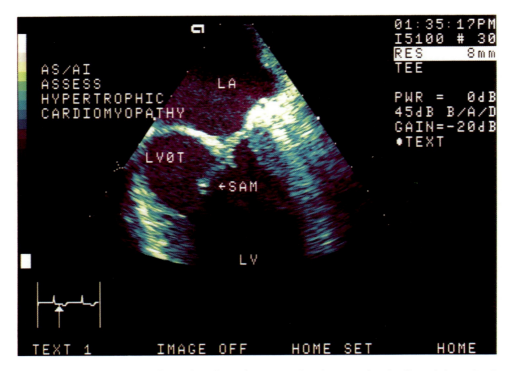

Figure 7-1B: Transverse four-chamber view, systole: the anterior leaflet of the mitral valve is drawm into the left ventricular outflow tract (LVOT). SAM = systolic anterior motion of the mitral valve; LA = left atrium; LV = left ventricle.

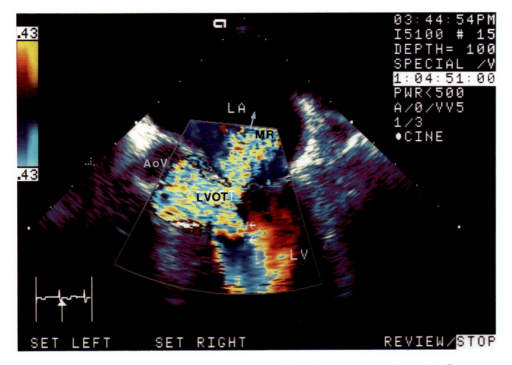

Figure 7-1C: Left ventricular outflow tract (LVOT) turbulence seen by color flow mosaic pattern begins below the aortic valve (AoV), where the mitral valve approaches the septum narrowing the LV outflow tract in systole. There is also mitral regurgitation (MR). LA = left atrium; LV = left ventricle.

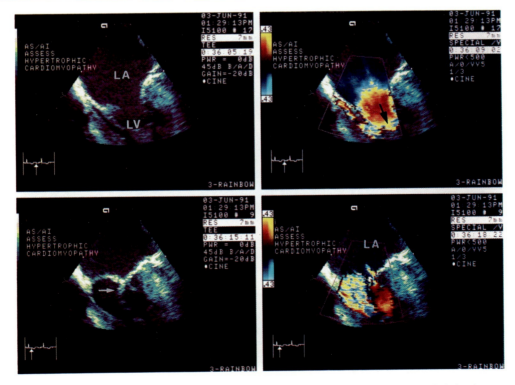

Figure 7-2: Multisequence of hypertrophic cardiomyopathy. Upper left and right demonstrates diastolic mitral inflow; lower left depicts systolic anterior motion of the mitral valve and lower right images outflow obstruction. LA = left atrium; LV = left ventricle.

Fig. 7-3.

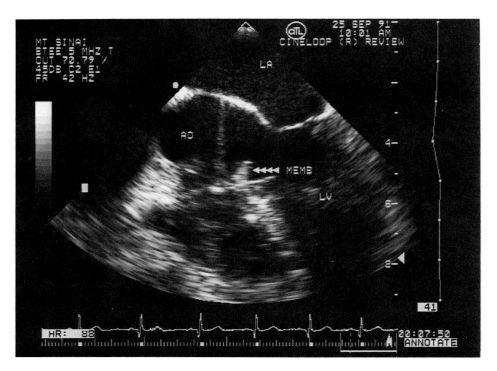

Figure 7-3A: Subaortic membrane. Another etiology of left ventricular outflow obstruction due to the growth of a membranous shelf (MEMB) below the aortic valve (AO) (arrow). LA = left atrium; LV = left ventricle.

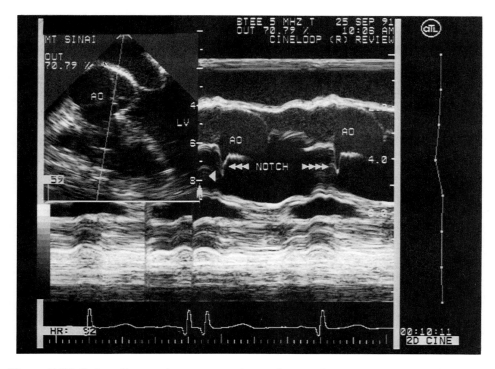

Figure 7-3B: Subaortic membrane generates early systolic notching (arrows, M-mode) of the aortic valve in contradistinction to the midsystolic obstruction created by hypertrophic cardiomyopathy. LV = left ventricle; AO = aorta.

Fig. 7-4.

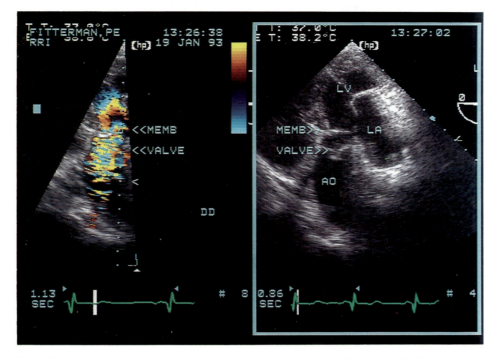

Figure 7-4: Longitudinal transgastric view (75° axis) of membrane (MEMB) in relation to the aortic valve (right figure) and the color Doppler systolic turbulence due to outflow obstruction (left side). LA = left atrium; LV = left ventricle.

Fig. 7-5.

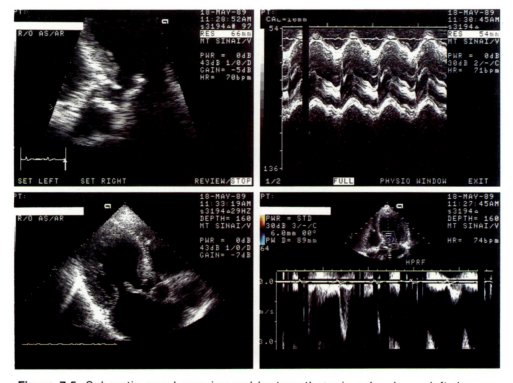

Figure 7-5: Subaortic membrane imaged by transthoracic echo: lower left demonstrates the fibrous membrane jutting out of the interventricular septum. Upper left highlights the membrane; the early notching is seen in the upper right. A 36 mm Hg systolic gradient is recorded in the lower right.

8

Coronary Artery Disease

Coronary Artery Anatomy

Coronary artery anatomy is best defined by coronary angiography. However, the proximal coronaries are occasionally seen with transthoracic echo, particularly the very proximal portions of the left main and the right coronary arteries.

Transesophageal echo can usually visualize segments of the proximal left coronary artery in 90% of patients, and the proximal right coronary in approximately 50% of patients. Color Doppler is valuable in differentiating normal from abnormal flow.

Bibliography

1. Zwicky P, Daniel WG, Mugge A, Lichtlen PR: Imaging of coronary arteries by color-coded transesophageal Doppler echocardiography. *Am J Cardiol* 62:639–640, 1988.
2. Yamagishi M, Miyatake K, Beppu S, Kumon K, Suzuki S, Tanaka N, Nimura Y: Assessment of coronary blood flow by transesophageal two-dimensional pulsed Doppler echocardiography. *Am J Cardiol* 65:641–4644, 1988.
3. Yoshida K, Yoshikawa J, Hozumi T, Yamaura Y, Akasaka T, Fukaya T, Kato, H: Detection of left main coronary artery stenosis by transesophageal color Doppler and two-dimensional echocardiography. *Circulation* 81: 1271–1276, 1990.
4. Arazoza E, Bowser M, Obeid A: Coronary artery fistula: Diagnosis by biplane transesophageal echocardiography. *J Am Soc Echocardiogr* 5: 277–280, 1992.
5. Iliceto S, Marangelli V, Memmwola C, Rizzon P: Transesophageal Doppler echocardiography evaluation of coronary blood flow velocity in baseline conditions and during dipyridamole-induced coronary vasodilation. *Circulation* 83:61–69, 1991.

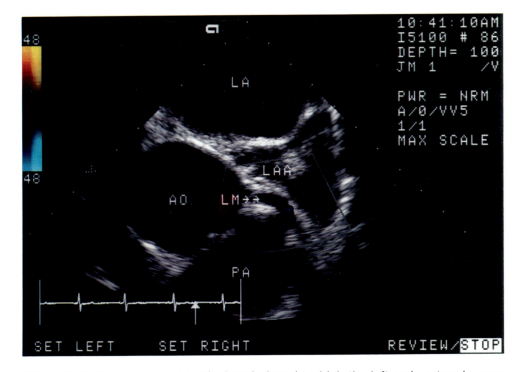

Figure 8-1: Transverse, short axis, basal plane in which the left main artery is seen between the aorta (AO) and the atrial appendage (LAA). There is a small thrombus in the appendage. The left main (LM) coronary artery (arrows) is seen to originate at approximately 3:00 from the left aortic sinus. The origin of coronary artery is usually several millimeters superior to the aortic valve plane. LA = left atrium; PA = pulmonary artery.

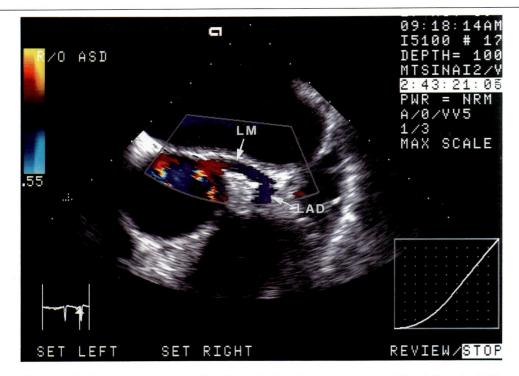

Figure 8-2: Demonstrates color flow Doppler in a longer segment of the left main (LM) and the proximal portion of the left anterior descending artery (LAD) as it takes a 90° turn to supply the septum and anterior left ventricular wall (transverse basal plane).

Fig. 8-3.

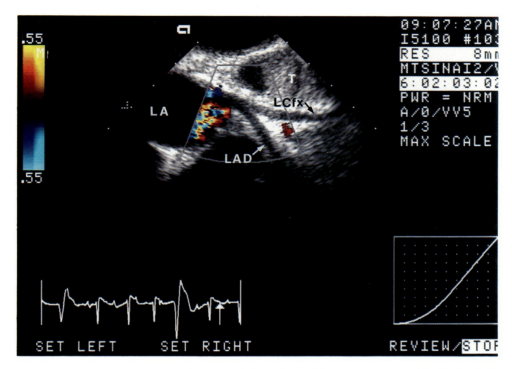

Figure 8-3: Horizontal plane of a short left main and long segments of both the left anterior descending (LAD) and left circumflex (LCfx) arteries. There is a thrombus (T) in the left atrial appendage. LA = left atrium.

Fig. 8-4.

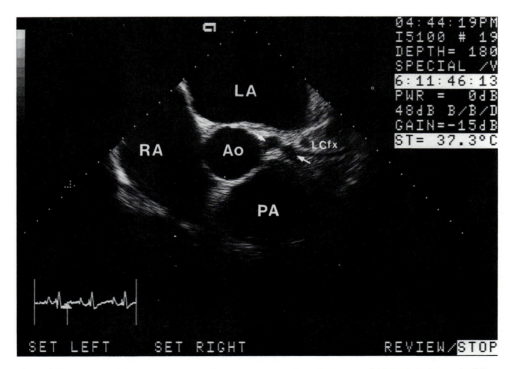

Figure 8-4: A calcified segment of the left main artery is seen with approximately 50% occlusion in its midportion (arrows). The left circumflex artery (LCfx) is seen coursing to the right. LA = left atrium; RA = right atrium; PA = pulmonary artery.

Fig. 8-5.

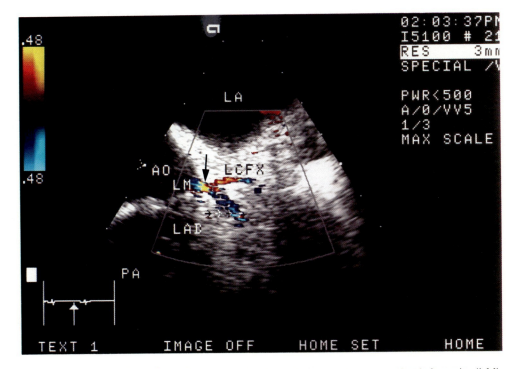

Figure 8-5: Color flow Doppler demonstrates mild turbulence in the left main (LM) artery (arrow) consistent with a mild stenotic lesion. The left circumflex (LCFX) and left anterior descending (LAD) flow are also seen. Color flow Doppler is useful in detecting a coronary artery that may be difficult to image directly. AO = aorta; LA = left atrium; PA = pulmonary artery.

Fig. 8-6.

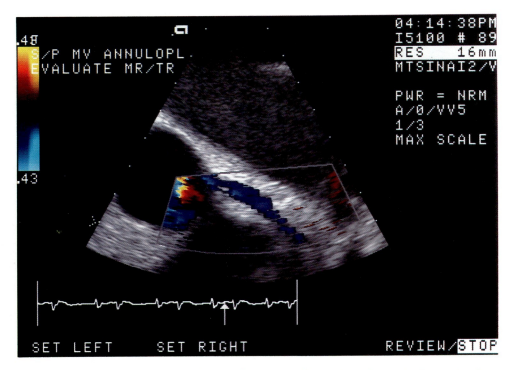

Figure 8-6: Color flow in the left anterior descending artery. By reducing color flow filters and aliasing velocity, coronary flow can be enhanced.

Coronary Artery Disease • 213

Fig. 8-7.

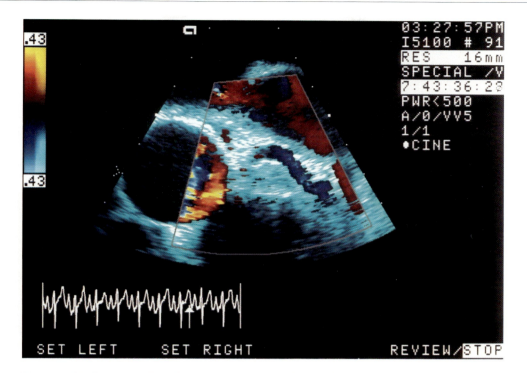

Figure 8-7A: The color flow in the coronary artery is highlighted by contrasting B-color of the myocardium. This may also improve visualization of low velocity coronary blood flow.

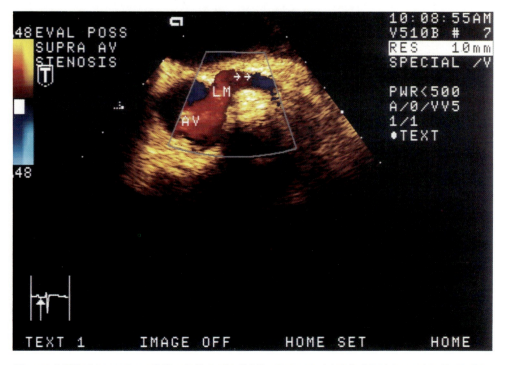

Figure 8-7B: Aneurysm of the left main (LM) coronary highlighted by color Doppler.

Fig. 8-8.

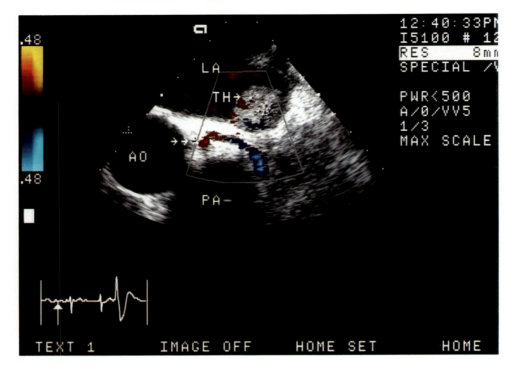

Figure 8-8: Occasionally, the coronary artery takes a superior course before burrowing into the myocardium. Here the Doppler red flow in the left main artery (arrows) courses superiorly before turning inferiorly (blue) in the LAD. There is a thrombus (TH, arrow) in the left atrial appendage. LA = left atrium; PA = pulmonary artery.

Fig. 8-9.

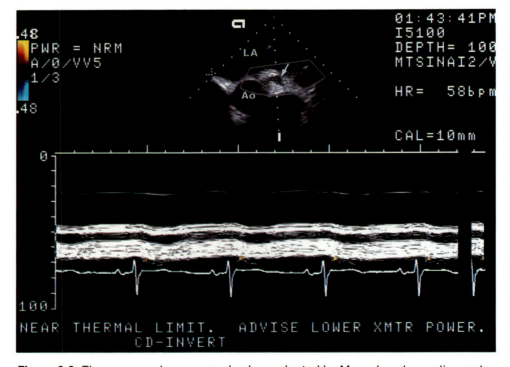

Figure 8-9: The coronary lumen can also be evaluated by M-mode echocardiography. This is an M-mode of an ectatic left main (arrow) in which the lumen appears to be slightly larger in systole than diastole. Coronary flow normally occurs predominantly in diastole. LA = left atrium; Ao = aorta.

Coronary Artery Disease • 215

Fig. 8-10.

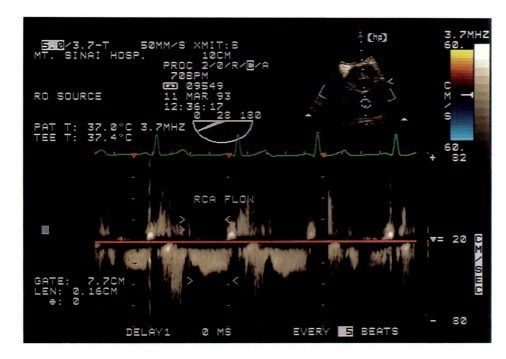

Figure 8-10: Pulsed Doppler flow of a coronary artery is difficult unless the sample volume is significantly reduced. Here diastolic flow is recorded from the right coronary artery (RCA flow outlined by arrows) obtained in a 28° axis.

Fig. 8-11.

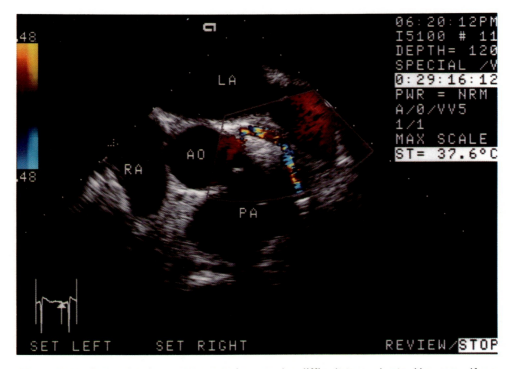

Figure 8-11: Stenosis of coronary arteries may be difficult to evaluate. However, if we visualize turbulent flow during our imaging, we report the finding. This patient has turbulence throughout the left main and left anterior descending artery. The patient had diffuse disease confirmed at a coronary angiography. LA = left atrium; RA = right atrium; Ao = aorta; PA = pulmonary artery.

Fig. 8-12.

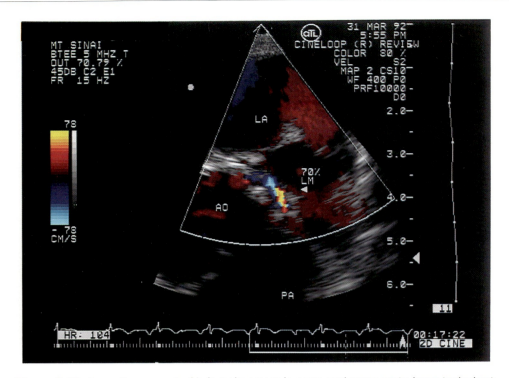

Figure 8-12: A small segment of left main artery is seen and appears to have turbulent flow. Significant left main (LM) coronary obstruction (70%) was confirmed by arteriography. LA = left atrium; Ao = aorta.

Fig. 8-13.

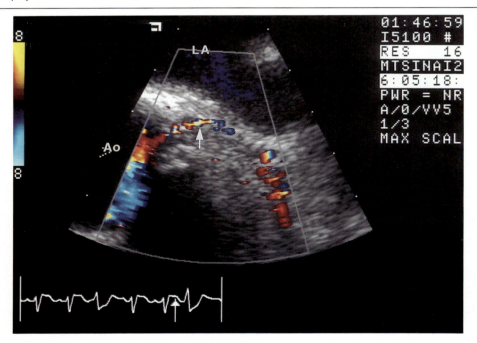

Figure 8-13: This patient has a significantly narrowed left main coronary artery identified by turbulent flow. This patient had prior aortic valve replacement and presented with recurrent ventricular tachycardia. Transesophageal echo demonstrated a normal functioning aortic prosthesis but narrowing in the left main coronary artery. Subsequent confirmation at cardiac catheterization led to surgery that demonstrated that a suture from the prior aortic replacement had compromised the origin of the left main coronary artery, which was now obstructed. This vessel was bypassed with resolution of the patient's arrhythmia. LA = left atrium; Ao = aorta.

Coronary Artery Disease • 217

Fig. 8-14.

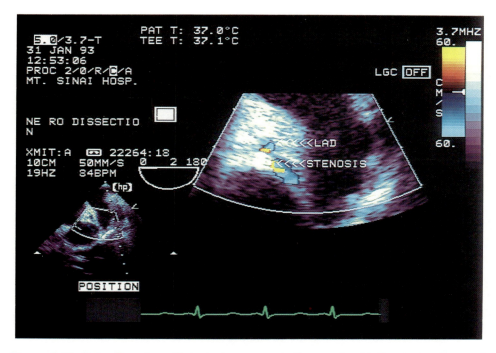

Figure 8-14: Color Doppler with turbulence was in the proximal left anterior descending (LAD) artery confirmed by subsequent angiography. AO = aorta; LAA = left atrial appendage.

Fig. 8-15.

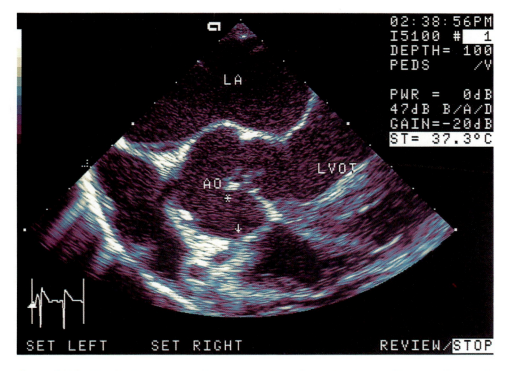

Figure 8-15: The right coronary artery (arrow) has its origin slightly higher in the aorta (AO) than the left main and is seen at approximately 6 to 7 o'clock in this transverse plane. LVOT = left ventricular outflow tract; LA = left atrium.

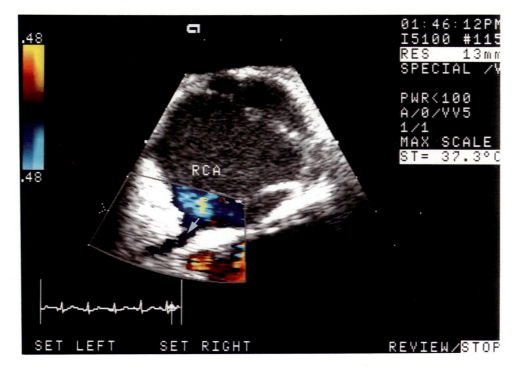

Figure 8-16: Flow in the right coronary artery (RCA, arrow).

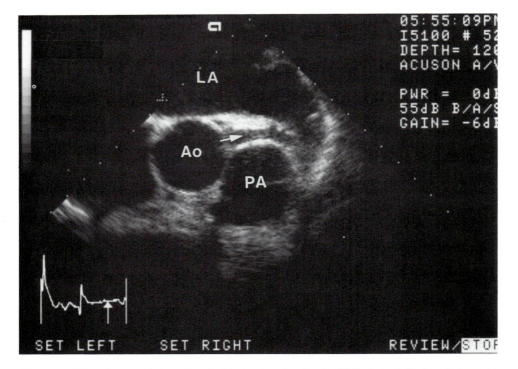

Figure 8-17A: The saphenous veins are usually more dilated and their origin may not be well visualized. This saphenous graft is seen coursing to the left circumflex distribution (arrow). LA = left atrium; Ao = aorta; PA = pulmonary artery.

Fig. 8-17. (cont'd)

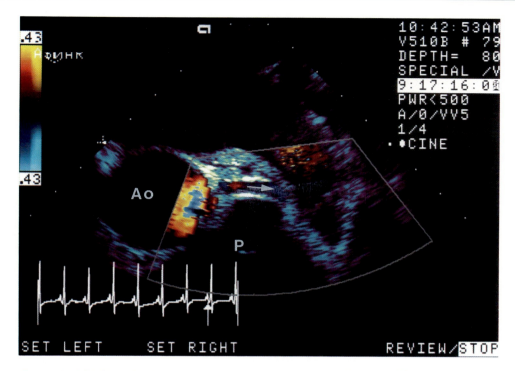

Figure 8-17B: Flow in the saphenous vein graft to the left circumflex. Ao = aorta; P = pulmonary artery.

Ischemic Heart Disease

The presence of coronary artery disease can be diagnosed before myocardial damage has occurred by either exercise or perfusion interventions or coronary angiography.

Once myocardial damage has occurred, wall motion is abnormal, which can be detected by either nuclear gated blood pool imaging (MUGA) or echocardiography. Usually routine transthoracic ultrasound will provide several adequate imaging planes to detect wall motion abnormalities (short axis mid-papillary muscle, and apical two- and four-chamber views). Occasionally, because of technical difficulties, transthoracic ultrasound may not be diagnostic and transesophageal echocardiography is performed. In the horizontal plane, the apex of the ventricle is not seen, though the short axis plane in the transgastric position and the four-chamber views facilitate evaluation of global and regional ventricular function. The apex can be better appreciated in the longitudinal transesophageal plane by either the transgastric two-chamber view or the two-chamber view above the diaphragm. Ventricular function is monitored intraoperatively during cardiac surgery or noncardiac surgery in high risk cardiac patients in these views.

Bibliography

1. Patel AM, Miller FA, Khanderia BK, et al: Role of transesophageal echocardiography in the diagnosis of papillary muscle rupture secondary to endocardial infarction. *Am Heart J* 118:1330, 1989.
2. Koenig K, Kasper W, Hofmann T, et al: Transesophageal echocardiography for diagnosis of rupture of the ventricular septum or left ventricular papillary muscle during acute myocardial infarction. *Am J Cardiol* 59:362, 1987.

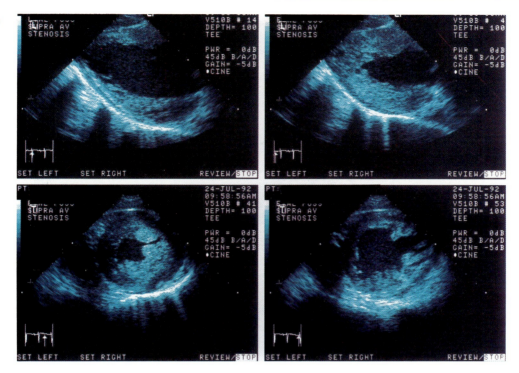

Figure 8-18A: Transgastric interrogation of ventricular function should be performed in both the longitudinal plane (upper left = diastole; upper right = systole) and the transverse plane (lower right = diastole; lower left = systole).

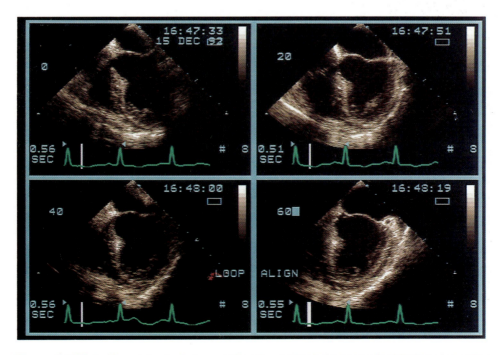

Figure 8-18B: Left ventricular interrogation by multiplane probe facilitates circumferential evaluation of left ventricular function (LV is imaged at 0° and 20° axis in the two upper frames, and 40° and 60° in the two lower frames.

Fig. 8-18. (cont'd)

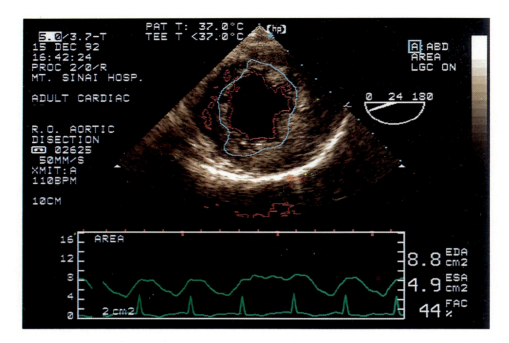

Figure 8-18C: Automated edge detection algorithms can evaluate beat-to-beat ventricular function. Accuracy of this method is dependent on the quality of the 2-D image (transgastric short axis view, 24° axis plane). This patient's LV fractional area change was normal at 44%. The end-diastolic area (EDA = 8.8 cm^2) and end-systolic area (4.9 cm^2) are tracked beat to beat in real time.

Fig. 8-19.

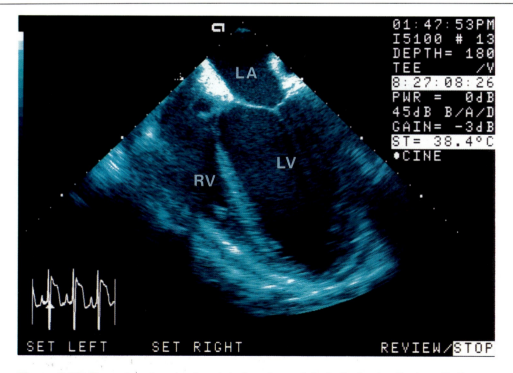

Figure 8-19: Four-chamber, horizontal plane in systole (mitral valve is closed) demonstrates a dilated ventricle with diffuse left ventricular dysfunction. Though patients with either ischemic or idiopathic dilated cardiomyopathy may present with a dilated ventricle, usually coronary artery disease is distinguished by the presence of regional wall motion abnormalities or discrepancies between left (LV) and right ventricular (RV) involvement.

Fig. 8-20.

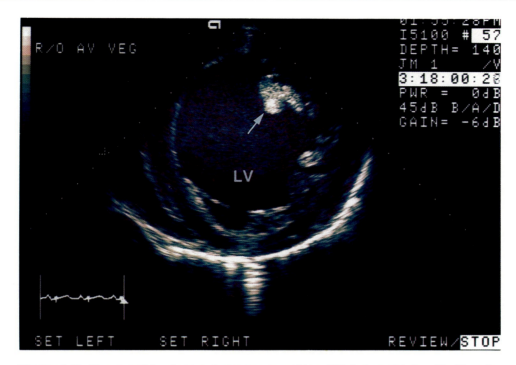

Figure 8-20: Transgastric short axis transverse plane. Dilated ventricle with fibrosis of the anterolateral medial papillary muscle (arrow), which can cause mitral regurgitation. The B-color mode highlights the echodensity of the myocardial fibrosis. This view can be utilized to monitor left ventricular function since all three coronary arteries perfuse regions imaged in this plane. (See Chapter 2.)

Fig. 8-21.

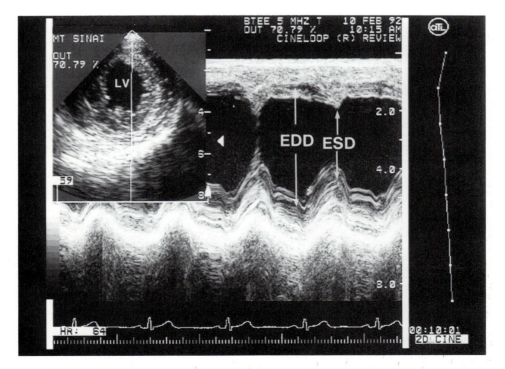

Figure 8-21A: The M-mode echocardiogram taken in the transgastric short axis plane faciliates assessment of ventricular function. This patient has normal systolic function. EDD = end-diastolic dimension; ESD = end-systolic dimension; LV = left ventricle.

Fig. 8-21. (cont'd)

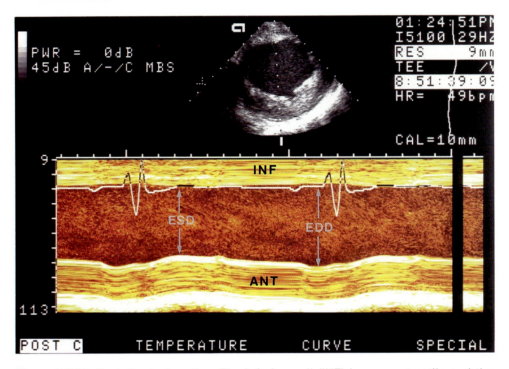

Figure 8-21B: Systolic dysfunction. The inferior wall (INF) is noncontractile and the anterior wall (ANT) is hypocontractile. The M-color picture demonstrates fine haze swirling in the left ventricular cavity, "spontaneous contrast" or "echogenic smoke," due to stasis of blood in a severely hypocontractile ventricle. EDD = end-diastolic dimension; ESD = end-systolic dimension.

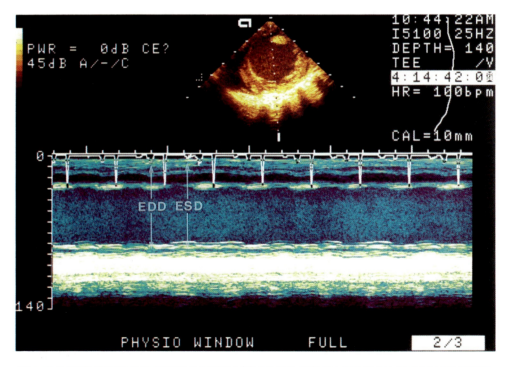

Figure 8-21C: Dilated cardiomyopathy with severe *diffuse,* not focal, hypocontractility. EDD = end-diastolic dimension; ESD = end-systolic dimension.

Fig. 8-22.

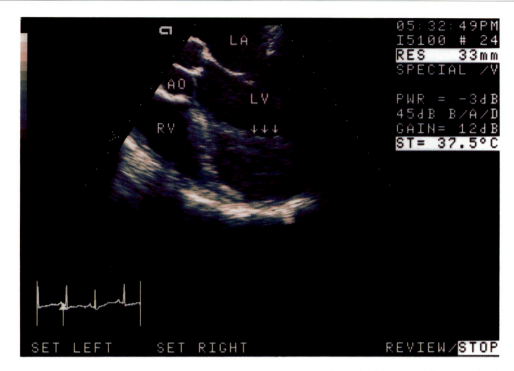

Figure 8-22A: Layers of spontaneous echo contrast or "smoke" (arrows) in an apical aneurysm due to low flow may predispose to thrombus formation. LA = left atrium; LV = left ventricle; RV = right ventricle; AO = aorta.

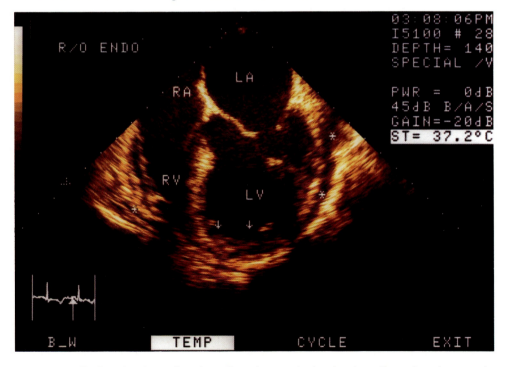

Figure 8-22B: B-color four-chamber view demonstrates laminar thrombus (arrows in the left ventricular, LV, apex) with a small pericardial effusion (asterisks). The thrombus is diagnosed by the presence of a different tissue density than the underlying muscle and its protrusion from the normal myocardial contour. The anteroapical area was also severely hypocontractile. Portions of the thrombus are pedunculated, which may connote higher embolic potential than sessile clots. RA = right atrium; RV = right ventricle; LA = left atrium.

Fig. 8-22. (cont'd)

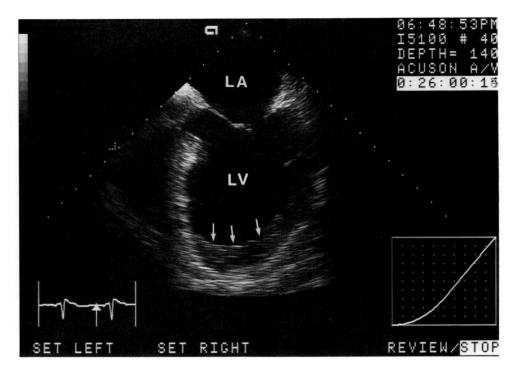

Figure 8-22C: Laminar apical thrombus (arrows). LA = left atrium; LV = left ventricle.

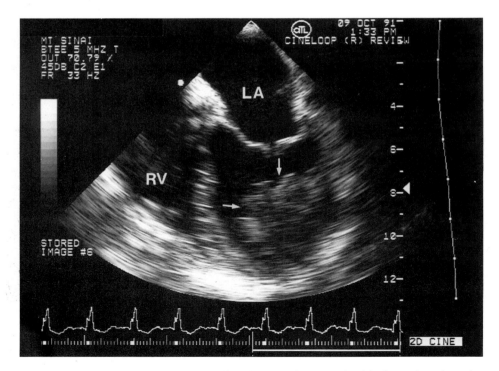

Figure 8-22D: Large multilobar mass fills the anterior apex in this four-chamber view. The underlying myocardial wall motion was only mildly hypocontractile. This mass was actually a leiomyosarcoma. LA = left atrium; RV = right ventricle.

Fig. 8-23.

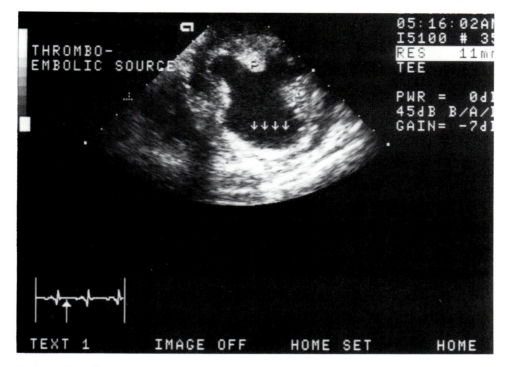

Figure 8-23A: Regional wall motion is usually appreciated best during real-time video sequences. However, in this short axis transgastric view, the normal oval systolic contour is distorted because the anterior wall (supplied by the left anterior descending artery) is scarred (arrows), manifested by the thin wall that was fibrosed and did not thicken.

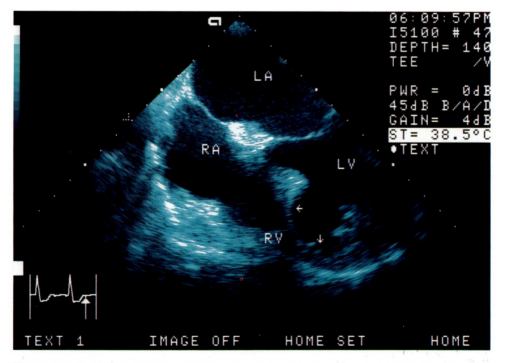

Figure 8-23B: Mid to apical septal thinning is seen in this four-chamber view (arrows) in a patient who had total occlusion of left anterior descending artery distal to the first septal artery. Notice that the basal septum thickens normally because it is proximal to the obstruction. LA = left atrium; LV = left ventricle; RA = right atrium; RV = right ventricle.

Fig. 8-24.

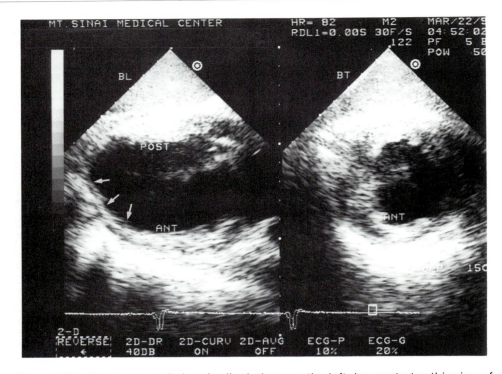

Figure 8-24: The transgastric longitudinal plane on the left demonstrates thinning of the anterior apex (arrows) in a patient with total occlusion of the left anterior descending artery. The transverse plane on the right did not detect the wall motion abnormality because the apex is not imaged in this view.

Fig. 8-25.

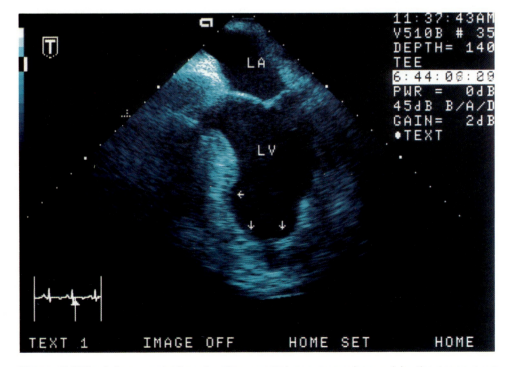

Figure 8-25A: A large apical and antero-septal aneurysm imaged in the transverse plane (arrows). LA = left atrium; LV = left ventricle.

Fig. 8-25. (cont'd)

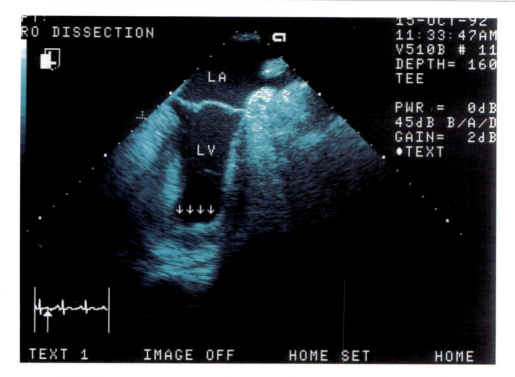

Figure 8-25B: The same aneurysm in the longitudinal plane (arrows). LA = left atrium; LV = left ventricle.

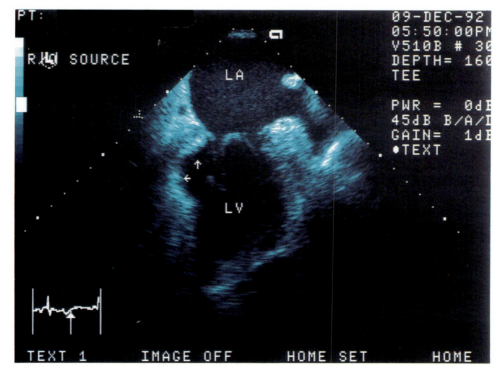

Figure 8-25C: A posterior aneurysm (arrows), longitudinal plane. LA = left atrium; LV = left ventricle.

Fig. 8-26.

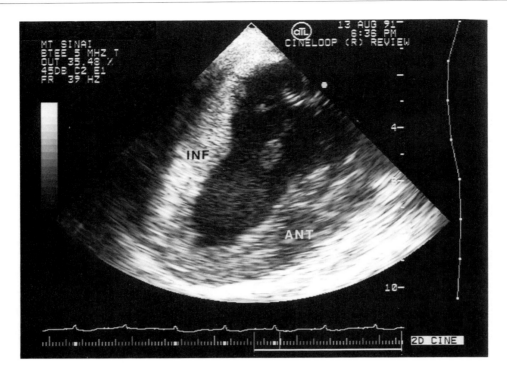

Figure 8-26A: Two-chamber view in the longitudinal plane demonstrates a hypertrophied left ventricle in diastole. INF = inferior wall; ANT = anterior wall.

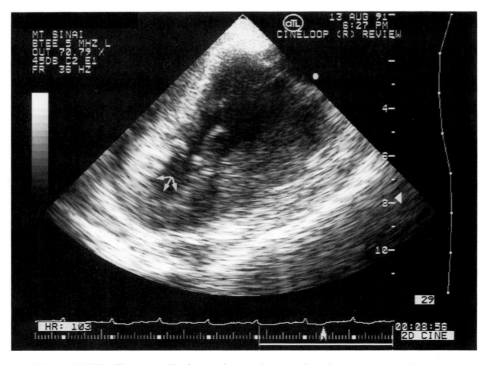

Figure 8-26B: The systolic frame imaged a small apical aneurysm (arrows).

Fig. 8-27.

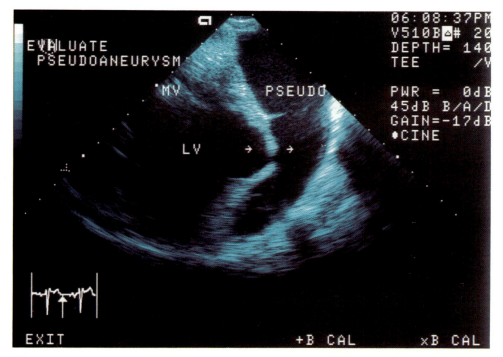

Figure 8-27A: A very serious complication of a myocardial infarction is pseudoaneurysm formation in which actual rupture of the myocardium occurs which is tamponaded by the surrounding adventitia preventing exsanguination and sudden death. Classically, the pseudoaneurysm is diagnosed by its thin neck separating it from the remaining ventricle in contradistinction to a normal aneurysm, which has a wide neck. Histopathology reveals that an aneurysm has residual cellular components, whereas in a psuedoaneurysm the wall consists of only adventitia. Distorted transverse plane of a pseudoaneurysm (PSEUDO) seen as an out pouching off the inferior wall of the left ventricle (LV). The thin neck is highlighted by arrows. MV = mitral valve.

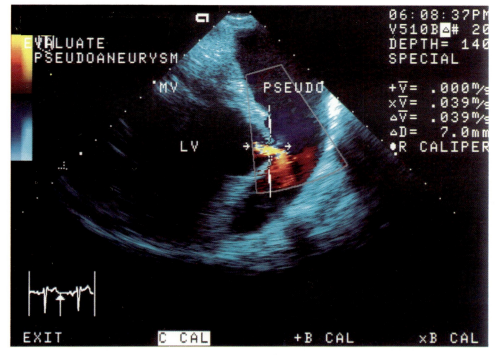

Figure 8-27B: Color flow Doppler demonstrates free communication between the ventricle and the pseudoaneurysm (PSEUDO) through the thin neck (arrows). MV = mitral valve; LV = left ventricle.

Fig. 8-28.

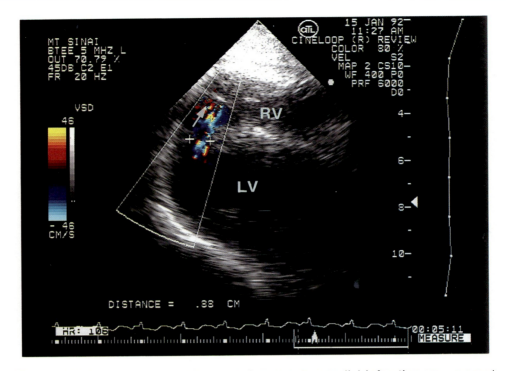

Figure 8-28A: Ventricular septal defect due to a myocardial infarction may present with hypotension, heart failure, a loud systolic murmur, and a precordial thrill. This transgastric longitudinal two-chamber view images the apical septal ventricular septal defect, which developed soon after a large anteroseptal infarct. RV = right ventricle; LV = left ventricle.

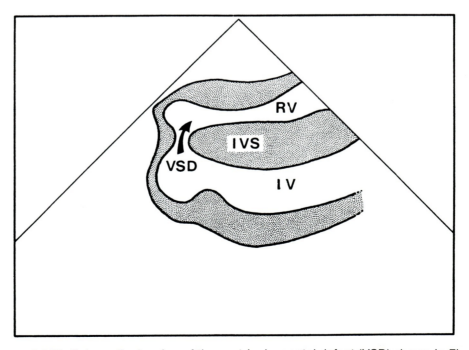

Figure 8-28B: Schematic drawing of the ventricular septal defect (VSD) shown in Fig. 8–28A. RV = right ventricle; IVS = intraventricular septum.

9

The Left Atrium

Left Atrial Myxomas

Left atrial myxomas, the most common primary cardiac tumors, can be either sessile or pedunculated and are usually attached to the intra-atrial septum. Though they occur in the left atrium three times more frequently than in the right atrium, myxomas may occasionally be biatrial. Therefore, the right atrium should be interrogated as carefully as the entire left atrium. Because the left atrial myxoma is frequently pedunculated, it may swing through the mitral orifice into the left ventricular inflow tract, partially obstructing mitral inflow and creating symptoms similar to mitral stenosis: dyspnea and orthopnea. Because of its systemic manifestations such as fever, embolization, weight loss, high sedimentation rate and anemia, a myxoma may be confused with endocarditis. A careful transthoracic echo in the long and short axis and apical view can usually reveal the presence or absence of myxoma. However, occasionally the transthoracic study may be technically difficult or inadequate to define the extent of the myxoma's base, possible damage to the mitral valve, and the complete right atrium. Therefore, transesophogeal echo may be utilized to confirm the presence of a myxoma and to define the extent of the involvement of the atrial septum. Since the myxoma may swing into the left ventricle during diastole, a ventriculogram is usually avoided when cardiac catheterization is performed to visualize the coronary arteries preoperatively.

Bibliography

1. Nomeir AM, Watts LE, Seagle R, Joyner CR, Corman C, Prichard RW: Intracardiac Myxomas: twenty-year echocardiographic experience with review of the literature. *J Am Soc Echocardiogr* 2:139–150, 1989.
2. Obeid AI, Marvasti M, Parker F, Rosenberg J: Comparison of transthoracic and transesophgeal echocardiography in diagnosis of left atrial myxoma. *Am J Cardiol* 63:1006–1008, 1989.
3. Dittman H, Volcker W, Karsch KR, Seipel L: Bilateral atrial myxomas detected by transesophageal two-dimensional echocardiography. *Am Heart J* 118:172–173, 1989.

4. Mugge A, Daniel WG, Haverich A, et al: Diagnosis of noninfective cardiac mass lesions by two-dimensional echocardiography. Comparison of the transthoracic and transesophageal approaches. *Circulation* 66: 1101–1109, 1991.
5. Reeder GS, Khanderia BK, Seward JB, Tajik AJ: Transesophageal echocardiography and cardiac masses. *Mayo Clin Proc* 66:1101–1109, 1991.

Fig. 9-1.

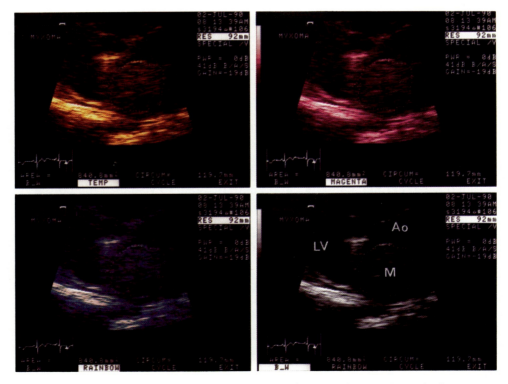

Figure 9-1A: A transthoracic long axis echocardiogram demonstrates in four-color B-mode frames a faint outline in the left atrium suggestive of a potential mass (M). LV = left ventricle; Ao = aorta.

Fig. 9-1. (cont'd)

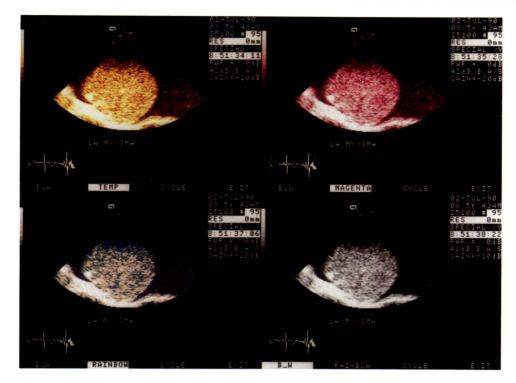

Figure 9-1B: These four-color B-mode frames demonstrate a large left atrial myxoma easily demonstrated in the transesophageal four-chamber view. Note the textural heterogeneity of the myxoma seen best in the lower left frame.

Fig. 9-2.

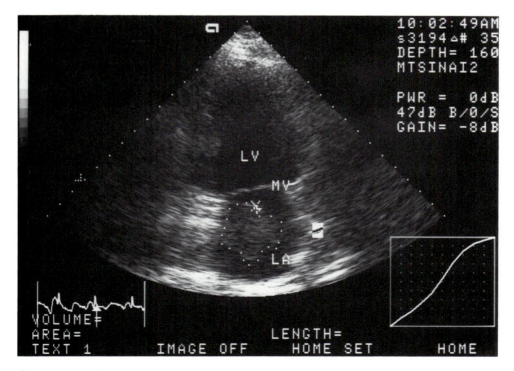

Figure 9-2A: Forty-four-year-old woman with a 2-year history of dyspnea and recent positional syncope. Transthoracic apical view imaged a faint outline of a left atrial mass (dotted outline). LV = left ventricle; LA = left atrium; MV = mitral valve.

236 • Clinical Atlas of Transesophageal Echocardiography

Fig. 9-2.
(cont'd)

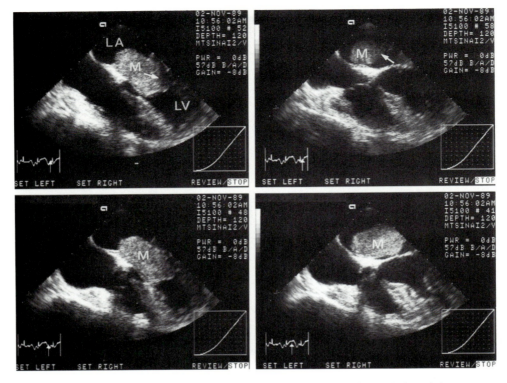

Figure 9-2B: Transesophageal dynamic sequence of the patient's left atrial myxoma (M) prolapsing into the left ventricle (LV) in diastole. LA = left atrium.

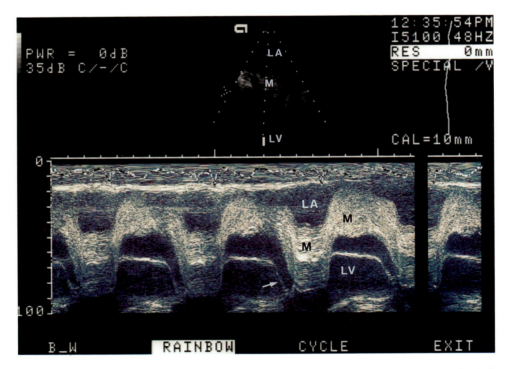

Figure 9-2C: Color M-mode demonstrates the myxoma (M) prolapsing into the left ventricle (LV) in distole. Note the lag between opening of the mitral valve (arrow) and the myxoma's entering the LV. LA = left atrium.

Fig. 9-2. (cont'd)

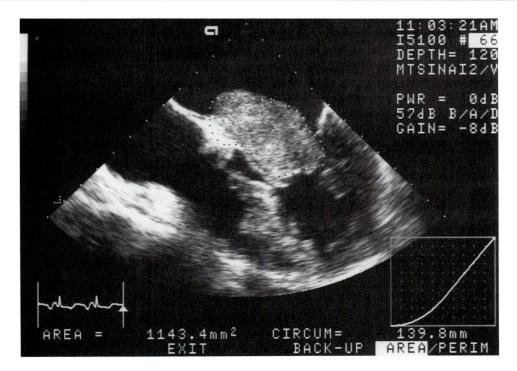

Figure 9-2D: The myxoma measures at least 11.43 cm² in this transesophageal transverse four-chamber view as it prolapses into the left ventricle from its left atrial stalk in disatole.

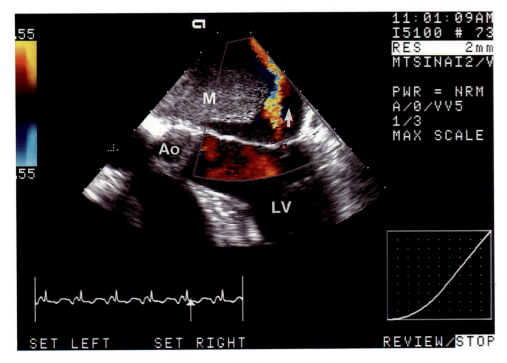

Figure 9-2E: There is mild mitral regurgitation, possibly due to traumatic damage due to the myxoma (M), which has swung back into the left atrium in systole. LV = left ventricle; Ao = aorta.

Fig. 9-3.

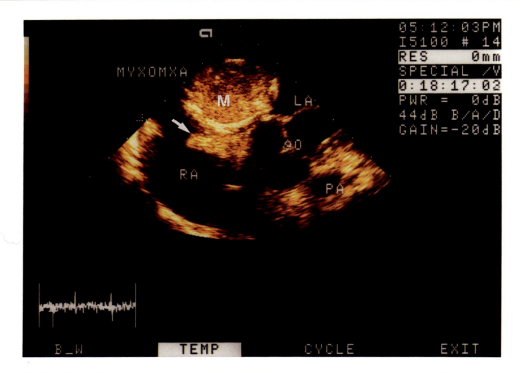

Figure 9-3: Biatrial myxoma (transverse basal view). A large left atrial (LA) myxoma (M) and smaller right atrial (RA) myxoma (arrow). AO = aorta; PA = pulmonary artery.

Fig. 9-4.

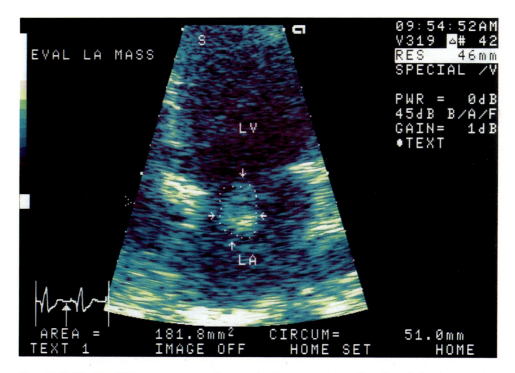

Figure 9-4A: Familial myxoma syndrome. A young woman who already had two prior operations for myxoma excision had this abnormal transthoracic echo with a mass on the atrial side of the anterior leaflet of mitral valve (arrows). LV = left ventricle; LA = left atrium; S = interventricular septum.

Fig. 9-4. (cont'd)

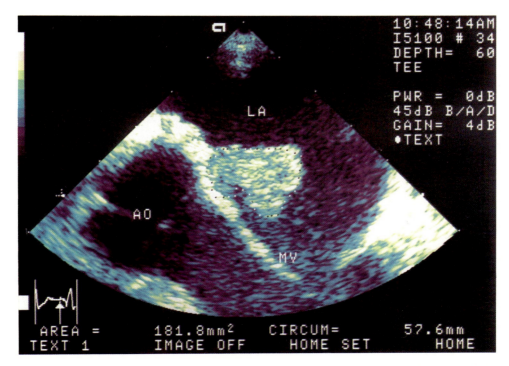

Figure 9-4B: TEE clearly outlined a 1.8 cm² mass on the atrial side of the base of the anterior leaflet of the mitral valve. LA = left atrium; MV = mitral valve; AO = aorta.

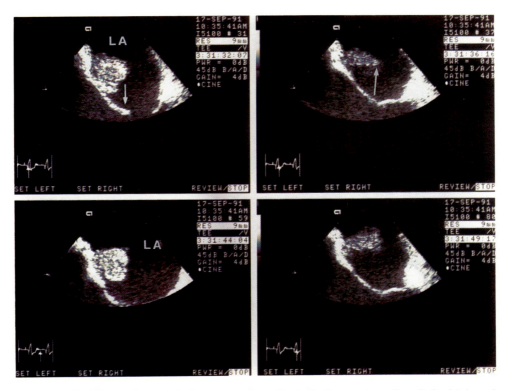

Figure 9-4C: The pedunculated myxoma has diastolic forward motion (left side) and swings back into the left atrium (LA) in systole (right).

Fig. 9-4. (cont'd)

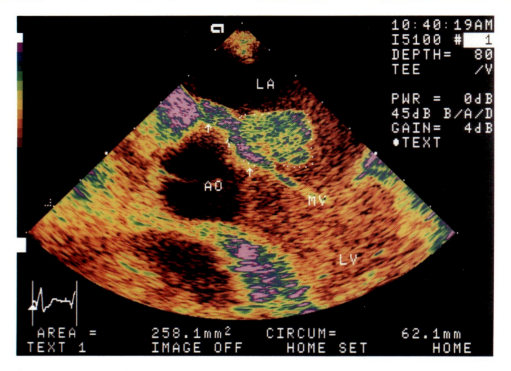

Figure 9-4D: B-color distinguishes the tumor (outlined = 2.58 cm², green/blue) from the underlying leaflet (purple) and blood (orange/red).

Fig. 9-5.

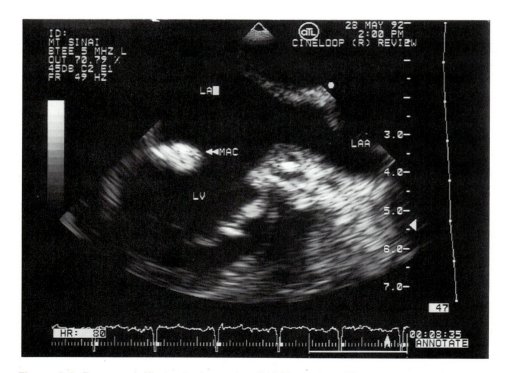

Figure 9-5: Dense calcified mitral annulus (MAC) can be difficult to differentiate from a tumor or vegetation. The calcium's density, lack of mobility, and location assist in confirming that this is annular. LA = left atrium; LAA = left atrial appendage; LV = left ventricle.

The Left Atrium • 241

Fig. 9-6.

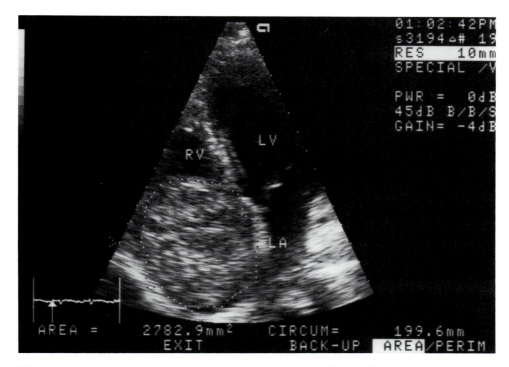

Figure 9-6: A massive right atrial myxoma (circled), 27.8 cm², completely fills the atrium and caused hepatic congestion and edema (transthoracic four-chamber apical view). RV = right ventricle; LV = left ventricle; LA = left atrium.

Fig. 9-7.

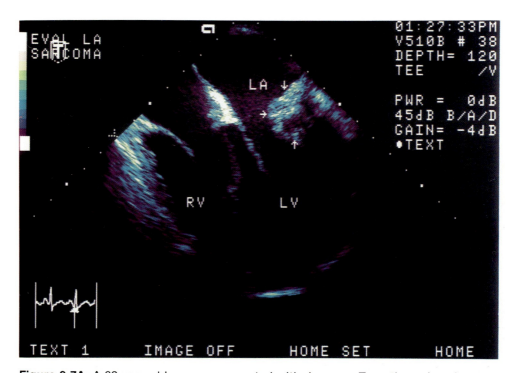

Figure 9-7A: A 63-year-old woman presented with dyspnea. Transthoracic echo suggested a calcific mitral annulus. TEE showed a large irregular-shaped, heterogeneous mass (arrows) extending from the annulus (arrows) (transverse plane). LA = left atrium; LV = left ventricle; RV = right ventricle.

Fig. 9-7. (cont'd)

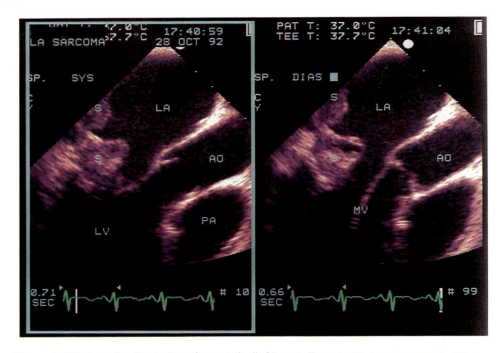

Figure 9-7B: Longitudinal plane in systole (left) and diastole (right) imaged multilobar mass which was a sarcoma (S). LA = left atrium; LV = left ventricle; PA = pulmonary artery; MV = mitral valve.

Fig. 9-8.

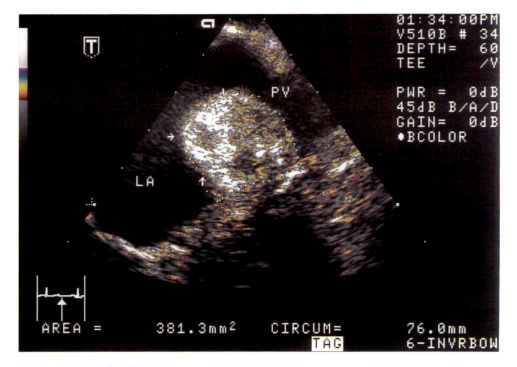

Figure 9-8: Mediastinal tumors can occasionally metastasize into a pulmonary vein as did this carcinoid tumor (arrows). PV = pulmonary valve; LA = left atrium.

Fig. 9-9.

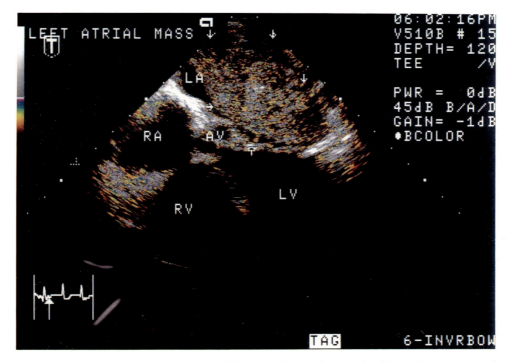

Figure 9-9: An 83-year-old woman in sinus rhythm and normal mitral valve presented with profound hypotension. The transesophageal echo demonstrated almost complete obliteration of the left atrium, sparing the left atrial appendage. Endocarditis of the mitral annulus with dissection and formation of an intramural hematoma filling the entire left atrium (LA) was discovered at postmortem examination. RA = right atrium; RV = right ventricle; LV = left ventricle; AV = aortic valve.

Left Atrial Appendage and Left Atrial Thrombi

The left atrial appendage (LAA) is a small outpouching off of the left atrium (described as dog-ear, peppercorn, conical-shaped), which is rarely seen adequately by routine transthoracic echocardiography. Autopsy studies have shown that the LAA may be multilobar and necessitate careful inspection in more than one plane. However, because of the predilection for thrombus formation in the left appendage in patients with atrial fibrillation and subsequent embolization, a thorough interrogation of the appendage is essential in the evaluation of patients with suspected embolic events.

The LAA can be visualized in the transverse basal plane at the level of the aorta and pulmonary artery. The conical-shaped appendage can also be seen in the longitudinal plane in the two-chamber view. A multiplane probe will facilitate circumferential evaluation of the LAA that may assist in tracking a suspected small thrombus.

The appendage is lined by small pectinate muscle ridges that may be difficult to differentiate from small thrombi. Echogenic "smoke," formed by an interaction between red blood cells and plasma in low-flow states, may be seen wafting up from the LAA into the left atrium in patients with atrial fibrillation. The LAA area ranges from 3 cm^2 to 5 cm^2 in normal patients and progressively dilates with diseases that dilate the left atrium.

Bibliography

1. Aschenberg W, Schluter M, Kremer P, Schroder E, Siglow V, Bleifeld W: Transesophageal two-dimensional echocardiography for the detection of left atrial appendage thrombus. *J Am Coll Cardiol* 7:163–166, 1986.
2. Daniel WG, Nellessen u, Schroder E, Nonnast-Daniel B, Bednarski P, Nikutta P, Lichtlen PR: Left atrial spontaneous echo contrast in mitral valve disease: an indicator for an increased thromboembolic risk. *J Am Coll Cardiol* 11:1204–1211, 1988.
3. Suetsugu M, Matsuzaki M, Toma Y, Anno Y, Maeda T, Okada T, Konishi M, Onos, Tanaka N, Hiro J, Nishimura Y, Kusukawa, R: Resection of mural thrombi and analysis of blood flow velocities in the left atrial appendage using transesophageal two-dimensional echocardiography and pulsed Doppler flowmetry. *J Cardiol* 18:385–394, 1988.
4. Black IW, Hopkins AD, Lee LL, Walsh WF, Jakobson BM: Left atrial spontaneous contrast: a clinical and echocardiographic analysis. *J Am Coll Cardiol* 18:398–404, 1991.
5. Pollick S, Taylor D: Assessment of left atrial appendage function by transesophageal echocardiography: implications for the development of thrombus. *Circulation* 84:223–231, 1991.
6. Wrisley D, Giambartolomei A, Lee I, Brownlee W: Left atrial ball thrombus: review of clinical and echocardiographic manifestations with suggestions for management. *Am Heart J* 1121:1784–1790, 1991.
7. Castello R, Pearson AC, Labovitz AJ: Prevalance and clinical implications of atrial spontaneous contrast in patients undergoing transesophageal echocardiography. *Am J Cardiol* 65:1149–1153, 1990.
8. Hoffman R, Lamberto H, Kress A, et al: Failure of trifluoperizine to resolve spontaneous echo contrast evaluated by transesophageal echocardiography. *Am J Cardiol* 66:648–649, 1990.

Embolic Source Bibliography

1. Pearson AC, Labovitz AJ, Tatineni S, Gomez ER: Superiority of transesophageal echocardiography in detecting cardiac source of embolism in patients with cerebral ischemia of uncertain etiology. *J Am Cardiol* 17:66–72, 1991.
2. Lee RJ, Bertzokis T, Yeoh T, Grogin HR, Choi D, Schmittger I: Enhanced detection of intracardiac sources of cerebral emboli by transesophageal echocardiography. *Stroke* 22:734–739, 1991.
3. Cujec B, Polasek P, Voli C, Shuaib A: Transesophageal echocardiography in the detection of potential cardiac source of embolism in stroke patients. *Stroke* 22:727–733, 1991.
4. Zenker G, Erbel R, Kramer G, et al: Transesophageal two-dimensional echocardiography in young patients with cerebral ischemic events. *Stroke* 19:345–348, 1988.
5. Pop G, Sutherland GR, Koudstaal PJ, et al: Transesophageal echocardiography in the detection of intracardiac embolic sources in patients with transient ischemic attacks. *Stroke* 21:560–565, 1990.

Fig. 9-10.

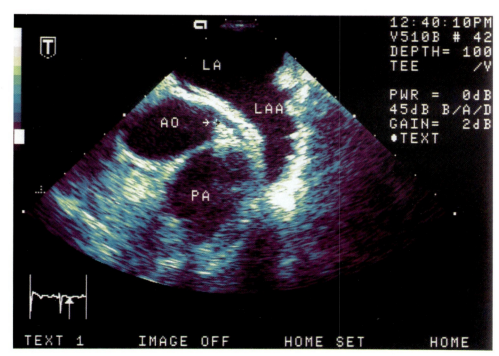

Figure 9-10: Transverse plane, basal level. The left atrial appendage (LAA) is lateral to the aorta (AO) and pulmonary artery (PA). LA = left atrium. Arrow points to the ostium of the left main coronary artery.

Fig. 9-11.

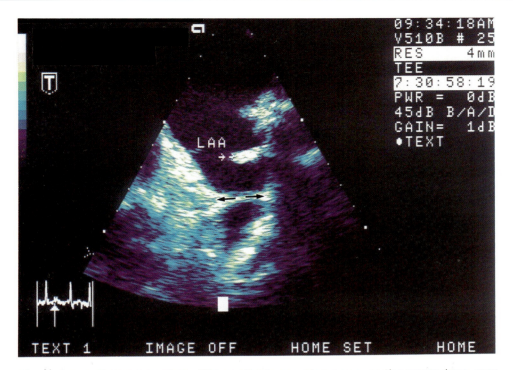

Figure 9-11A: Transverse plane. The pectinate muscles may span the appendage, may stud the lateral wall, and have the same tissue density as the underlying wall. LAA = left atrial appendage.

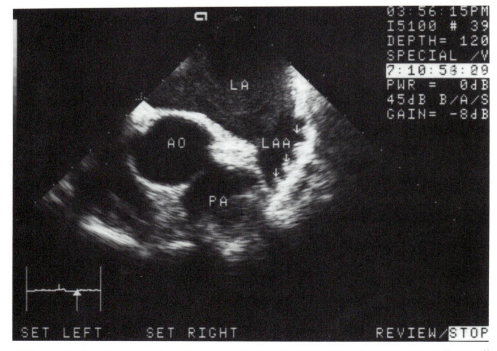

Figure 9-11B: Pectinate muscles in the left atrial appendage (LAA) are usually small and multiple arrows. LA = left atrium; AO = aorta; PA = pulmonary artery; LUPV = left upper pulmonary vein.

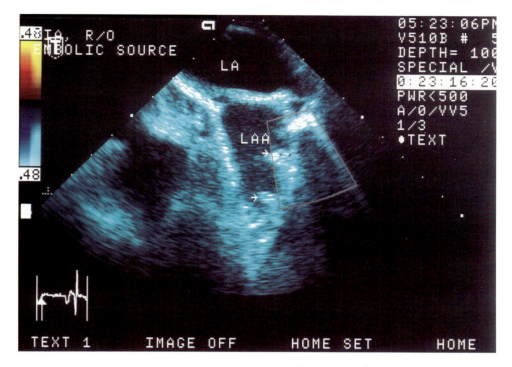

Figure 9-11C: B-color confirms that the lateral pectinate muscles have the same tissue echodensity as the left atrial appendage (LAA) wall.

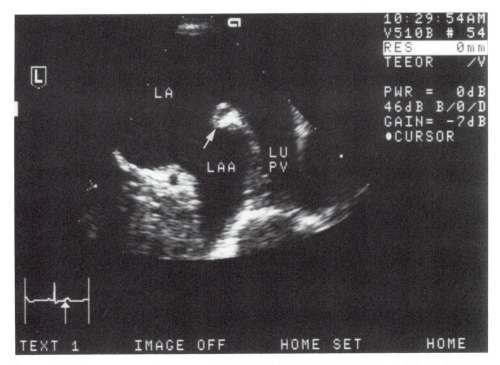

Figure 9-12: The septum betweeen the left atrial appendage (LAA) and the left upper pulmonary vein (LVPV) may have a bulbous, dense tip (arrow) that may be confused with a thrombus.

Fig. 9-13.

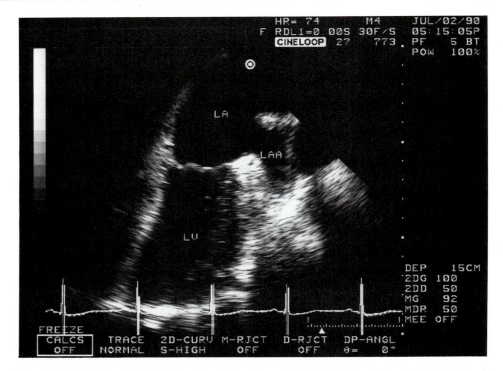

Figure 9-13A: Longitudinal two-chamber view. The left atrial appendage (LAA) is an anterolateral structure that is occasionally seen better in this plane than in the transverse plane. LV = left ventricle.

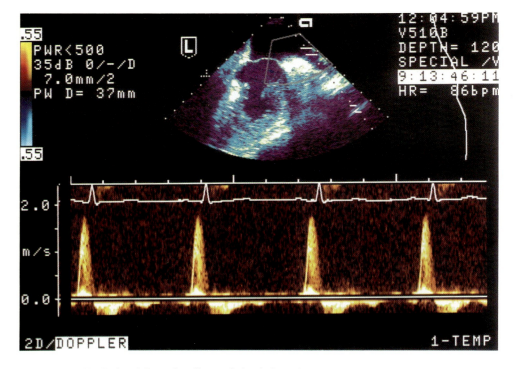

Figure 9-13B: Pulsed Doppler flow of the left atrial appendage in a patient in sinus rhythm demonstrates a single positive Doppler spike immediately following the "p" wave (longitudinal plane).

Fig. 9-14.

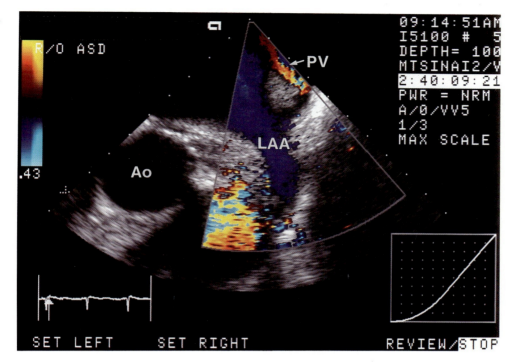

Figure 9-14: Color Doppler can assist in identifying the left atrial appendage (LAA) and the left upper pulmonary vein. Ao = aorta; PV = pulmonary vein.

Fig. 9-15.

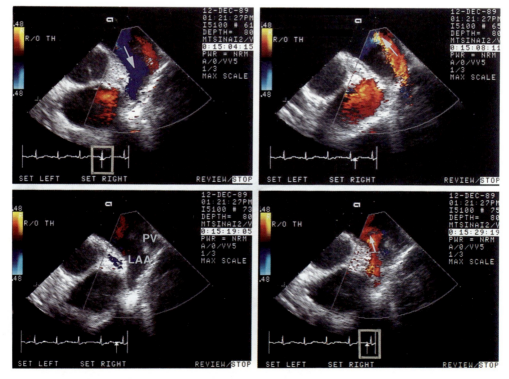

Figure 9-15A: Flow sequence. Lower right, active contraction of the appendage (late diastole, see ECG below) propels blood toward the transducer (orange-red flow); upper right, systolic flow into the left atrium (LA) from the pulmonary vein; upper left, with onset of the QRS, low velocity flow fills the appendage (arrow, blue). PV = pulmonary valve.

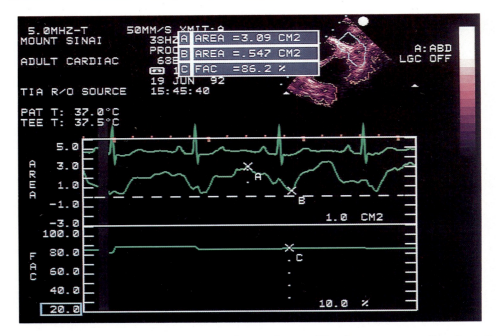

Figure 9-15B: Automatic edge detection and quantification measures the diastolic and systolic areas of the left atrial appendage (3.09 cm^2 and 0.547 cm^2, respectively) and documents an 86% change in area in this vigorously contracting LAA.

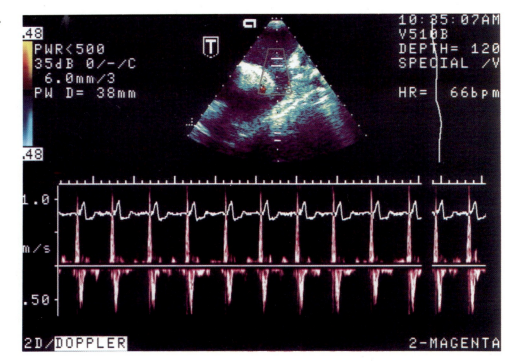

Figure 9-16A: Pulsed Doppler of the LAA demonstrates active contraction of the appendage with a sharp, positive spike immediately following the electrocardiographic "p" wave. Peak velocity is 0.75 m/s.

Fig. 9-16. (cont'd)

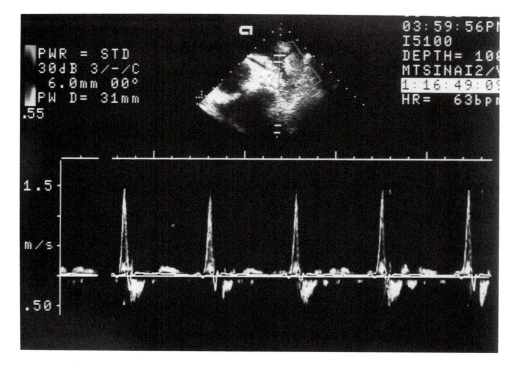

Figure 9-16B: A more vigorous contraction of the left atrial appendage generates a velocity of 1.5 m/s.

Fig. 9-17.

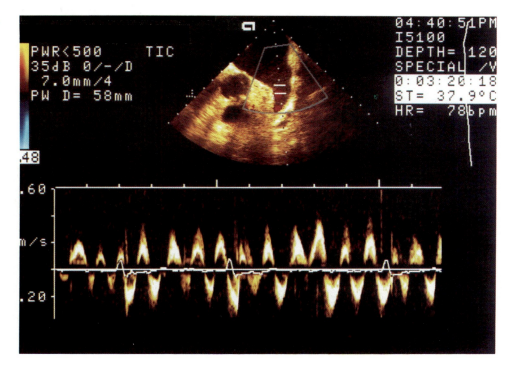

Figure 9-17A: In atrial fibrillation, pulsed Doppler of the left atrial appendage will demonstrate chaotic, rapid, lower velocity deflections (atrial rate = 360 beats/min).

Fig. 9-17. (cont'd)

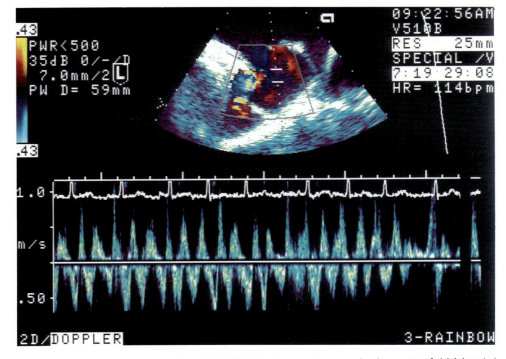

Figure 9-17B: This patient with atrial fibrillation had a ventricular rate of 114 beats/min, but had an atrial rate of 600 contractions/min.

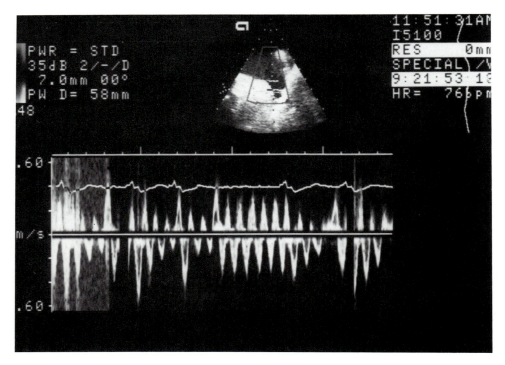

Figure 9-17C: Fibrillatory waves in the appendage can be very rapid (900 deflections/min).

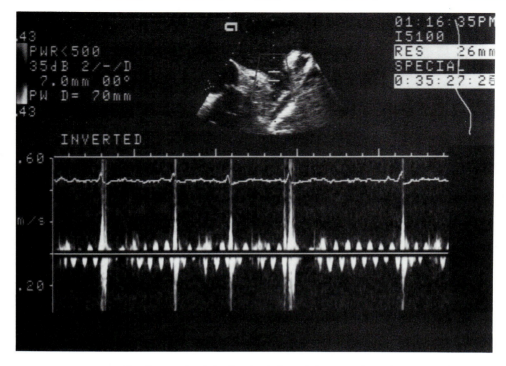

Figure 9-17D: This fibrillatory activity in the left atrial appendage is generating very low velocity (less than 0.1 m/s).

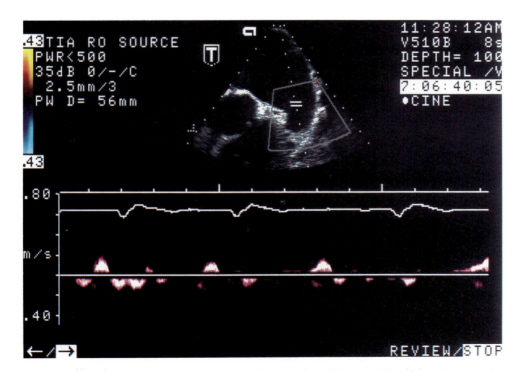

Figure 9-17E: A patient in atrial fibrillation with virtually no active appendage contractions. The low velocity flow in this patient and in the patient in Fig. 9–17D may connote a severe stasis with greater predisposition to thrombus formation.

Fig. 9-18.

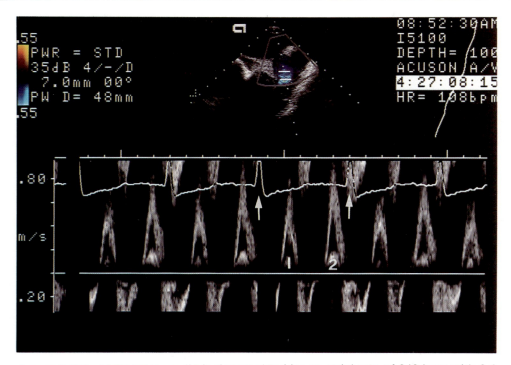

Figure 9-18A: Atrial tachycardia is documented by an atrial rate of 240 bpm with 2:1 atrioventricular conduction.

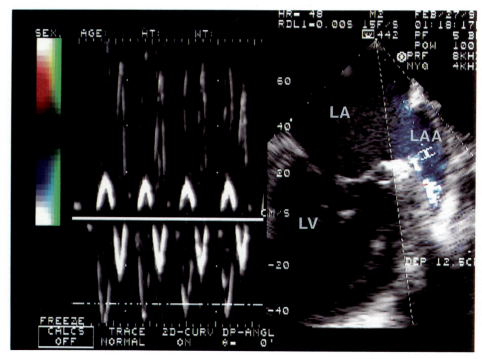

Figure 9-18B: Atrial flutter is confirmed by interrogating the left atrial appendage (LAA) in the longitudinal plane. LA = left atrium; LV = left ventricle.

Fig. 9-19.

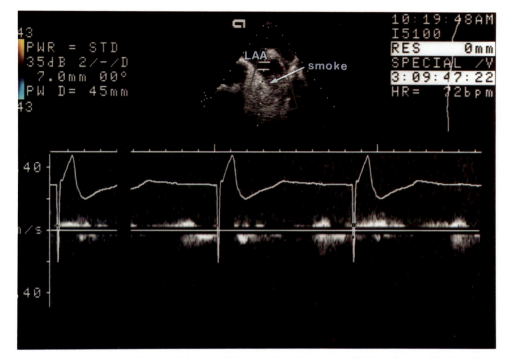

Figure 9-19: Stasis of blood in the left atrial appendage (LAA) of a patient with a pacemaker rhythm, manifested by no detectable Doppler flow, may predispose to "smoke" generation and thrombus formation.

Fig. 9-20.

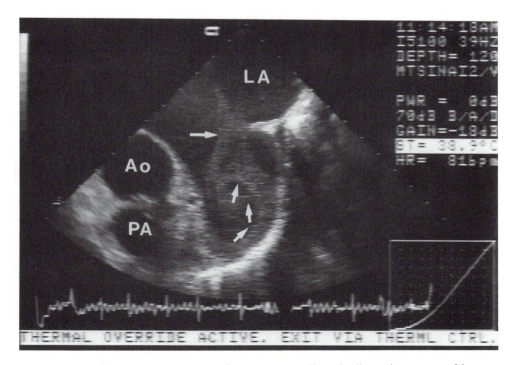

Figure 9-20A: Spontaneous echogenic contrast, or "smoke," can be seen wafting up in this appendage in a patient with afibrillation.

Fig. 9-20. (cont'd)

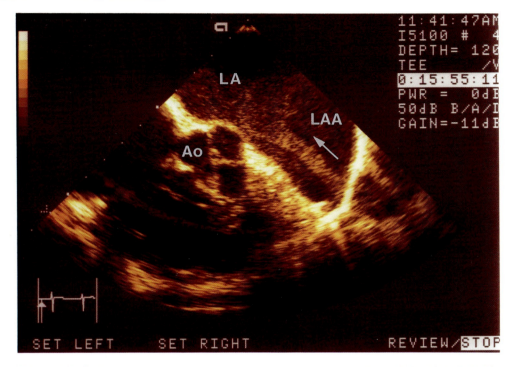

Figure 9-20B: Echogenic contrast, or "smoke," is seen in the dilated left atrial appendage (LAA). B-color may enhance smoke detection. LA = left atrium; Ao = aorta.

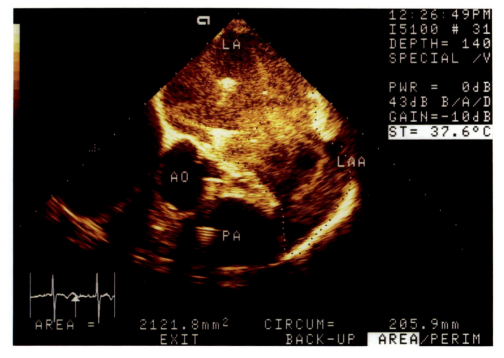

Figure 9-20C: Denser, more extensive smoke in a very dilated left atrial appendage (LAA) (21 cm²). AO = aorta; PA = pulmonary artery.

The Left Atrium • 257

Fig. 9-21.

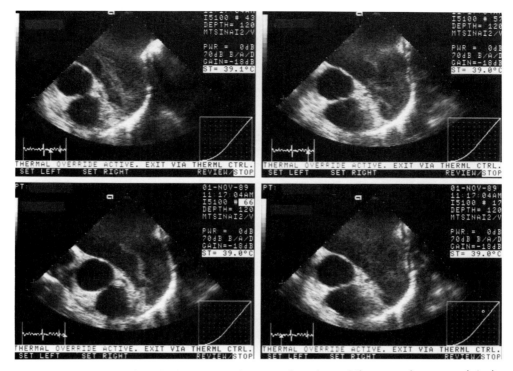

Figure 9-21: The dynamic nature of smoke, seen best in real time, can be appreciated in this multisequence figure. The gray wisps of "smoke" seen on the left are not seen in the frames on the right.

Fig. 9-22.

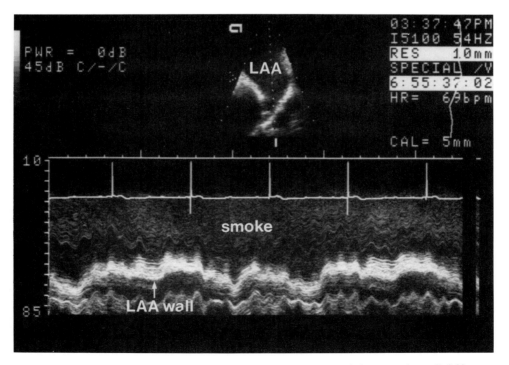

Figure 9-22A: An M-mode through a "smoke"-filled left atrial appendage (LAA) may more graphically demonstrate the dynamic haziness of the waves of "smoke" that remains in the LAA throughout the cardiac cycle in this patient with a ventricular pacemaker rhythm and underlying atrial fibrillation.

Fig. 9-22. (cont'd)

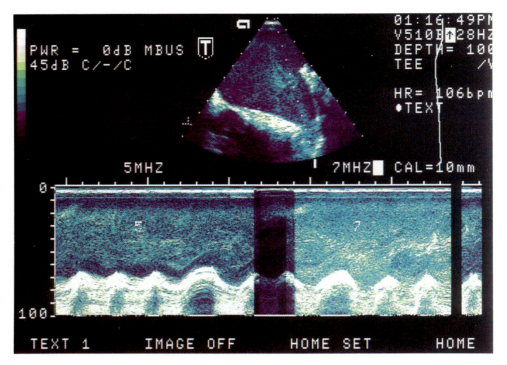

Figure 9-22B: Increased transducer frequency can enhance "smoke" detection. A 5 mHz probe was used on the left on the bottom M-mode through the appendage, while a 7 mHz probe frequency was used on the right.

Fig. 9-23.

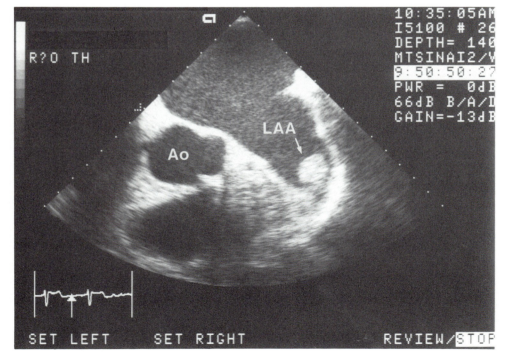

Figure 9-23: Stasis and "smoke" predispose to thrombus (arrow) development in the left atrial appendage (LAA), which frequently occurs at the apex. Ao = aorta.

Fig. 9-24.

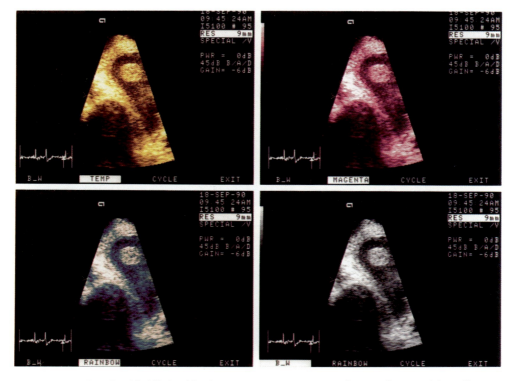

Figure 9-24: B-color highlights the heterogeneous nature of a small, round free-floating thrombus near the outlet of the left atrial appendage.

Fig. 9-25.

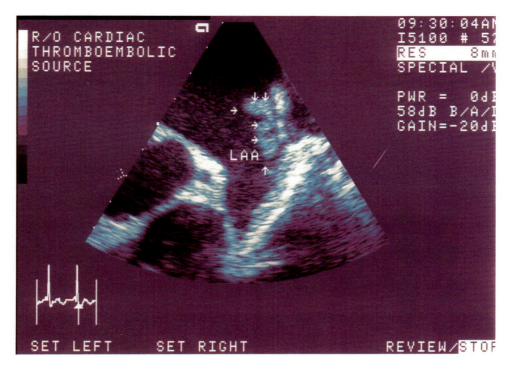

Figure 9-25: A multilobulated thrombus high on the lateral appendage wall (arrows) is less density than the underlying wall. LAA = left atrial appendage (B-color-enhanced).

Fig. 9-26.

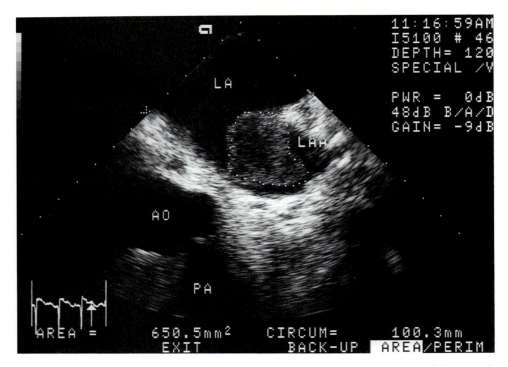

Figure 9-26A: A large thrombus (outlined, 6.5 cm²) fills most of the left atrial appendage (LAA). AO = aorta; PA = pulmonary artery.

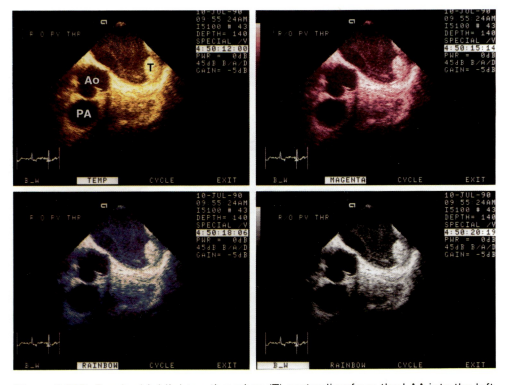

Figure 9-26B: B-color highlights a thrombus (T) protruding from the LAA into the left atrium (LA), which is "smoke"-filled. Ao = aorta; PA = pulmonary artery.

Fig. 9-27.

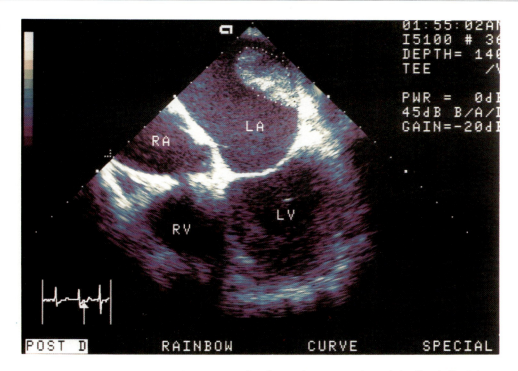

Figure 9-27A: A large thrombus protrudes from the appendage into the left atrium (LA). LV = left ventricle; RA = right atrium; RV = right ventricle.

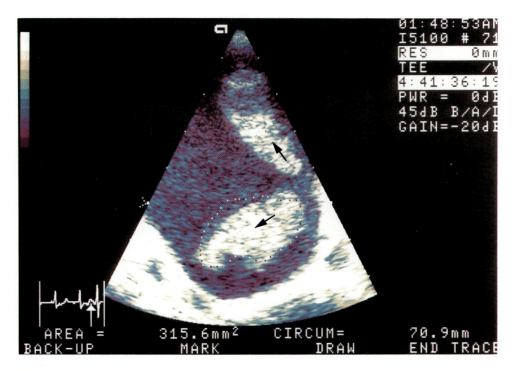

Figure 9-27B: Anterior inspection of the left atrium (LA) revealed two pedunculated lobes of the thrombus (arrows) that extended into the LA from the appendage. One lobe measured 3.15 cm^2.

Fig. 9-27. (cont'd)

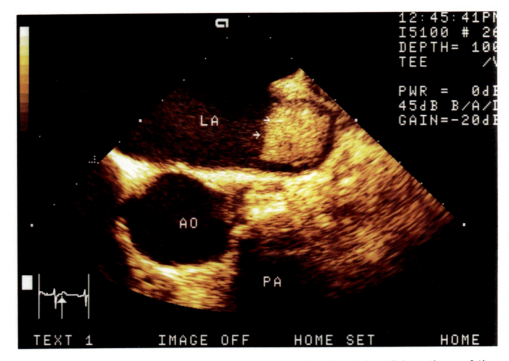

Figure 9-27C: Following 3 months of anticoagulation, the left atrial portions of the complex thrombus had dissolved with only the appendage portion remaining (arrows). LA = left atrium; AO = aorta; PA = pulmonary artery.

Fig. 9-28.

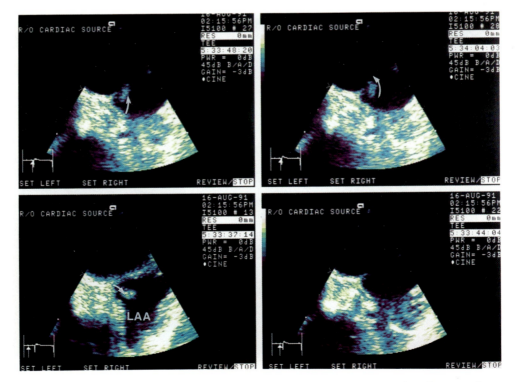

Figure 9-28: Documentation of embolization of a small pedunculated appendage thrombus (arrows track its motion), which is no longer seen in the lower right frame.

The Left Atrium 263

Fig. 9-29.

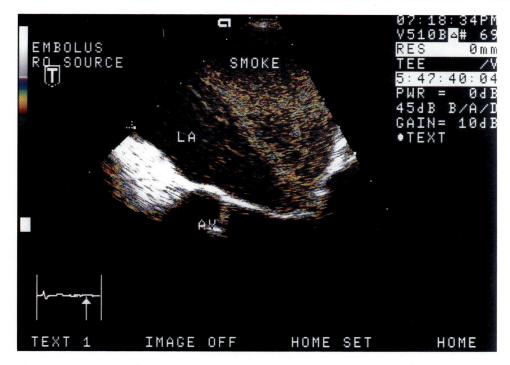

Figure 9-29A: Color B-mode can increase "smoke" detection. LA = left atrium; AV = aortic valve.

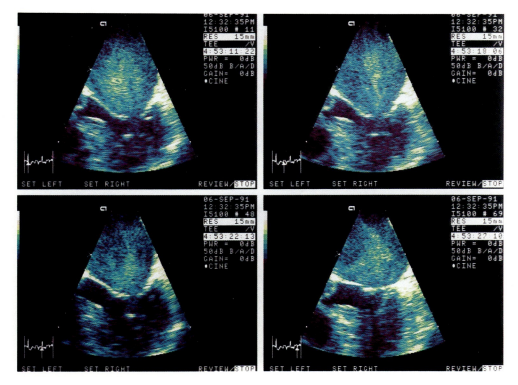

Figure 9-29B: Low flow in the left atrium (LA) due to atrial fibrillation can lead to "smoke" formation. AV = atrial valve.

Fig. 9-30.

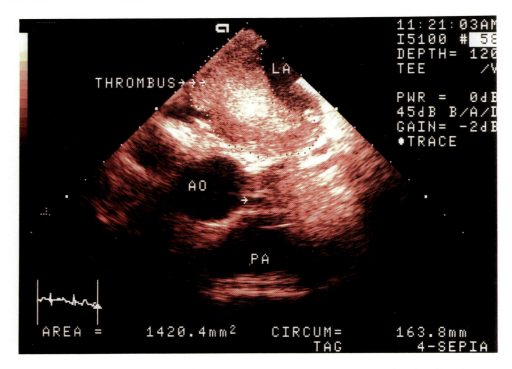

Figure 9-30: Almost the entire superior aspect of the left atrium (LA) is filled by thrombus (14.2 cm²). PA = pulmonary artery; AO = aorta.

Fig. 9-31.

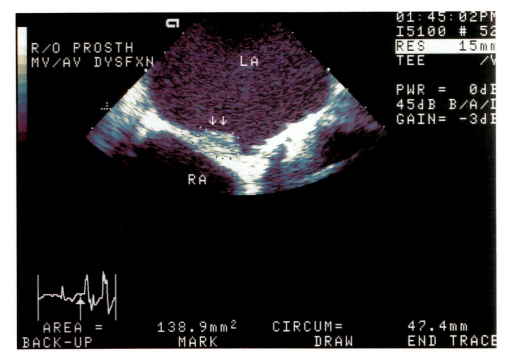

Figure 9-31: The entire left atrium (LA) should be interrogated carefully for thrombus. This small thrombus (1.4 cm²) was located on the interatrial septum in a patient in atrial fibrillation following mitral valve replacement. RA = right atrium.

Fig. 9-32.

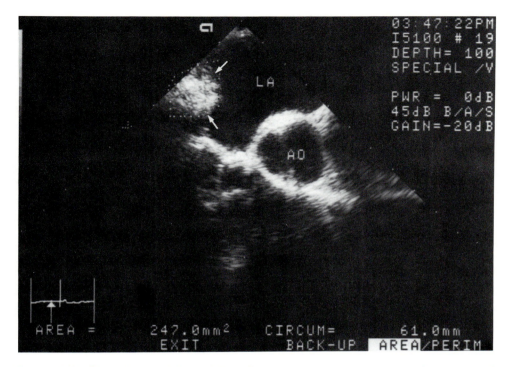

Figure 9-32: Thrombus (outlined, 2.5 cm²) located on the medial superior aspect of the left atrium (LA). AO = aorta.

Fig. 9-33.

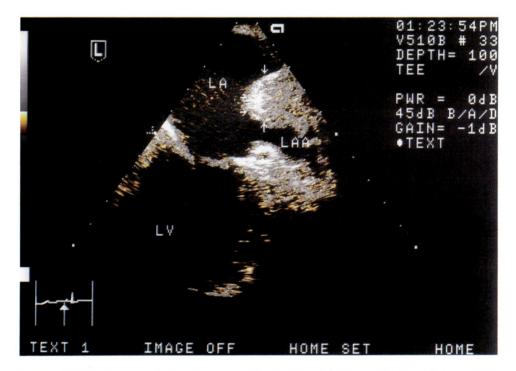

Figure 9-33: This mass (arrows) seen on the longitudinal two-chamber view was not a thrombus but a malignant carcinoid tumor indenting the left atrium (LA) from without. LAA = left atrial appendage; LV = left ventricle.

Pulmonary Veins

The four pulmonary veins convey oxygenated blood from the lungs into the left atrium. Both the left and the right sides of the left atrium each have an upper and a lower pulmonary vein. Pulmonary vein flow is pulsatile and is affected by left atrial compliance, mitral stenosis, and/or regurgitation and left ventricular function.

The pulmonary veins can be imaged in the transthoracic apical four-chamber view, but Doppler interrogation may be technically difficult. However, transesophageal echocardiography can image the pulmonary veins very well. The Doppler flow profile of pulmonary vein flow may provide indirect hemodynamic information on the left atrium.

Bibliography

1. Castello R, Pearson AC, Lenzen P, Labovitz AJ: Effect of mitral regurgitation on pulmonary venous velocities derived from transesophageal color-guided pulsed Doppler imaging. *J Am Coll Cardiol* 17:1499–1506, 1991.
2. Klein AL, Obarski TP, Stewart WJ, Casale PN, Pearce GL, Husbands K, Cosgrove DM, Salcedo EE: Transesophageal Doppler echocardiography of pulmonary venous flow: a new marker of mitral regurgitation severity. *J Am Coll Cardiol* 18:518–526, 1991.
3. Keucherer HF, Muhiudeen IA, Kusumoto FM, Lee E, Moulinier LE, Cahalan MK, Schiller NB: Estimation of mean left atrial pressure from transesophageal pulsed Doppler echocardiography of pulmonary venous flow. *Circulation* 82:1127–1139, 1990.
4. Nishimura RA, Abel MD, Hatle LK, Tajik AJ: Relation of pulmonary vein to mitral flow velocities by transesophageal Doppler echocardiography. *Circulation* 81:1488–1497, 1990.

Fig. 9-34.

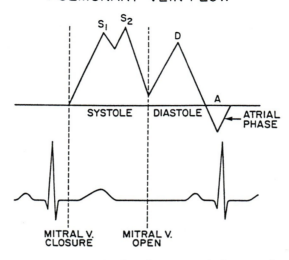

Figure 9-34: Pulmonary vein Doppler flow has several phases reflecting left atrial and left ventricular function. With the onset of ventricular systole, the mitral valve closes and the left atrium relaxes following its active contraction, contributing to early systolic pulmonary vein inflow (S_1). More importantly, ventricular contraction draws the mitral annulus towards the apex, creating a suctioning affect drawing pulmonary vein blood into the left atrium (S_2). The systolic phase of pulmonary flow may be monophasic or biphasic, depending on the heart rate and if atrial relaxation and annular displacement coincide with the onset of diastole. The mitral valve opens and the left atrium empties into the left ventricle, drawing pulmonary vein blood toward and into left atrium (D flow). The last phase of pulmonary venous flow coincides with active atrial contraction (following the ECG "p" wave), which propels blood forward across the mitral valve as well as retrograde into the pulmonary vein (A phase).

Fig. 9-35.

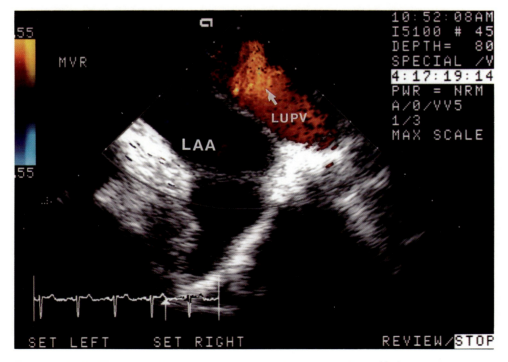

Figure 9-35A: The normal anatomic relationship between the left atrial appendage (LAA) and left upper pulmonary vein (LUPV), separated by a thin septum (transverse basal view).

Fig. 9-35. (cont'd)

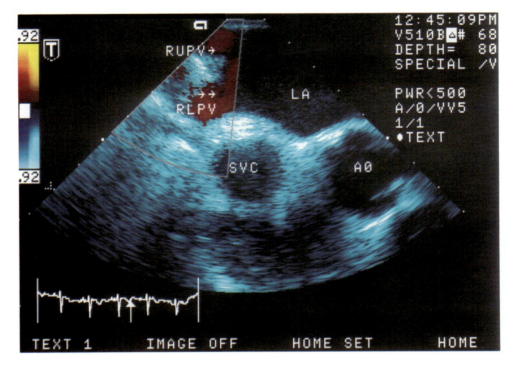

Figure 9-35B: The location of the right upper (RUPV) and right lower (RLPV) pulmonary veins (transverse plane). LA = left atrium; AO = aorta; SVC = superior vena cava.

Fig. 9-36.

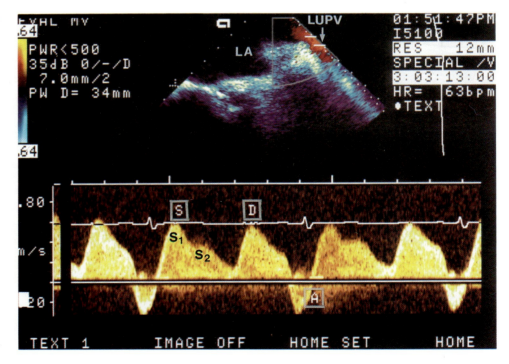

Figure 9-36: Color Doppler identifies Doppler sample volume in the the left upper pulmonary vein (LUPV). Doppler interrogation reveals normal biphasic forward systolic phases (S_1 and S_2), monophasic diastolic forward flow (D), and a small atrial phase of reverse flow (A). LA = left atrium.

Fig. 9-37.

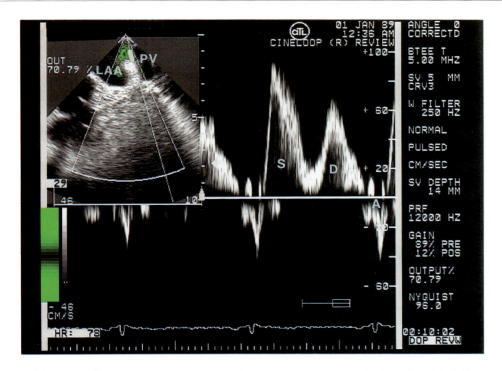

Figure 9-37: Monophasic systolic phase of a left upper pulmonary vein (PV) inflow. The systolic (S) peak and velocity time integral is normally greater than the diastolic (D). LAA = left atrial appendage.

Fig. 9-38.

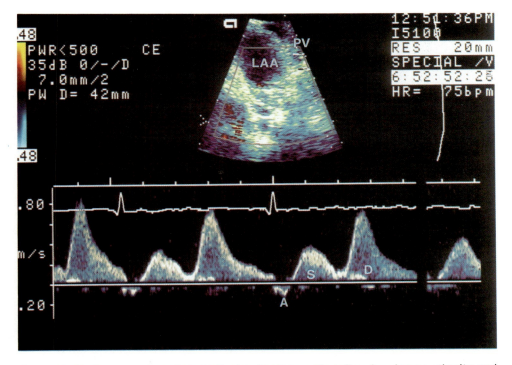

Figure 9-38: The systolic component of pulmonary vein inflow has lower velocity and a smaller velocity time integral than the diastolic phase which may be seen when the left atrial systolic pressure is elevated (i.e., mitral regurgitation, restrictive heart disease, myocardial ischemia). PV = pulmonary vein; LAA = left atrial appendage.

Fig. 9-39.

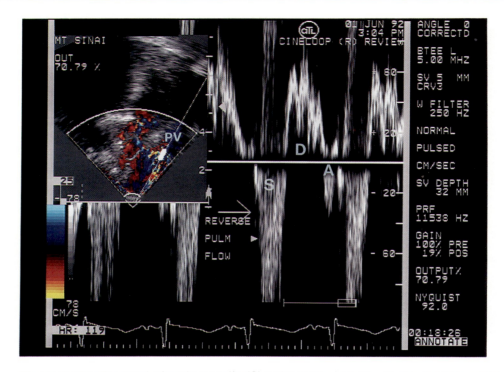

Figure 9-39A: Reversal of early systolic (S) pulmonary vein flow is due to retrograde flow into the vein rather than out into the left atrium. This pattern is seen in significant (4+) mitral regurgitation (MR). Patients with 2+ or less MR have normal pulmonary vein flow, while >3+ MR causes blunted or reversal systolic inflow.

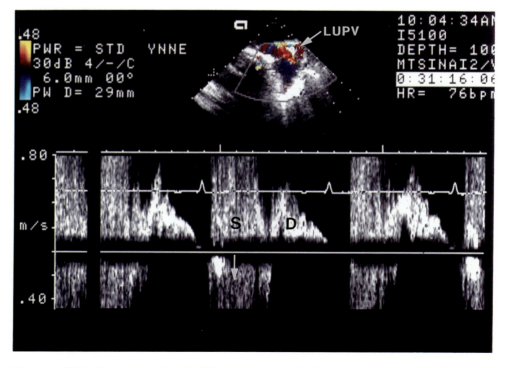

Figure 9-39B: Turbulent systolic (S) pulmonary vein flow due to an eccentric mitral regurgitation jet directed into the left upper pulmonary vein (LUPV).

Fig. 9-40.

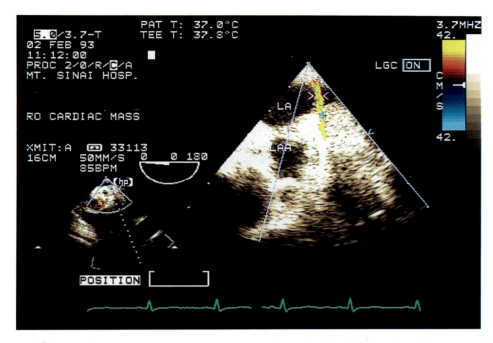

Figure 9-40: Left upper pulmonary vein flow is constricted (therefore narrow and turbulent) due to extrinsic compression from a mediastinal tumor.

Intra-Atrial Septal Aneurysms

Intra-atrial septal aneurysms (ASA) are a congenital aneurysmal formation of the thin portion (fossa ovalis) of the inter-atrial septum. This can be seen occasionally on the transthoracic apical four-chamber view but is better appreciated in the transverse plane in the low four-chamber plane or in the longitudinal plane at the left atrial-right atrial level. By definition, at least a 1.5 cm length of the interatrial septum should swing at least 1.1 cm into either atrium or a total excursion of 1.1 cm. Usually, with inspiration, cough or Valsalva, the ASA swings into the right atrium (see also pp 332–333).

Bibliography

1. Pearson AC, Nagelhout D, Castello R, et al: Atrial septal aneurysm and stroke: a transesophageal echocardiography study. *J Am Coll Cardiol* 18: 1223–1229, 1991.
2. Hanley PC, Tajik J, Hynes JK, et al: Diagnosis and classification of atrial septal aneurysm by two-dimensional echocardiography: report of 80 consecutive cases. *J Am Coll Cardiol* 6:1370–1282, 1985.
3. Fyke FE, Tajik AJ, Edward WD, Seward JB: Diagnosis of lipomatous hypertrophy of the atrial septum by two-dimensional echocardiography *J Am Coll Cardiol* 1:1352–1357, 1953.
4. Hellenbrand WE, Fehey JT, McGowan FX, Weltin GG, Kleinman CS: Transesophageal echocardiography guidance of transcatheter closure of atrial septal defect. *Am J Cardiol* 66:207–213, 1990.
5. Morimoto K, Matsuzaki M, Tohma Y, Ono S, Tanaka N, Michishige H, Murata K, Anno Y, Kusukawa R: Diagnosis and quantitative evaluation of secundum-type atrial septal defect by transesophageal Doppler echocardiography. *Am J Cardiol* 66:85–91, 1990.
6. Scheider D, Hanrath P, Vogel P, Meinertz T: Improved morphologic characterization of atrial septal aneurysm hy transesophageal echocardiography: relation to cerebrovascular events. *J Am Coll Cardiol* 16:1000–1007, 1990.
7. Schwinger M, Gindea A, Freedberg R, Kronzon I: The anatomy of the interatrial septum: a transesophageal echocardiography study. *Am Heart J* 119:1401–1405, 1990.

The Left Atrium • 273

Fig. 9-41.

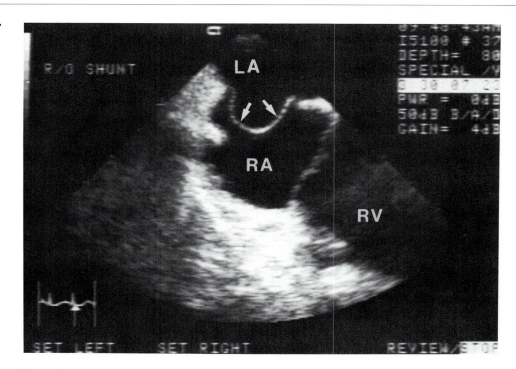

Figure 9-41: In the low four-chamber view (transverse plane), the intra-atrial septum (arrows) is seen bowing into the right atrium. LA = left atrium; RA = right atrium; RV = right ventricle.

Fig. 9-42.

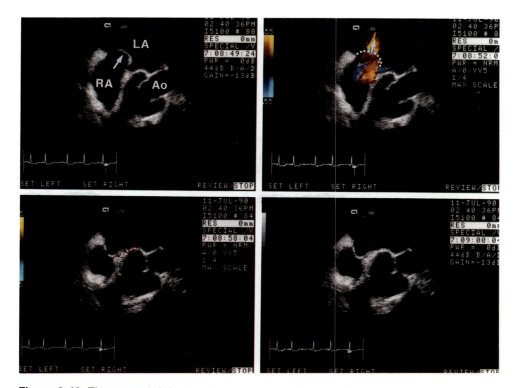

Figure 9-42: The upper left frame demonstrates atrial septal bowing into the left atrium (LA). The right and the left lower images demonstrate bowing into the right atrium (RA). Importantly, the upper right figure demonstrates a patent foramen ovale (arrow) associated with the atrial aneurysm. Ao = aorta.

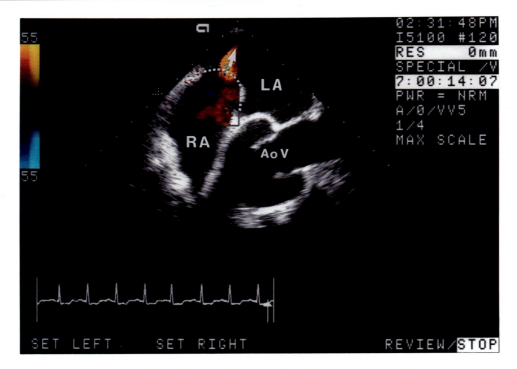

Figure 9-43: A patent foramen ovale (arrow) is frequently associated with a septal aneurysm. If the atrial septum bows towards the left atrium and the right-sided pressures are transiently elevated such as with a Valsalva or straining maneuver, there can be shunting across a patent foramen ovale. Therefore, interrogation of the atrial septum is required during investigation for a potential cardioembolic source (dotted lines outline the intra-atrial septal aneurysm. LA = left atrium; RA = right atrium; AoV = aortic valve.

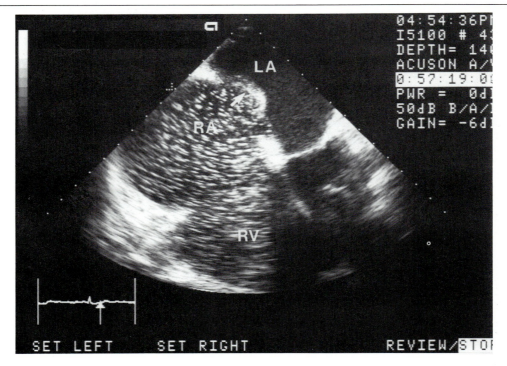

Figure 9-44: Contrast echo is utilized to interrogate an intra-atrial septal aneurysm for a possible patent foramen ovale. In this patient, contrast fills the right atrium (RA), the bowing atrial septal aneurysm, and right ventricle (RV). There was no shunt at the atrial level. RA = right atrium.

Fig. 9-45.

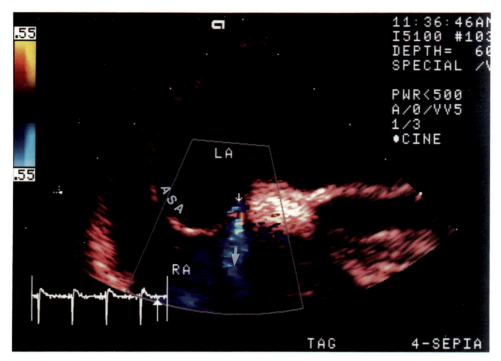

Figure 9-45: In the transverse plane, the patent foramen ovale facilitates a small left-to-right shunt as the atrial septal aneursym (ASA) bows into the right atrium (RA). LA = left atrium.

10

Right Atrial Masses

The right atrium can be easily visualized by routine transthoracic two-dimensional echocardiography, particularly the right ventricular inflow, four-chamber, and subxiphoid views. However, there are occasionally structures seen in the right atrium which present diagnostic problems that can be better visualized by transesophageal echocardiography (TEE). The right atrium is usually a little smaller than the left atrium and it has three inflow vessels: the inferior and superior vena cavae and the coronary sinus. It has one outlet: into the right ventricle through the tricuspid valve. Anatomically, the right atrium may have small pectinate muscles on its free wall, has a small appendage, and is separated from the left atrium by the thin interatrial septum. Pathology that may affect the interatrial septum include congenital abnormalities such as the interatrial septal aneurysm (IASA), patent foramen ovale (PFO), atrial septal defect (ASD), and iatrogenic abnormalities such as the septal defect created during mitral balloon valvuloplasty or through surgical procedures, including cardiac transplantation. Most cardiac tumors affect the left side of the heart. An atrial myxoma occurs in the left atrium three times more commonly than in the right atrium. Metastatic tumors commonly infiltrate the pericardium and solid tissue tumors occur more frequently in left ventricle. However, occasionally tumors can involve the right atrium and can be fully defined by transesophageal echocardiography.

This chapter will focus on abnormalities in the right atrium that may be congenital, normal variants, or pathological.

Fig. 10-1.

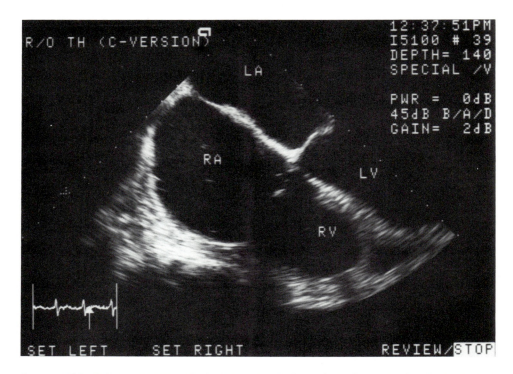

Figure 10-1: This demonstrates the transverse view of the four cardiac chambers as the transducer is raised above the diaphragm. The right atrium (RA) is separated from the left atrium (LA) by an interatrial septum, which is usually a thin membranous structure that may have bulbous distal and proximal segments and a thin area in the middle (fossa ovalis) where the foramen ovale was patent during the fetal circulation. LV = left ventricle; RV = right ventricle.

Fig. 10-2.

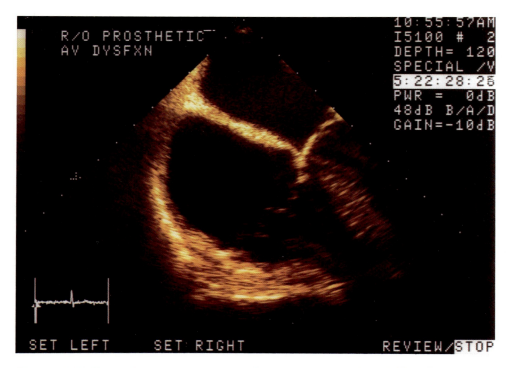

Figure 10-2: The interatrial septum may be uniformly thickened. This B-color 2-D picture highlights the interatrial septum well.

Fig. 10-3.

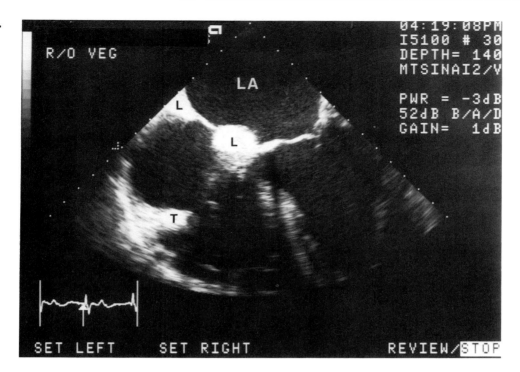

Figure 10-3A: This four-chamber transverse view demonstrates a round echogenic mass with some shadowing that represents lipomatous infiltration (L) of the interatrial septum near the atrial ventricular junction. This is a common variant that can be mistaken for a myxoma. The tricuspid annulus (T) is also lipomatous. LA = left atrium.

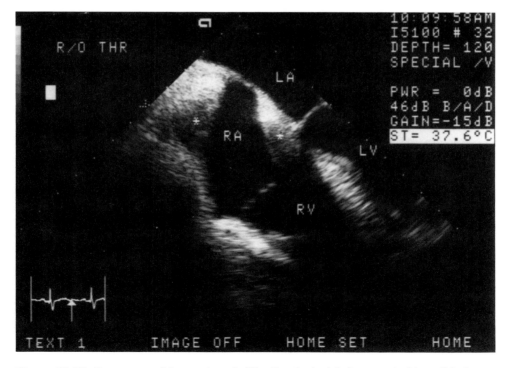

Figure 10-3B: Two areas of lipomatous infiltration (asterisks) separated by a thin fossa ovalis. LA = left atrium; LV = left ventricle; RA = right atrium; RV = right ventricle.

Fig. 10-3. (cont'd)

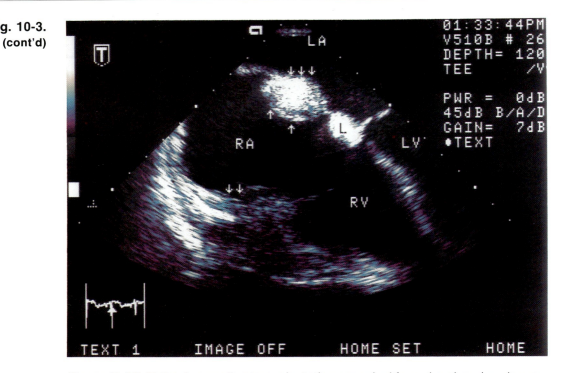

Figure 10-3C: Following cardiac transplantation, an apical four-chamber view demonstrates a lipomatous basal septum and thickened suture sites (arrows) on the interatrial septum and free wall of the right atrium (RA) where the donor heart was anastomosed to the native RA. LA = left atrium; LV = left ventricle; RV = right ventricle.

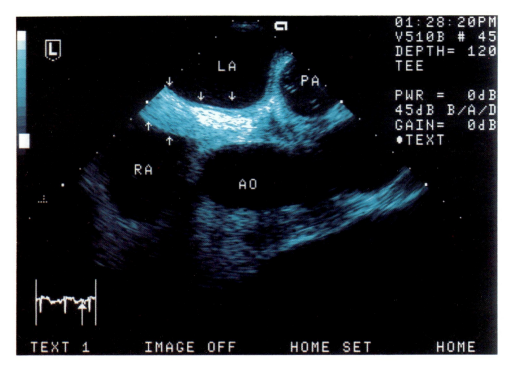

Figure 10-3D: Longitudinal plane of the thickened interatrial septum (arrows) following cardiac transplantation.

Fig. 10-4.

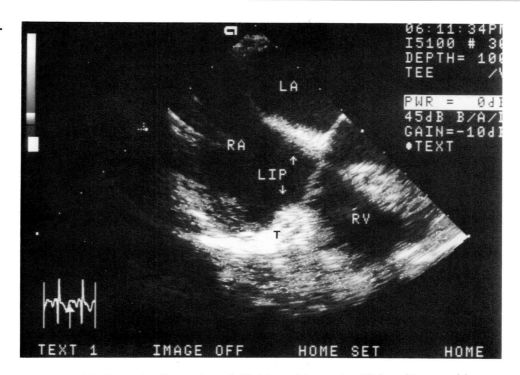

Figure 10-4A: Extensive lipomatous (LIP) tricuspid annulus (T) in a 28-year-old pregnant patient who was referred to exclude a possible right atrial (RA) tumor. LA = left atrium; RV = right ventricle.

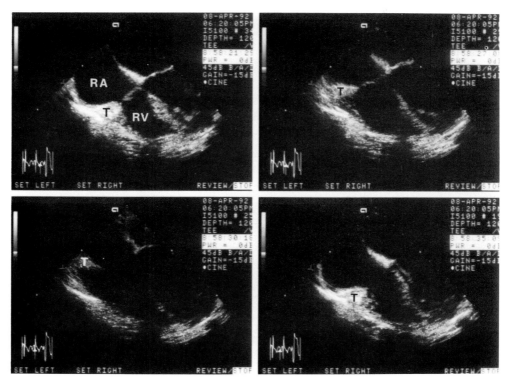

Figure 10-4B: Dynamic sequence confirming the lipomatous tricuspid annulus (T). The patient had an uneventful normal delivery. Follow-up echo was unchanged 6 months later. RA = right atrium; RV = right ventricle.

Fig. 10-5.

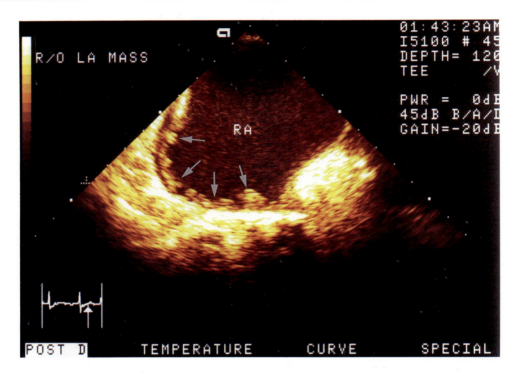

Figure 10-5A: The normal right atrial (RA) free wall in this B-color figure demonstrates small ridges and elevations consistent with the pectinate muscles (arrows). These can be differentiated from thrombi because they are usually multiple, small and line the free wall of the atria, have the same density as the underlying tissue, and may thicken during atrial contraction.

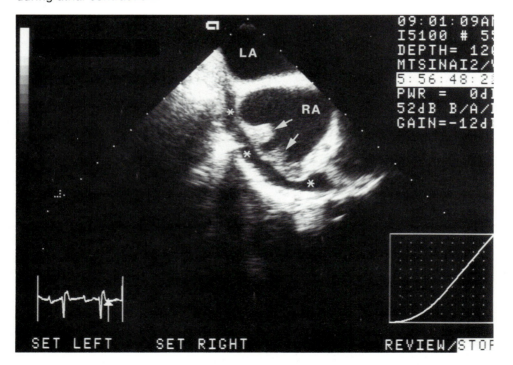

Figure 10-5B: Pectinate muscles (arrows) on the free wall of the right atrium (RA) outlined more prominently because of a small pericardial effusion (asterisks) separating the parietal pericardium from the free wall of the right atrium. One particular ridge is denser, but the real time picture demonstrated the atria to contract and the patient was in sinus rhythm, making this very unlikely to be a thrombus. LA = left atrium.

Fig. 10-6.

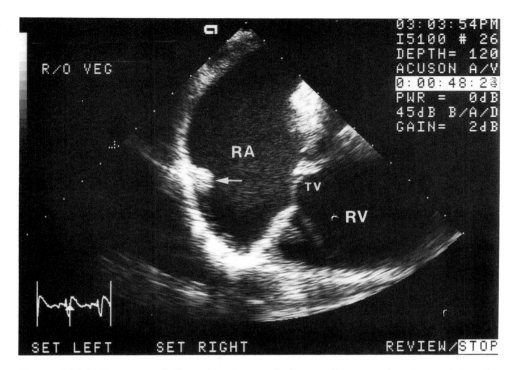

Figure 10-6A: Transverse inflow view demonstrates another prominent round density which is a small thrombus (arrow) in a dilated right atrium (RA) in a patient with paroxysmal atrial fibrillation. TV = tricuspid valve; RV = right ventricle.

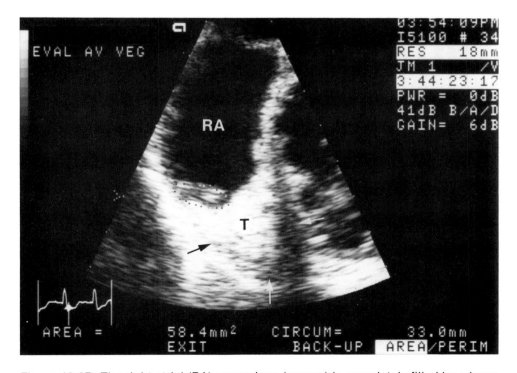

Figure 10-6B: The right atrial (RA) appendage (arrows) is completely filled by a large white dense thrombus (T) with a softer, less dense superior portion (outlined, 0.58 cm^2) protruding from the appendage. This patient was in atrial fibrillation. (Transverse inflow view).

Fig. 10-7.

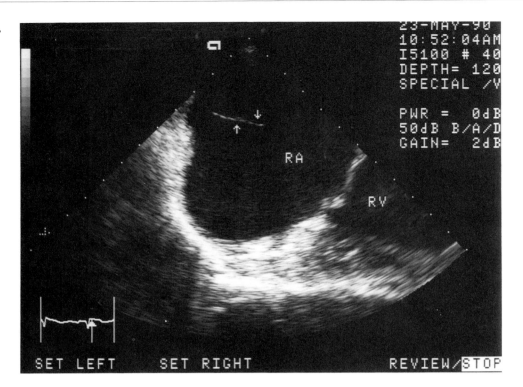

Figure 10-7A: Occasionally there are UFOs (unidentified floating objects) in the right atrium (RA) that need to be defined. In up to 25% of patients, the eustachian valve may be seen at the junction of the inferior vena cava and the right atrium. This is a thin filamentous membrane (arrows) that is a vestigial organ serving as a valve separating the two chambers. Occasionally, it may be highly mobile, extending into the right atrium and undulating with flow. Color flow Doppler will demonstrate that there is no obstruction created by this flap. Transverse right ventricular (RV) inflow view.

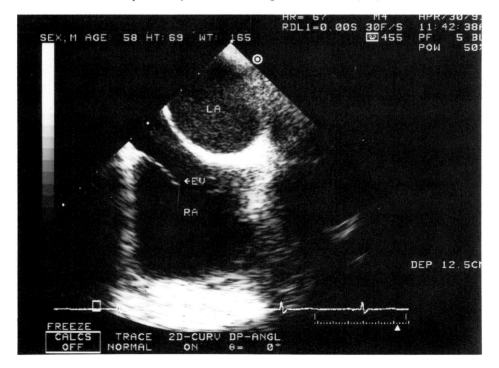

Figure 10-7B: In the right ventricular inflow view in the longitudinal plane, the eustachian valve (EV) can be plainly seen (arrow) as the inferior vena cava enters into the right atrium (RA). RV = right ventricle.

Fig. 10-8.

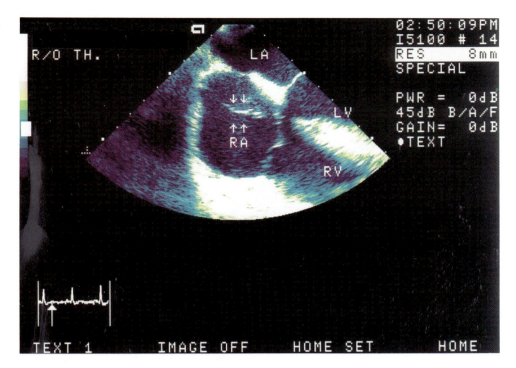

Figure 10-8A: The Chiari network is a filamentous membranous network in the right atrium (RA). This rarely causes obstruction and may undulate with blood flow. In this transverse view, the Chiari network is outlined by the B-color mode (arrows). Note that the interatrial septum is thickened by lipomatous infiltration. RV = right ventricle; LV = left ventricle.

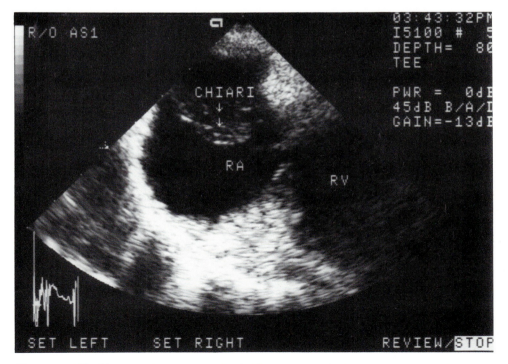

Figure 10-8B: The chaotic motion of the Chiari network is demonstrated, and may mimic a pathological mass. RA = right atrium; RV = right ventricle.

Fig. 10-9.

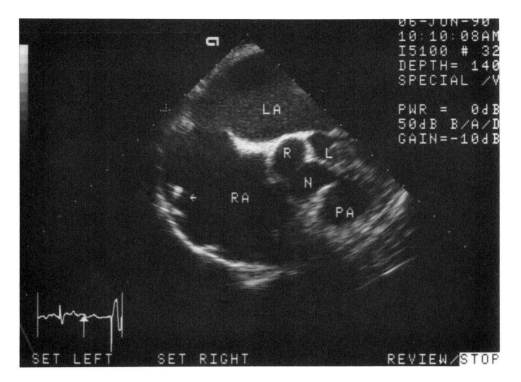

Figure 10-9A: The right atrium (RA) serves as a conduit for many other structures such as pacemakers and catheters. In this figure, a right atrial pacemaker wire is seen (arrow on the free wall of the right atrium). It was differentiated from the normal ridges of the free wall right atrium by its motion and density. Transverse basal view. LA = left atrium; PA = pulmonary artery; aortic valve cusps: L = left; N = noncoronary; R = right.

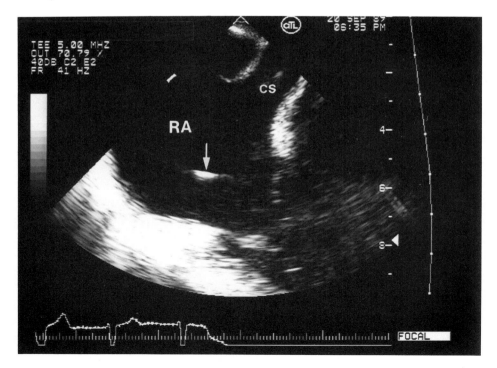

Figure 10-9B: At the level of a dilated coronary sinus (CS), there is a pacemaker wire traversing the right atrium (RA) on its way into the right ventricle. Because two-dimensional echo presents a single plane, the full extent of the pacemaker wire through the right atrium into the right ventricle was not appreciated.

Fig. 10-9.
(cont'd)

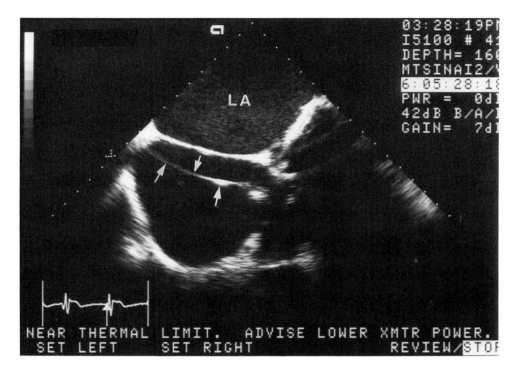

Figure 10-9C: A pacemaker wire (arrows) is seen coursing the right atrium and entering the right ventricle. LA = left atrium.

Fig. 10-10.

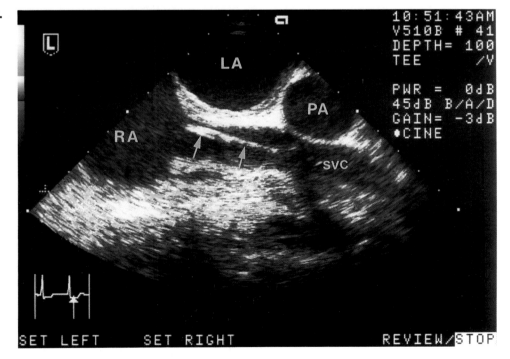

Figure 10-10A: A central venous pressure catheter (arrows) is seen in the superior vena cava (SVC), in the longitudinal plane. LA = left atrium; RA = right atrium; PA = pulmonary artery.

288 • Clinical Atlas of Transesophageal Echocardiography

Fig. 10-10. (cont'd)

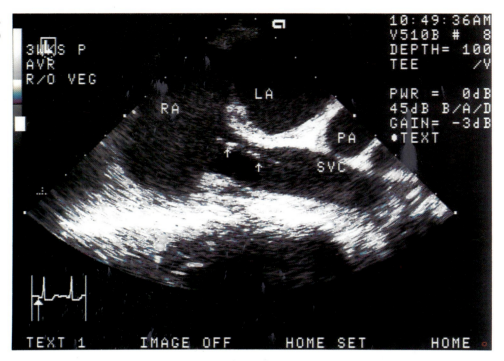

Figure 10-10B: The same catheter (arrows) at a different angle.

Fig. 10-11.

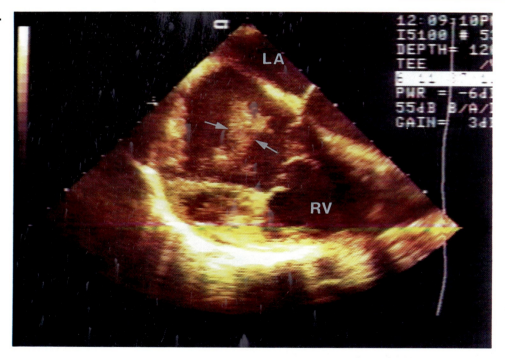

Figure 10-11A: An amorphous floating structure in the middle of the right atrium as well as a denser structure along the free wall of the right atrium presented in a more interesting fashion. This very active person had several episodes of acute shortness of breath which warranted more extensive work-up including a chest wall echocardiogram that demonstrated a possible mass in the right atrium. The transesophageal echocardiogram in this right atrial four-chamber view, transverse plane, demonstrated a large mass along the free wall of the right atrium with a pedunculated floating portion (arrows) in the middle of the right atrium. LA = left atrium; RV = right ventricle.

Fig. 10-11.
(cont'd)

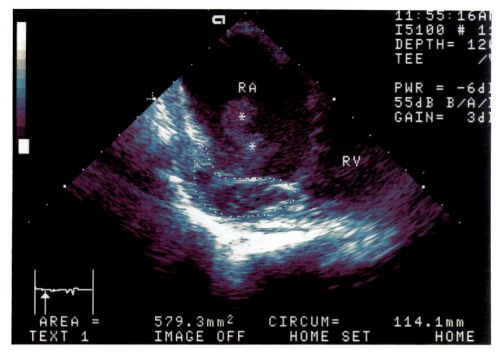

Figure 10-11B: The B-color highlights the softer nature of the floating portion of the mass in the middle of the right atrium (RA). Surgical excision of this malignant tumor (leiomyosarcoma) required reconstruction of the right atrium. RV = right ventricle.

Fig. 10-12.

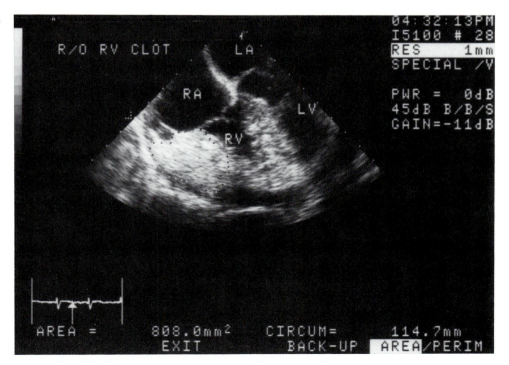

Figure 10-12A: A large mass in the area of the tricuspid annulus protruding outside of the normal contour of the heart and surrounded by a small pericardial effusion. This was a malignant tumor metastatic to the pericardium indenting the free wall of the right atrium (RA)/right ventricle (RV). LV = left ventricle; LA = left atrium.

Fig. 10-12. (cont'd)

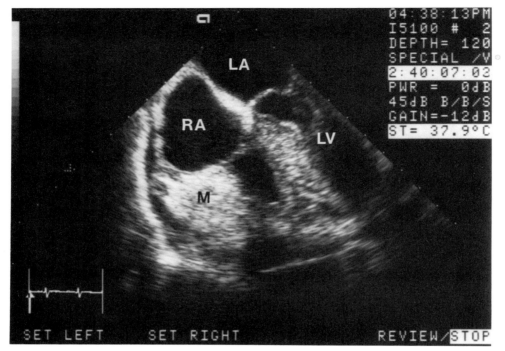

Figure 10-12B: The same abnormal mass (M) from a slightly different angle appears as a spade-like structure outside of the normal contour of the right ventricle. The patient's primary tumor was breast cancer and this mass decreased in size with chemotherapy. LA = left atrium; RA = right atrium; LV = right ventricle.

Fig. 10-13.

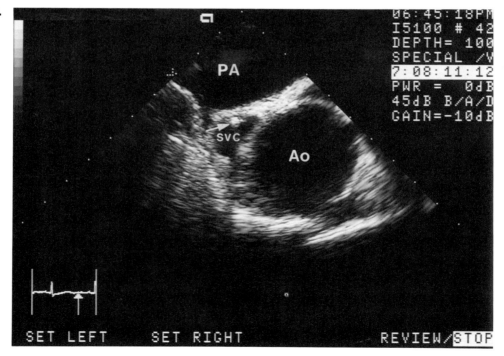

Figure 10-13: A catheter (arrow) entering into the right atrium can be seen in the superior vena cava (SVC) in this transverse plane at the aortic (Ao) level. PA = pulmonary artery.

Fig. 10-14.

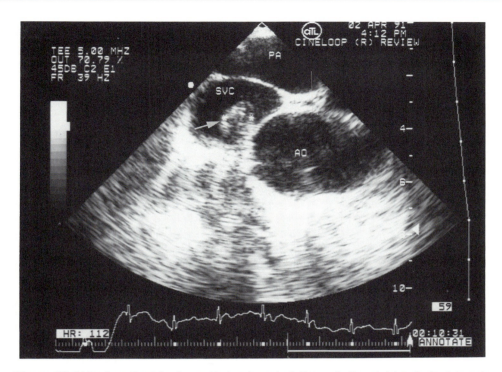

Figure 10-14A: A patient had a catheter inserted through the right subclavian vein into the right atrium for antibiotic infusion. Two weeks later, the patient developed a superior vena cava (SVC) syndrome with edema of the neck and upper extremities. A transesophageal echocardiogram in the transverse plane at the aorta and superior vena cava level demonstrated a density suggestive of a thrombus (arrow). AO = aorta; PA = pulmonary artery.

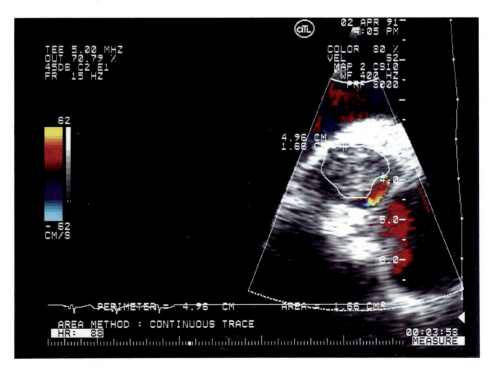

Figure 10-14B: As the transducer was directed more superiorly, almost the entire superior vena cava was occluded by the thrombus (encircled, measuring 1.66 cm^2) and only a small area of flow was seen by color Doppler. This thrombus was felt to be obstructing the patient's superior vena cava. The patient was given heparin for several weeks which led to the disappearance of this abnormal mass and the edema.

Fig. 10-15.

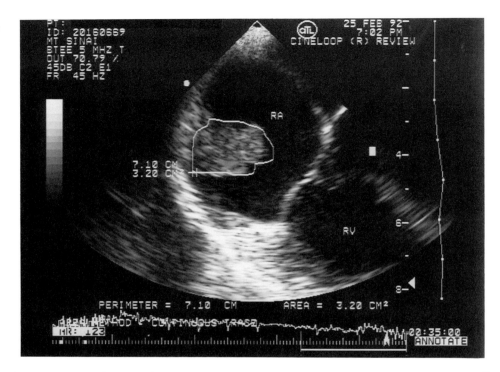

Figure 10-15A: Right atrial (RA) sarcoma in the transverse plane measuring 3.2 cm^2. RV = right ventricle.

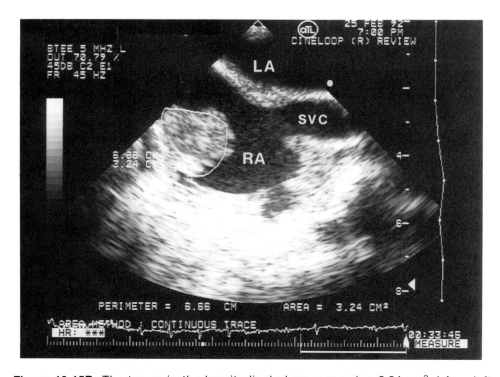

Figure 10-15B: The tumor in the longitudinal plane measuring 3.24 cm^2. LA = left atrium; RA = right atrium; SVC = superior vena cava.

Fig. 10-16.

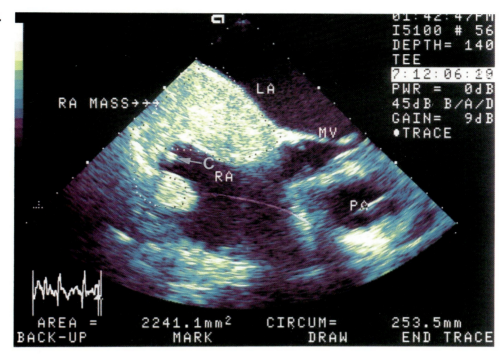

Figure 10-16A: This woman presented with ascites and edema. Transesophageal imaging revealed a large refractile mass filling most of the right atrium (RA), which seemed to be contiguous with the interatrial septum. B-color imaging gave the impression that the density and refractile character of a lipoma measuring at least 22.4 cm². C = catheter; LA = left atrium; MV = mitral valve.

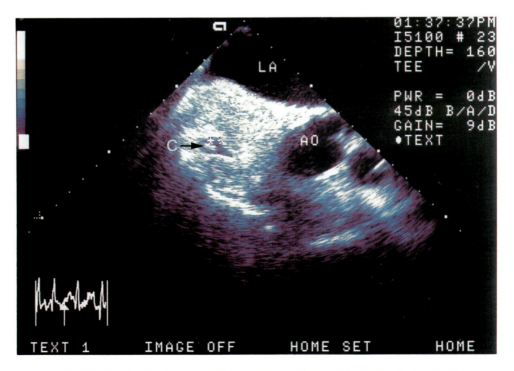

Figure 10-16B: As the probe was raised, we saw that the pulmonary artery catheter (C) was entirely surrounded by the mass. Surgical excision of this mass confirmed that it was a massive lipoma. LA = left atrium; AO = aorta.

Fig. 10-17.

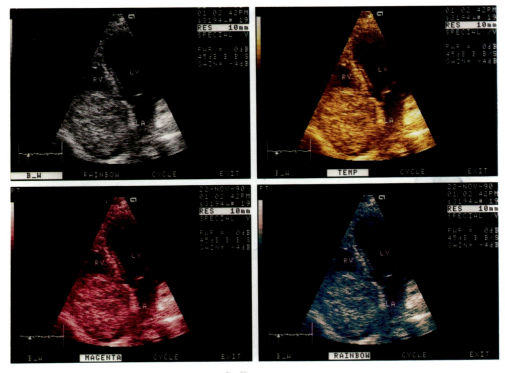

Figure 10-17: Massive right atrial myxoma filling the entire chamber, diagnosed by B-color transthoracic echo, four-chamber view.

Fig. 10-18.

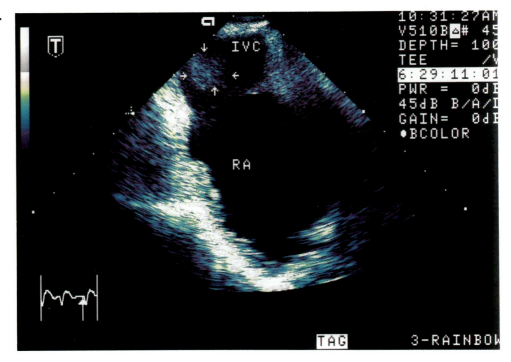

Figure 10-18A: A rare, but significant mass (arrows) was detected ascending the inferior vena cava (IVC) reaching the junction of the right atrium (RA).

Fig. 10-18. (cont'd)

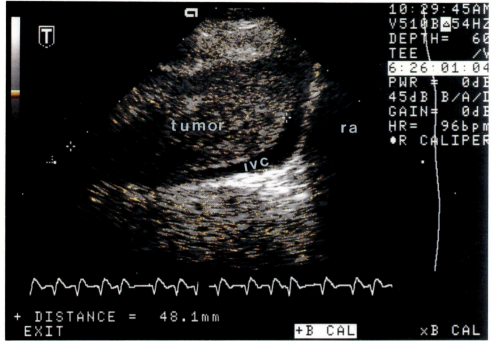

Figure 10-18B: The mass was a renal cell carcinoma which had metastasized up the inferior vena cava (IVC). RA = right atrium.

11

Pericardial Disease

Effusions

Pleural and pericardial effusions can usually be diagnosed by x-ray or transthoracic echocardiograms. However, they can also be seen by transesophageal echo, particularly following open heart surgery.

Fig. 11-1.

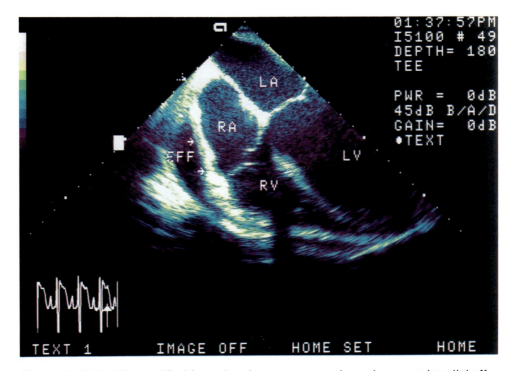

Figure 11-1A: In this modified four-chamber transverse plane view, a pericardial effusion (EFF) was seen anterior to the right atrium (RA) and right ventricle (RV) (arrows). LA = left atrium; LV = left ventricle.

Fig. 11-1. (cont'd)

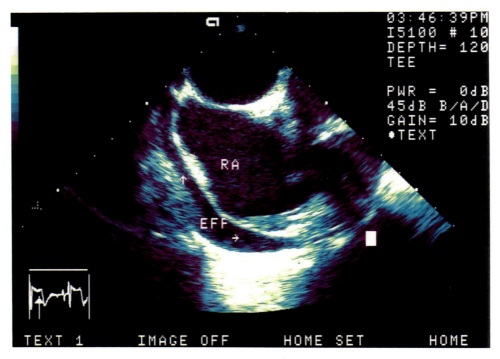

Figure 11-1B: A small pericardial effusion (EFF) anterior to the right atrium (RA).

Fig. 11-2.

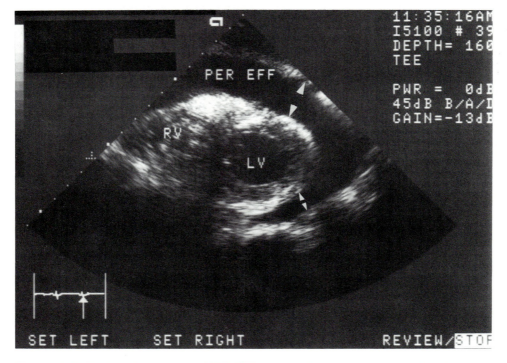

Figure 11-2: Pericardial effusion (PER EFF, arrows) is seen anterior and posterior to the heart in this transverse short axis transgastric plane. RV = right ventricle; LV = left ventricle.

Fig. 11-3.

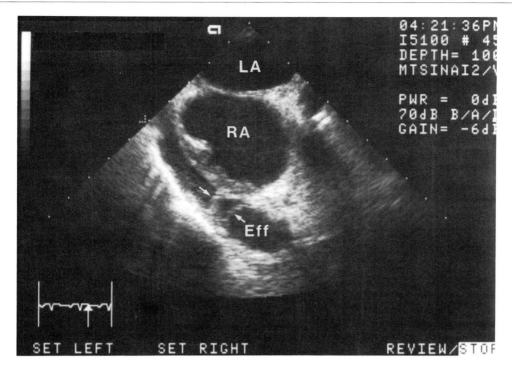

Figure 11-3: A pericardial effusion (Eff) seen anterior to the right atrium (RA) with fibrous adhesions (arrows) spanning the pericardial fluid. LA = left arium.

Fig. 11-4.

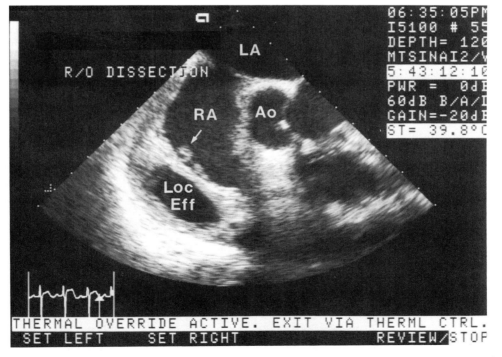

Figure 11-4: A pericardial effusion developed in a patient after open heart surgery. This transesophageal echocardiogram demonstrated fibrous thickening of the pericardium with loculated pericardial effusion (Loc Eff) anterior to the right atrium. Arrow points to pectinate muscles in the right atrium (RA). LA = left atrium; Ao = aorta.

Fig. 11-5.

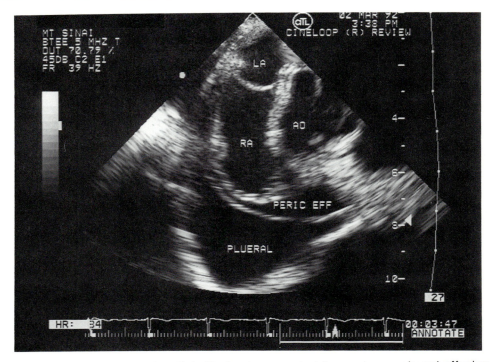

Figure 11-5: A small pericardial effusion is separated from a larger pleural effusion. RA = right atrium; LA = left atrium; AO = aorta.

Fig. 11-6.

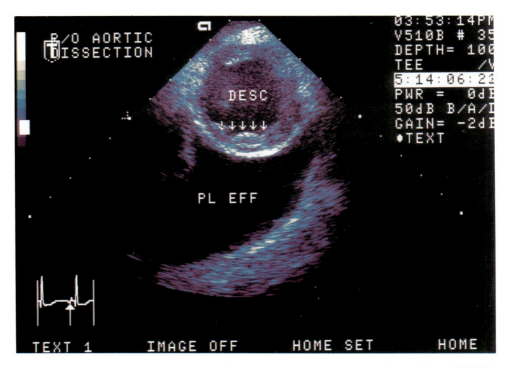

Figure 11-6: A pleural effusion (PL EFF) is seen adjacent to the descending (DESC) aorta in the transverse plane. Arrows point to plaque in the aorta.

Fig. 11-7.

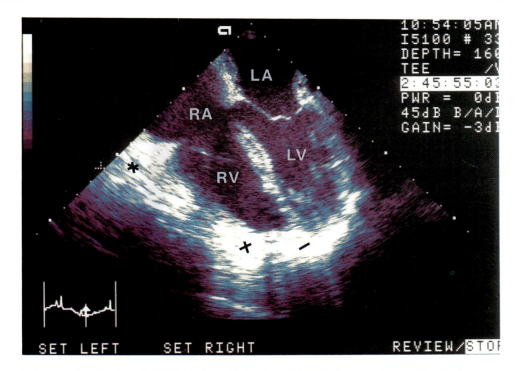

Figure 11-7: Pericardial thickening, fibrosis, and calcification in a patient who presented with symptoms consistent with pericardial constriction. This B-color transverse four-chamber view demonstrates significant echo-density of the entire pericardium (asterisks) compared to the myocardium of the intraventricular septum. This patient had pericardial constriction confirmed at surgery. LA = left atrium; RA = right atrium; LV = left ventricle; RV = right ventricle.

Fig. 11-8.

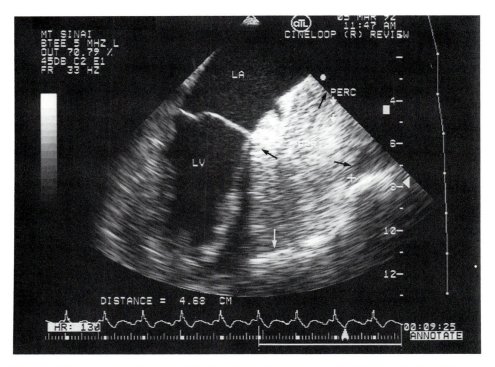

Figure 11-8: A large anterior mediastinal hematoma (arrows) collected following open heart surgery (longitudinal plane). LA = left atrium; LV = left ventricle.

12

Congenital Heart Disease in the Adult

Atrial Septal Defects

Atrial septal defects (ASD) are one of the most common congential cardiac anomalies and, excluding mitral valve prolapse, may be the most common congenital heart disease in adults.

There are three major locations of the atrial septal defects:

1. Ostium Secundum Type: The most common ASD is the ostium secundum type which is in the midseptal area and superior to the fossa ovalis. The septum primum forms the left side of the atrial septum and the septum secundum forms the right side. The septum primum usually fuses with the septum secundum to seal the foramen ovale. The foramen may serve as a unidirectional valve facilitating a small intracardiac shunt particularly with obstructive lesions of the right heart and increased right-sided pressures. (See diagram in the following section on Patent Foramen Ovale, pp 327). Importantly, the ostium secundum is a defect in the septum primum and is distinct from a patent foramen ovale (PFO), an open flap.

2. Sinus Venosus Type: The sinus venosus defect is located high in the atrial septum in close proximity to the superior vena cava entry into the right atrium. A venosus defect is frequently associated with partial anomalous pulmonary venous return from the right lung at the junction of superior vena cava and right atrium which facilitates a large shunt of deoxygenated blood into the left atrium through the defect.

3. Ostium Primum Type: This type of ASD is associated with an endocardial cushion defect and is at the level of the atrioventricular valves.

The volume of flow through the ASD is dependent upon the size of the defect and the relative compliance of the left and right ventricle as well as the pulmonary and systemic vascular resistances. The pressures across the ASD and in all four chambers of the heart should be similar during diastole. However, a left-to-right shunt can occur in three phases, late ventricular systole, early diastole, and with atrial contraction. Transiently, there may be a right-to-left shunt during the onset of ventricular systole. Increasing intrathoracic and right-sided pressure as with Valsalva maneuver or during deep cough may also cause a right to left shunt. Eventually, if the left-to-right shunt is large, it causes enlargement of the right atrium, right ventricle, as well as the left atrium. Pulmonary vascular flow increases and there is a plethora of the pulmonary arteries and pulmonary vascular seen on chest x-ray.

Patients with ASD may present late in life with cardiac symptoms because the volume overload is well tolerated for many years. They may develop atrial arrhythmias, mild congestive heart failure, pulmonary hypertension, exertional dyspnea, or a paradoxical embolic event.

The physical exam in patients with ASD may include a fixed second heart sound, a diastolic rumbling murmur due to increase flow of the tricuspid valve, and evidence of pulmonary hypertension.

The electrocardiogram may demonstrate atrial arrhythmias, particularly atrial fibrillation. Ostium secundum may cause right axis deviation, right ventricular hypertrophy with a rSR^1 in V_1. A sinus venosus defect may be associated with a negative P wave in lead III. A primum defect may have left axis deviation. All defects may cause a prolonged P-R interval. Routine transthoracic echo may suggest ASD by the presence of dilated left and right atria and right ventricle and abnormal septal motion consistent with right ventricular volume overload.

The transesophageal echo is extremely valuable in locating the ASD, measuring the size of the defect, documenting shunt direction, as well as evalvating pulmonary venous return. Frequently, patients without symptoms or risk factors of coronary artery disease may not require cardiac catheterization before undergoing surgical repair of an ASD if a noninvasive evaluation has been thorough.

PFO should not be confused with an atrial septal defect. The PFO is lack of fusion of the septum secundum to septum primum facilitating right to left shunting. The foramen is important in the fetus to shunt blood from the right to left atrium, avoiding the nonfunctioning lungs, and seals quickly post partum with the neonate's first breaths. A probe patent foramen ovale is present in up to 28% of autopsied hearts and in 10% of patients studied by TEE. The presence of a a PFO may be an important source of a paradoxical embolus causing a transient ischemic attack or stroke. Contrast injections are more sensitive than color flow Doppler alone to detect a PFO.

Fig. 12-1.

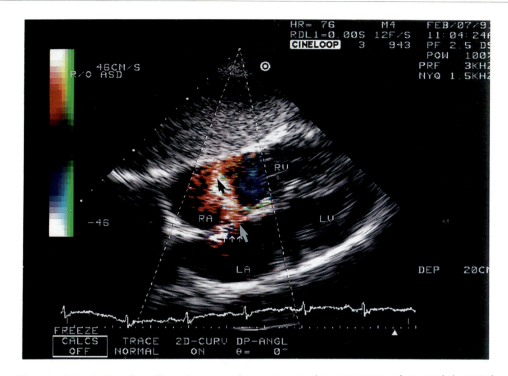

Figure 12-1: Color flow Doppler may demonstrate the presence of an atrial septal defect by transthoracic echo, particularly the subxiphoid view. A contrast study done transthoracically may also demonstrate transient right-to-left shunt or negative contrast. (The right atrium is filled with microbubbles except where the blood enters from the left atrium through the defect). RV = right ventricle; RA = right atrium; LV = left ventricle; LA = left atrium.

Fig. 12-2.

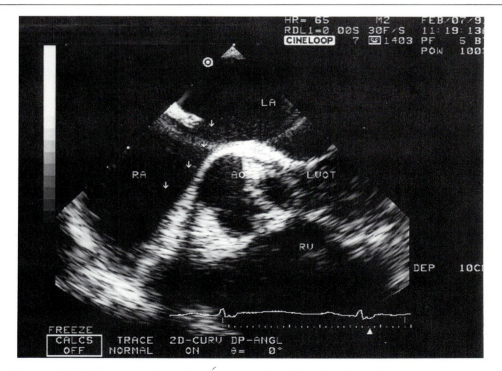

Figure 12-2A: Transesophageal transverse plane five-chamber view demonstrates a 1 cm atrial septal defect (arrows) secundum type. RV = right ventricle; RA = right atrium; LA = left atrium; AO = aorta; LVOT = left ventricular outflow tract.

Fig. 12-2.
(cont'd)

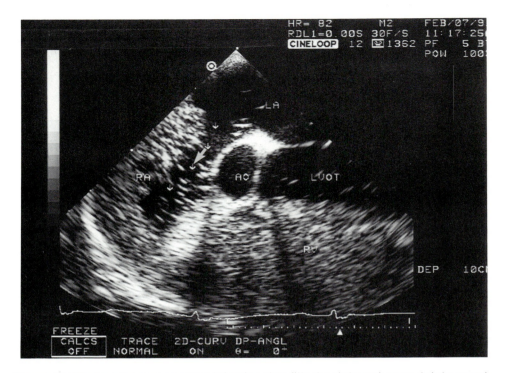

Figure 12-2B: A peripheral contrast injection that fills the right atrium and right ventricle demonstrates the negative contrast effect from flow entering the left atrium into the right atrium. Microbubbles were also seen in the left ventricular outflow tract (LVOT) and left atrium (LA) consistent with the bidirectional nature of most atrial septal defects even though there is usually very little right-to-left flow. RA = right atrium; AO = aorta.

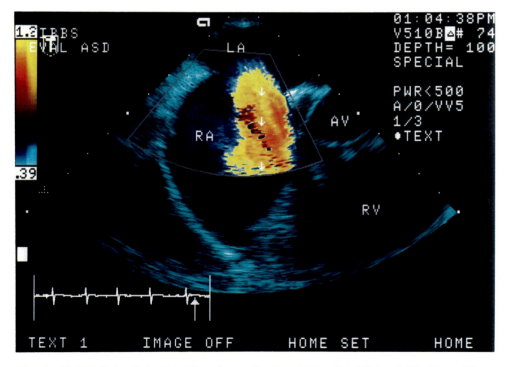

Figure 12-2C: Color flow Doppler clearly demonstrates the left-to-right shunt. RA = right atrium; RV = right ventricle; AV = atrial valve; LA = left atrium.

Fig. 12-3.

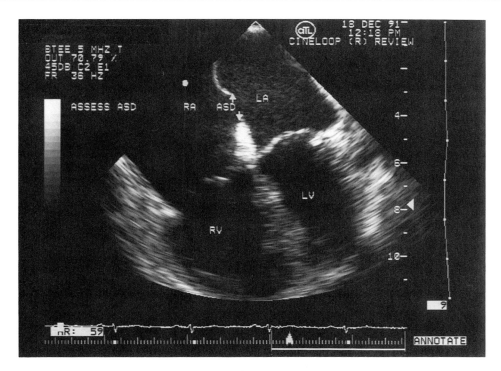

Figure 12-3A: By definition, an atrial septal defect (ASD) is a lack of atrial septal tissue. This should be confirmed visually to differentiate an ASD from a patent foramen ovale. This transverse four-chamber view identifies a 1.1 cm secundum ASD (arrows). RV = right ventricle; RA = right atrium; LV = left ventricle; LA = left atrium.

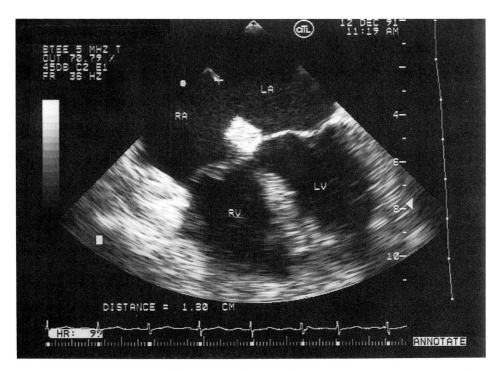

Figure 12-3B: A larger secundum atrial septal defect (1.8 cm) in the transverse four-chamber view. RV = right ventricle; RA = right atrium; LV = left ventricle; LA = left atrium.

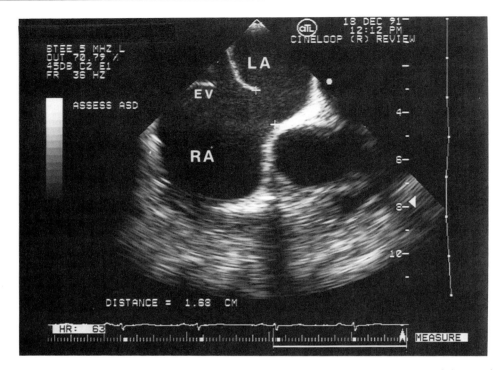

Figure 12-3C: The longitudinal plane can also localize this secundum atrial septal defect (1.68 cm). The eustachian valve (EV) is seen at the junction of the inferior vena cava and right atrium (RA). LA = left atrium.

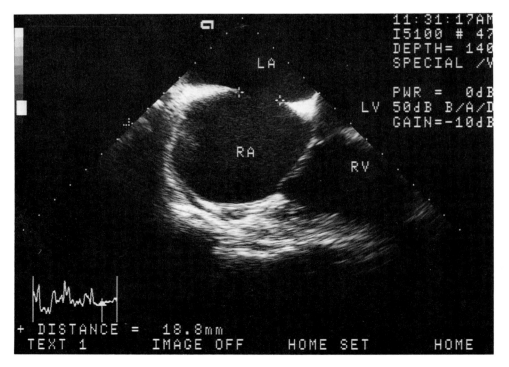

Figure 12-3D: The same defect as in Fig. 3C seen in the transverse plane. RV = right ventricle; RA = right atrium; LV = left ventricle; LA = left atrium.

Fig. 12-3.
(cont'd)

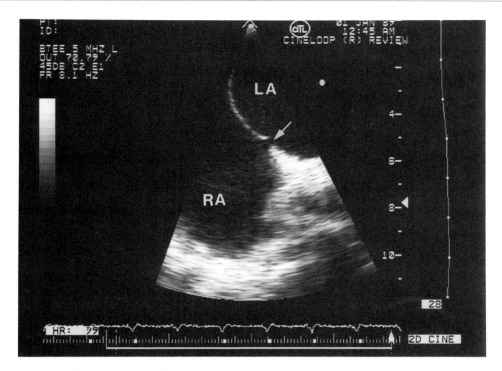

Figure 12-3E: A very small secundum defect (arrow) seen only in the longitudinal view. RA = right atrium; LA = left atrium.

Fig. 12-4.

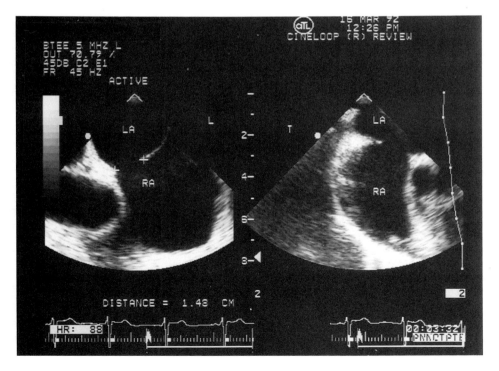

Figure 12-4A: Both imaging planes should be utilized to interrogate for a defect. The secundum atrial septal defect is seen on both the longitudinal (left) and the transverse (right) plane. RA = right atrium; LA = left atrium.

Fig. 12-4. (cont'd)

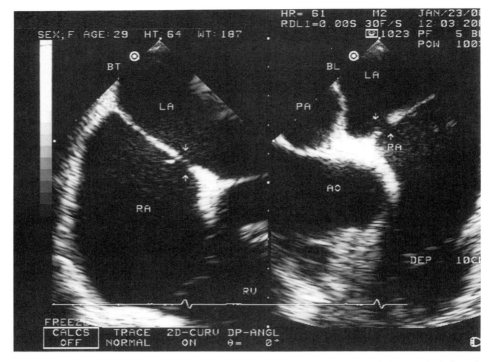

Figure 12-4B: The actual dropout of tissue of this secundum atrial septal defect is visualized better in the longitudinal plane (right) than in the transverse (left). RA = right atrium; LA = left atrium; PA = pulmonary artery; AO = aorta.

Fig. 12-5.

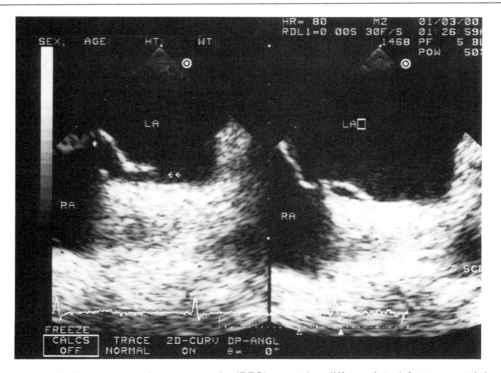

Figure 12-5A: A patent foramen ovale (PFO) must be differentiated from an atrial septal defect. A PFO is a persistence of the fetal communication from the right (RA) to left atrium (LA) through the septae secundum and primum. If the septae do not fuse, there may be a flaplike membrane that lifts off, facilitating a small intra-atrial shunt that may be predominantly right to left, but may be bidirectional. The right-side longitudinal plane depicts the closed foramen which lifts off in the left-sided frame.

Fig. 12-5. (cont'd)

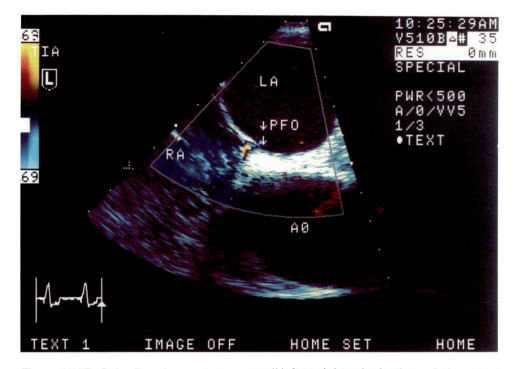

Figure 12-5B: Color flow demonstrates a small left-to-right color jet through the patent foramen ovale (PFO) (longitudinal plane). RA = right atrium; LA = left atrium; AO = aorta.

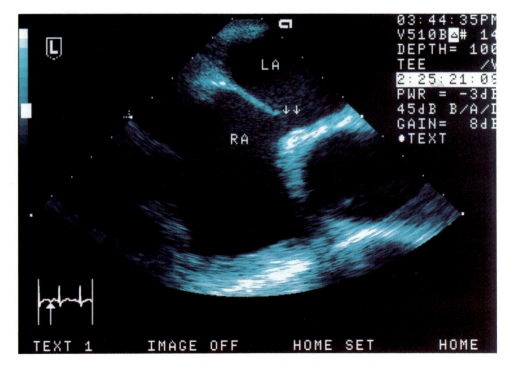

Figure 12-5C: Compare the patent foramen ovale "flap" to the actual atrial septal defect seen in the longitudinal view. LA = left atrium; RA = right atrium.

Fig. 12-5. (cont'd)

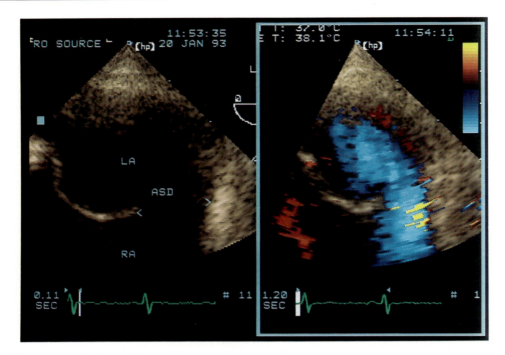

Figure 12-5D: Color flow demonstrating a left-to-right shunt through a secundum atrial septal defect (ASD) (longitudinal plane, 70° axis). LA = left atrium; RA = right atrium.

Fig. 12-6.

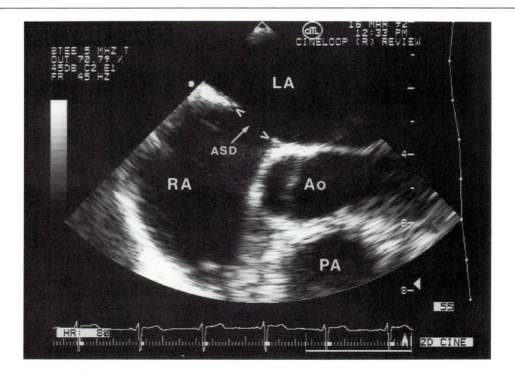

Figure 12-6A: Contrast studies are performed by injecting commercially available precision microbubbles (all uniform size, 5–7 μm) or agitated saline into the right antecubital vein or another large vein. The injection generates echogenic microbubbles that normally pass through the right atrium (RA) and right ventricle and are almost completely filtered in the lungs. In this figure, the large (1.64 cm) secundum defect is identified (transverse plane). ASD = atrial septal defect; LA = left atrium; Ao = aorta; PA = pulmonary artery.

Fig. 12-6. (cont'd)

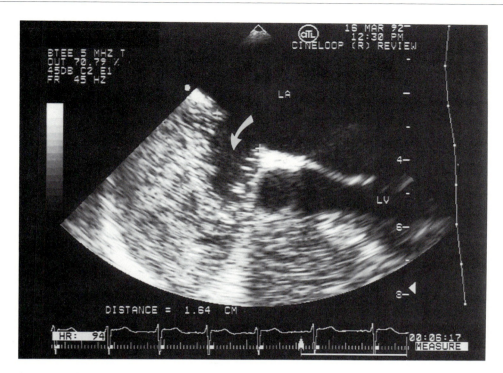

Figure 12-6B: "Negative contrast" effect. The right atrium and right ventricle are completely opacified by the injected contrast microbubbles except for the area in which "noncontrast" left atrial (LA) blood shunts through the atrial septal defect into the right atrium. LV = left ventricle.

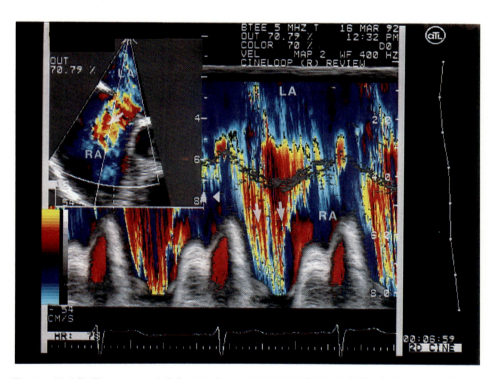

Figure 12-6C: The upper left inset shows transesophageal 2-D of the color Doppler demonstrates left-to-right flow through the secundum defect. The right side is color flow M-mode confirming the left-to-right shunt. RA = right atrium; LA = left atrium.

Fig. 12-7.

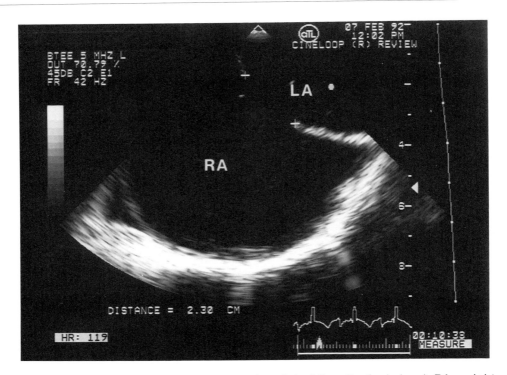

Figure 12-7A: A large (2.3 cm) atrial secundum defect (longitudinal plane). RA = right atrium; LA = left atrium.

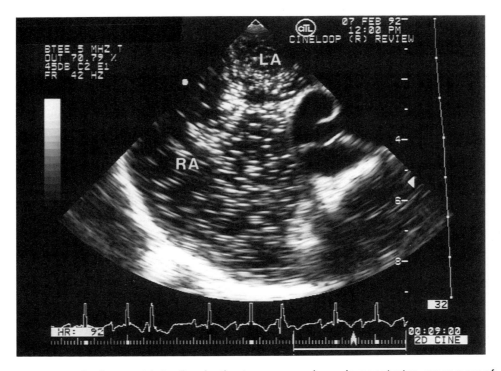

Figure 12-7B: Contrast injection in the transverse plane demonstrates crossover of microbubbles from right (RA) to left atrium (LA) through the defect. Most atrial septal defects will manifest transient right-to-left shunt, especially with cough or Valsalva.

Fig. 12-7.
(cont'd)

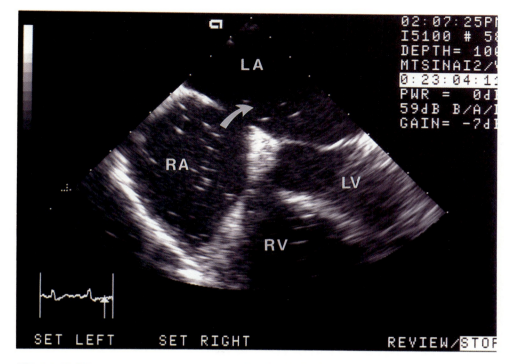

Figure 12-7C: In another patient, residual microbubbles freely cross a secundum defect (arrow). RV = right ventricle; RA = right atrium; LV = left ventricle; LA = left atrium.

Fig. 12-8.

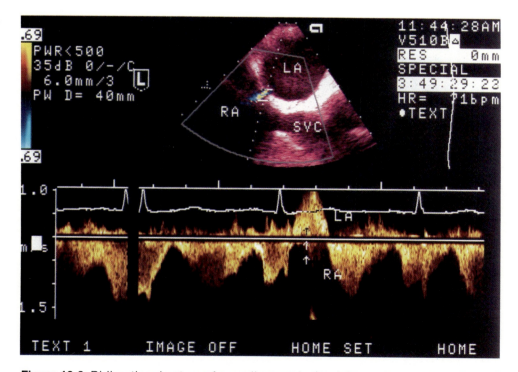

Figure 12-8: Bidirectional nature of a small secundum atrial septal defect (longitudinal plane) is demonstrated by pulsed Doppler (below), though predominantly left-to-right atrial flow is documented. Transient elevated right-sided pressures create a right-to-left shunt (arrows). RA = right atrium; LA = left atrium; SVC = superior vena cava.

Fig. 12-9.

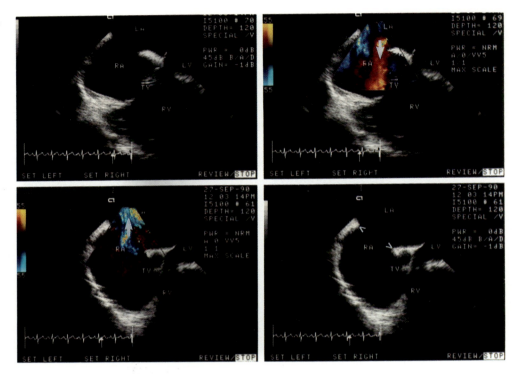

Figure 12-9A: Multiframe sequence demonstrating bidirectional shunting across a large secundum atrial septal defect by color flow Doppler. Lower right images the large defect. Upper right demonstrates diastolic left-to-right shunting, while the lower left depicts early systolic right to left shunting. RV = right ventricle; RA = right atrium; LV = left ventricle; LA = left atrium; TV = tricuspid valve.

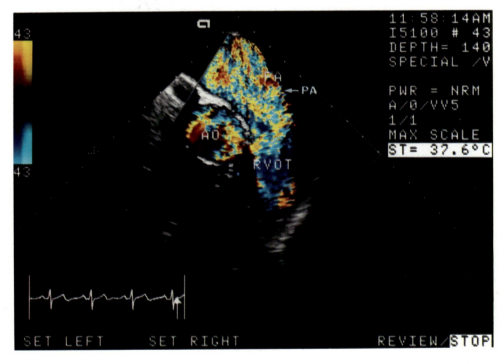

Figure 12-9B: The large shunt causes a dilated pulmonary artery with increased volume and turbulent flow. PA = pulmonary artery; AO = aorta; RVOT = right ventricluar outflow tract.

Fig. 12-10.

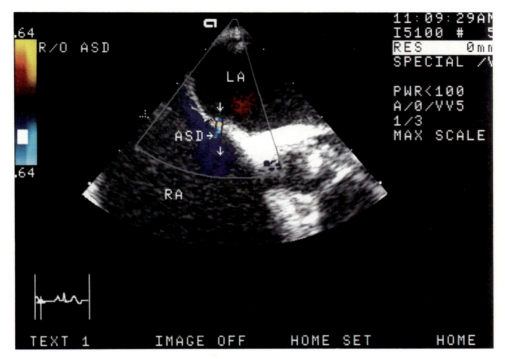

Figure 12-10A: Color Doppler is very sensitive and can detect tiny atrial septal defects (ASD) (secundum type, transverse plane). RA = right atrium; LA = left atrium.

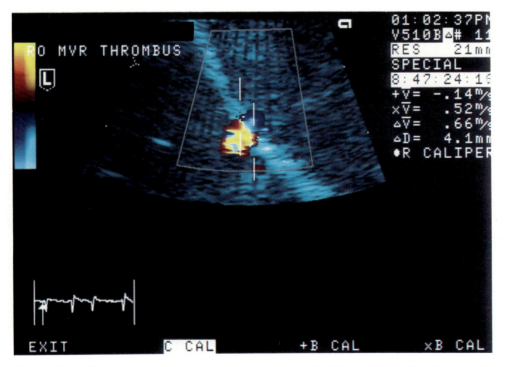

Figure 12-10B: A small (4 mm) secundum atrial septal defect detected only by color flow Doppler (longitudinal plane).

Fig. 12-10. (cont'd)

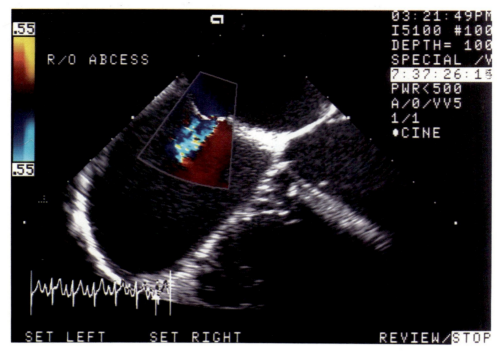

Figure 12-10C: Another small secundum defect seen by color Doppler (transverse plane).

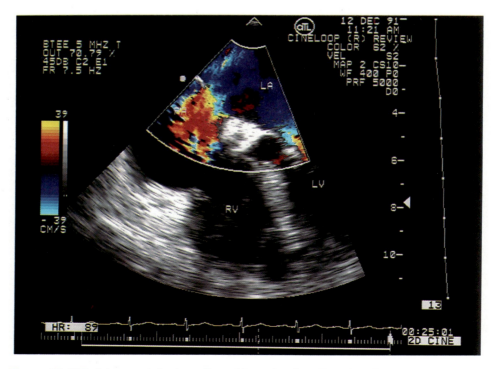

Figure 12-10D: A larger defect confirmed by color flow Doppler. RV = right ventricle; LV = left ventricle; LA = left atrium.

Fig. 12-10. (cont'd)

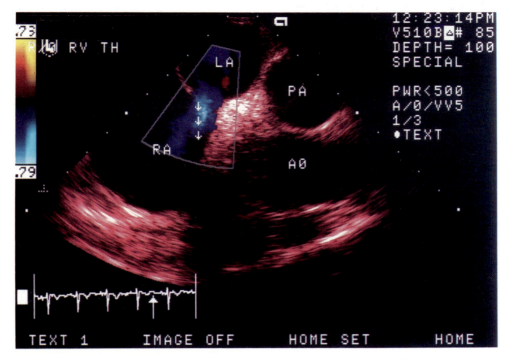

Figure 12-10E: A 1.2 cm secundum defect in the longitudinal plane. RA = right atrium; LA = left atrium; PA = pulmonary artery; AO = aorta.

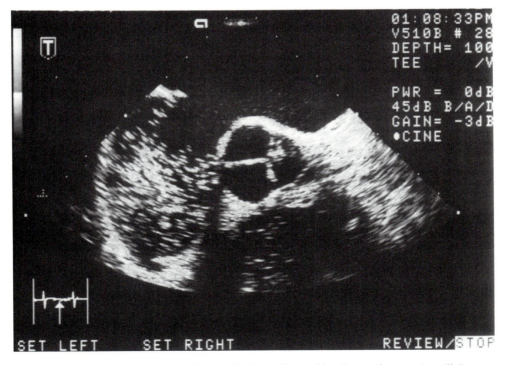

Figure 12-10F: A 2.0 cm secundum defect confirmed by "negative contrast" (transverse plane).

Fig. 12-11.

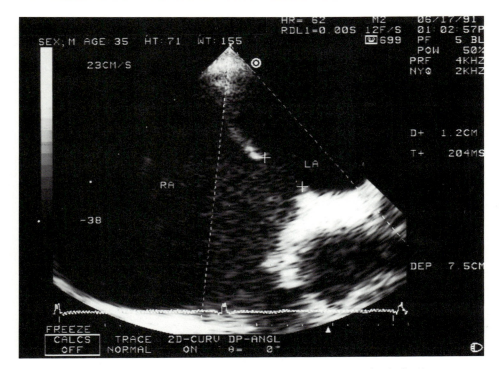

Figure 12-11A: Atrial septal defects may appear to be the same size in both transverse and longitudinal planes. A 1.2 cm defect is seen in the longitudinal plane. RA = right atrium; LA = left atrium.

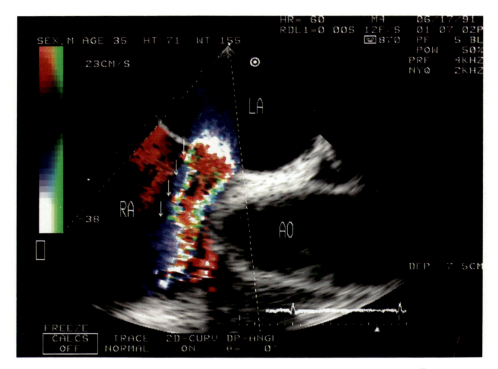

Figure 12-11B: Color flow in the longitudinal plane confirms the large defect. RA = right atrium; LA = left atrium; AO = aorta.

Fig. 12-11. (cont'd)

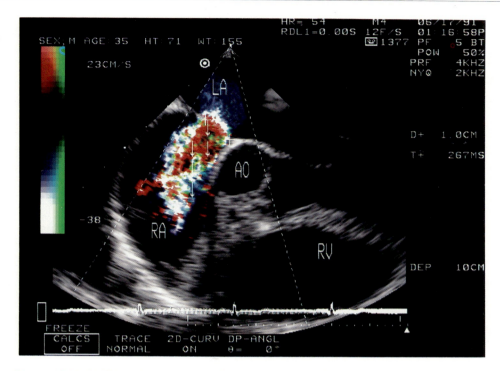

Figure 12-11C: The atrial septal defect appears smaller (1.0 cm) in the transverse plane. RV = right ventricle; RA = right atrium; LA = left atrium; AO = aorta.

Fig. 12-12.

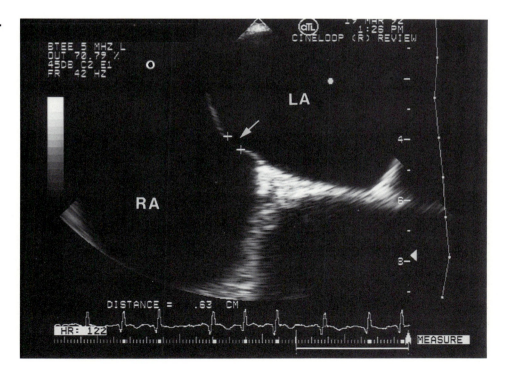

Figure 12-12A: A small atrial septal defect (0.63 cm) imaged in the longitudinal plane. RA = right atrium; LA = left atrium.

Fig. 12-12.
(cont'd)

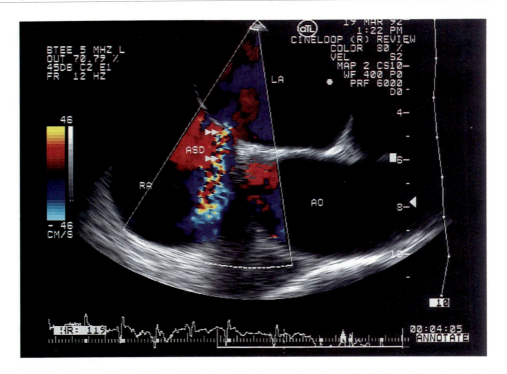

Figure 12-12B: Corresponding color Doppler in the longitudinal plane demonstrates a clearly defined left-to-right shunt. ASD = atrial septal defect; RA = right atrium; LA = left atrium; AO = aorta.

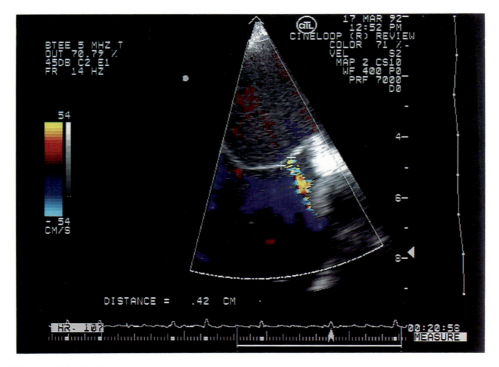

Figure 12-12C: The jet is much smaller and was difficult to document in the transverse plane.

Fig. 12-13.

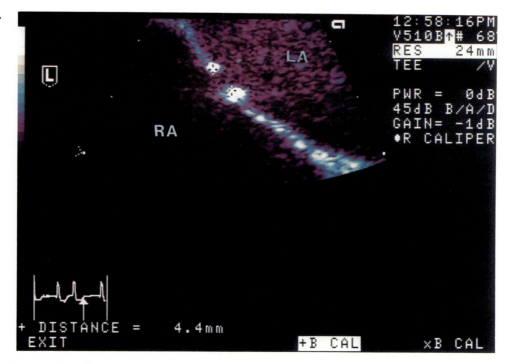

Figure 12-13A: High resolution imaging and B-color identify a 4.4 cm secundum defect. RA = right atrium; LA = left atrium.

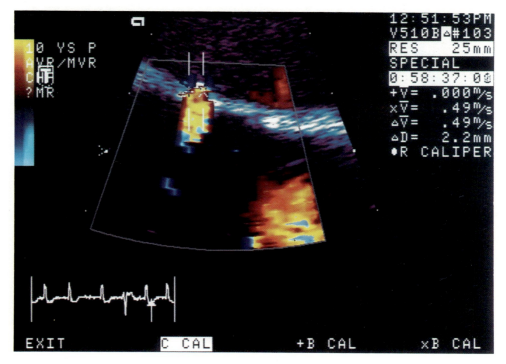

Figure 12-13B: A very small color flow jet is seen in the transverse plane.

Fig. 12-13.
(cont'd)

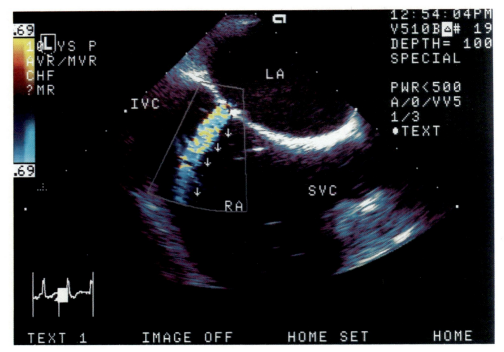

Figure 12-13C: The longitudinal plane detects a larger jet. RA = right atrium; LA = left atrium; SVC = superior vena cava; IVC = inferior vena cava.

Fig. 12-14.

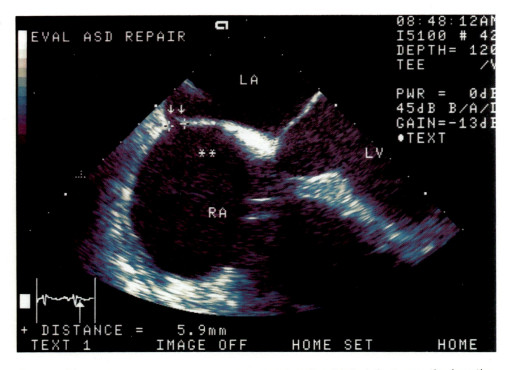

Figure 12-14A: A sinus venosus atrial septal defect is a high defect near the junction of the superior vena cava with the right atrium (RA). A small 5.9 mm venous atrial septal defect (arrows) (transverse plane). LV = left ventricle; LA = left atrium.

Fig. 12-14. (cont'd)

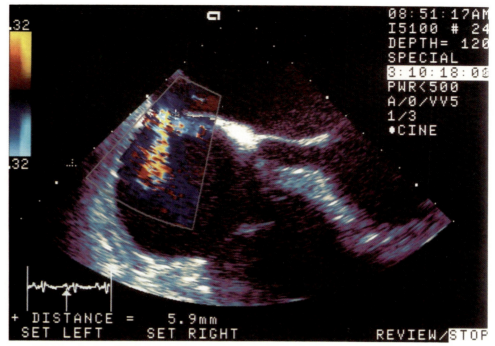

Figure 12-14B: Color flow Doppler confirms the presence of the atrial septal defect.

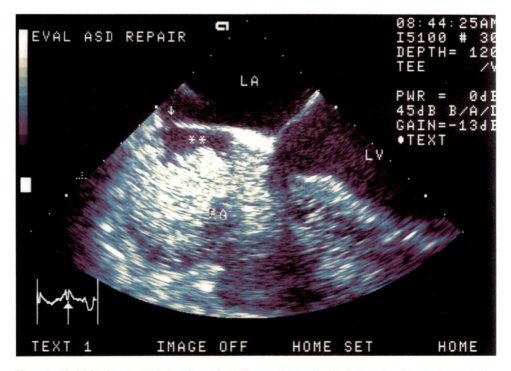

Figure 12-14C: Contrast injection identifies a "negative" defect in the region of the left-to-right shunt at the level of the septal defect (asterisks). RA = right atrium; LV = left ventricle; LA = left atrium.

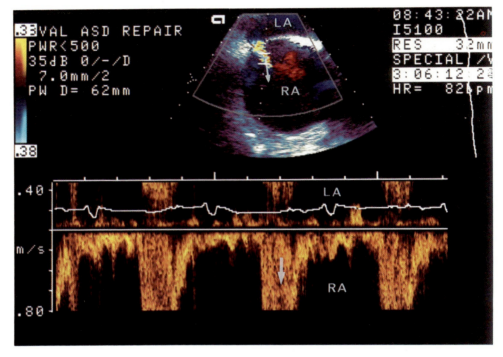

Figure 12-14D: Pulsed Doppler through the venosus defect demonstrates a predominant left-to-right shunt. RA = right atrium; LA = left atrium.

Patent Foramen Ovale

The interatrial septum forms through a complex embryological development. The septum primum appears first by 30 days and is duplicated by the septum secundum shortly thereafter. A communication in the septum secundum, the *foramen ovale,* leads to an opening in the septum primum called the *ostium secundum,* which facilitates shunting of fetal blood from the vena cava into the left atrium (see diagram below). In the newborn, the ostium

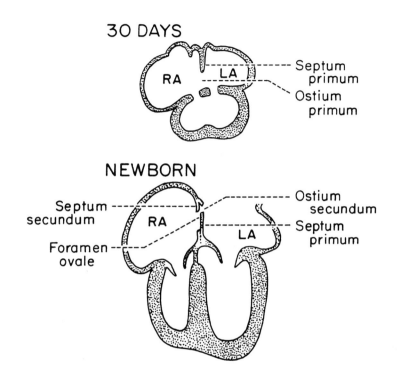

secundum seals as does the foramen ovale by a thin membrane called the fossa ovalis. In pathological studies, a "probe patent" foramen ovale may be detected in up to 25% of patients. In 1,000 consecutive TEEs performed at Mt. Sinai, we found a 9.2% incidence of PFO. Clinically, the foramen ovale may be a potential source of right atrial to left atrial shunting if there is transient elevation of right atrial pressures (i.e., during cough or Valsalva). A thrombus or mass originating in the lower or upper extemity veins, in the right atrium or on an indwelling catheter may embolize through a patent foramen ovale (PFO) under fortuitous circumstances. Though initially thought to be a more important risk factor for central emboli in younger patients, PFOs are actually larger in size in older patients. The presence of a PFO in itself does not confirm the source of an embolic event without confirmation of a thrombolic source (i.e., femoral vein or pelvic vein thrombus). Interrogation for a PFO requires peripheral contrast injections that opacify the right atrium and the right ventricle. In the presence of a PFO, three or more microbubbles pass through the PFO into the left atrium within three cardiac cycles. An atrial septal aneurysm swinging into the left atrium may force open a patent foramen ovale (see pp. 273–276 and 310–312).

Bibliography

1. Hagen PT, Scholz DG, Edwards WD: Incidence and size of patent foramen ovale during the first 10 decades of life: an autopsy study of 965 normal hearts. *Mayo Clinic Proc* 59:17–20, 1984.
2. Lechat PH, Mas JL, Lascault G, et al: Prevalence of patent foramen ovale in patients with stroke. *N Engl J Med* 318:1148–1152, 1988.
3. Mugge A, Daniel WG, Klopper JW, Litchlen PR: Visualization of patent foramen ovale by transesophageal color-coded Doppler echocardiography. *Am J Cardiol* 62:837–838, 1988.
4. Movsowitz C, Podolsky L, Meyerowitz CB, Jacobs L, Kottler MN: Patent foramen ovale: a nonfunctional embryological remnant or a potential cause of significant pathology. *J Am Soc Echocardiogr* 5:259–270, 1991.
5. Langholz D, Louie EK, Konstadt SN, Rao TLK, Scanlon PJ: Transesophageal echocardiography demonstration of distinct mechanism for right and left shunting across a patent foramen ovale in the absence of pulmonary hypertension. *J Am Coll Cardiol* 18:111–117, 1991.
6. Konstadt SN, Louie EK, Blaek S, Rao TLK, Scanlon P: Intraoperative detection of patent foramen ovale by transesophageal echocardiography. *Anesthesiology* 74:212–216, 1991.
7. Siostrzonek P, Zangeneh M, Gossinger H, et al: Comparison of transesophageal and transthoracic contrast echocsrdiography for detection of a patent foramen ovale. *Am J Cardiol* 68:1247–1249, 1991.

Fig. 12-15.

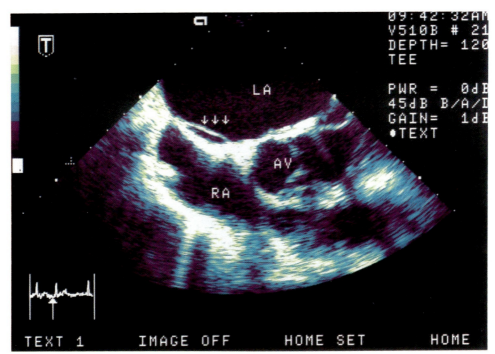

Figure 12-15A: A small fluid-filled space separates the thinner septum primum (arrows) from the thicker septum secundum of the interatrial septum. LA = left atrium; RA = right atrium; AV = aortic valve.

Fig. 12-15. (cont'd)

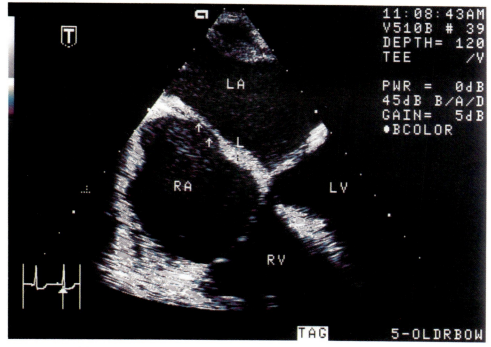

Figure 12-15B: The thin valve of the fossa ovalis (arrows) is superior to the limbus (L) of the atrial septum in this transverse plane. LA = left atrium; LV = left ventricle; RA = right atrium; RV = right ventricle.

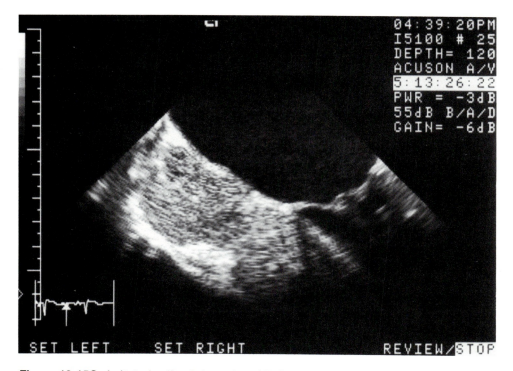

Figure 12-15C: Agitated saline injected rapidly into a peripheral vein generates microbubbles that fully opacify the right atrium and right ventricle. There is no evidence of shunting into the left atrium.

Fig. 12-16.

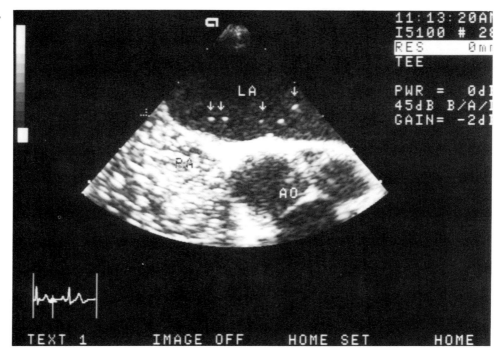

Figure 12-16A: Following opacification of the right atrium (RA) with the patient performing a Valsalva maneuver, microbubbles are seen in the left atrium (LA). AO = aorta.

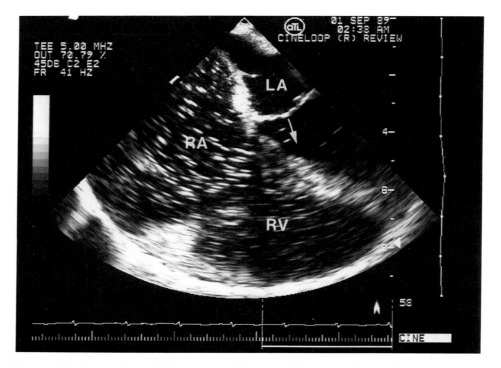

Figure 16B: Single microbubbles are visible in the left atrium (LA) and ventricle following their passage through a patent foramen ovale (arrow). RA = right atrium; RV = right ventricle.

Fig. 12-16. (cont'd)

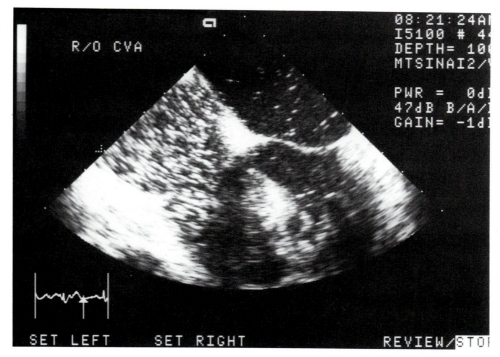

Figure 12-16C: Following a Valsalva maneuver or cough which transiently increases right-sided pressure, more bubbles are visible on the left side of the heart.

Fig. 12-17.

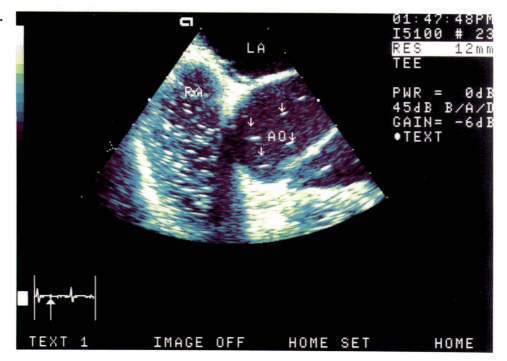

Figure 12-17: Occasionally though bubbles may not be seen in the left atrium (LA), they may be seen exiting out the aorta (AO, arrows). RA = right atrium.

Fig. 12-18.

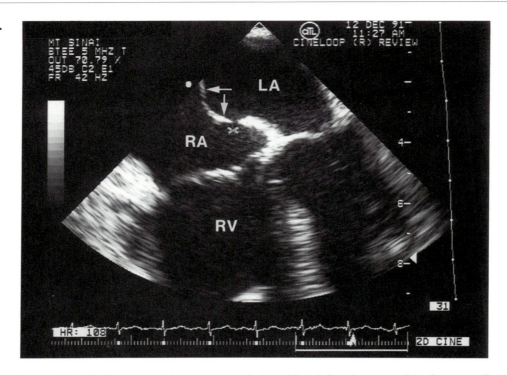

Figure 12-18A: An atrial septal aneurysm (arrows) involving the area of the fossa ovalis is at least 1.5 cm in length and either protrudes 1.1 cm into either atrial chamber or has a total excursion of 1.1 cm. The swinging of the aneurysm may open a patent foramen ovale (asterisk). LA = left atrium; RA = right atrium; RV = right ventricle.

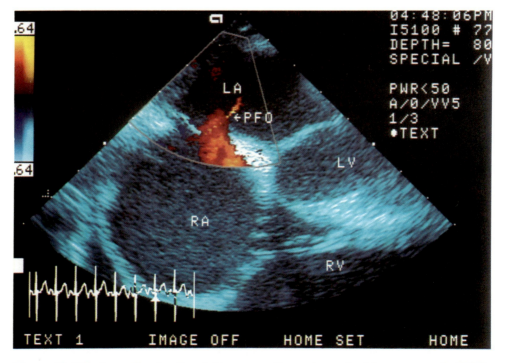

Figure 12-18B: A small color flow jet traverses through a patent foramen ovale (PFO). The red flow area below the patent foramen ovale outlines a localized septal aneurysm. LA = left atrium; LV = left ventricle; RA = right atrium; RV = right ventricle.

Fig. 12-18. (cont'd)

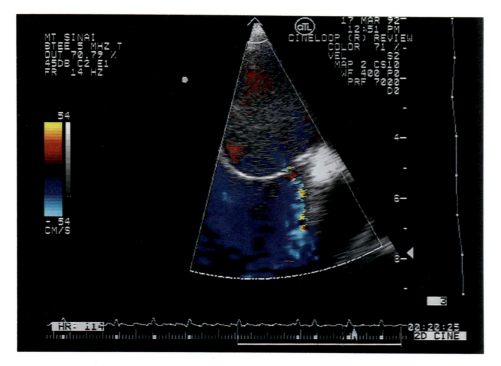

Figure 12-18C: As the atrial septal aneurysm swings into the right atrium, a small left-to-right shunt is seen through the patent foramen ovale.

Fig. 12-19.

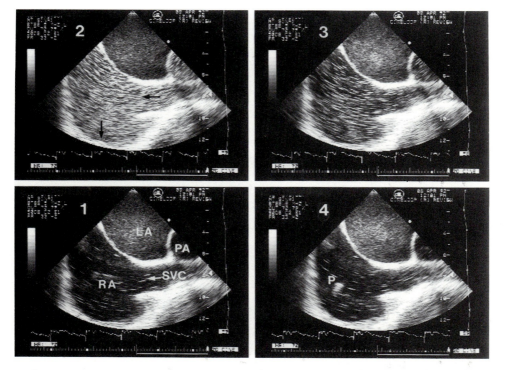

Figure 12-19: Sequence of a contrast injection through the right heart (frames 1–4) in the longitudinal plane. The bubbles enter through the superior vena cava (SVC) (frame 1, botom left), exit the right atrium out the pulmonary artery (PA) (frames 2–4). A pacemaker artifact (P) is seen in frame 4. There was no shunt. There is spontaneous echogenic contrast in the left atrium. LA = left atrium; RA = right atrium.

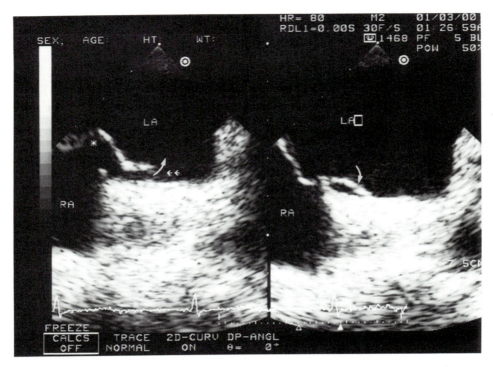

Figure 12-20: The "flap" of the patent foramen ovale is seen undulating in the longitudinal plane. LA = left atrium; RA = right atrium.

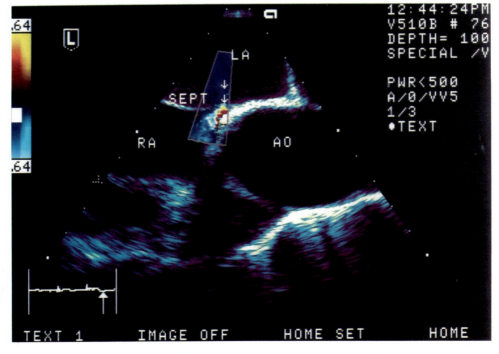

Figure 12-21A: A small color Doppler jet documents a left-to-right shunt through a patent foramen ovale (PFO) in the longitudinal plane. LA = left atrium; RA = right atrium; AO = aorta.

Fig. 12-21. (cont'd)

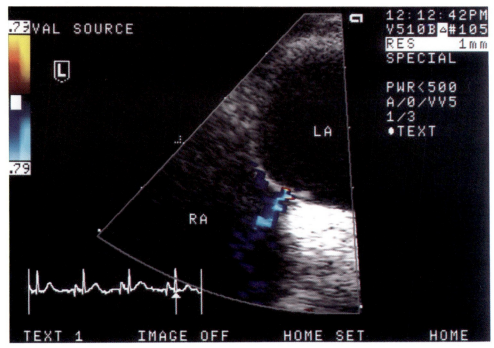

Figure 12-21B: A tiny patent foramen ovale is seen in light blue. LA = left atrium; RA = right atrium.

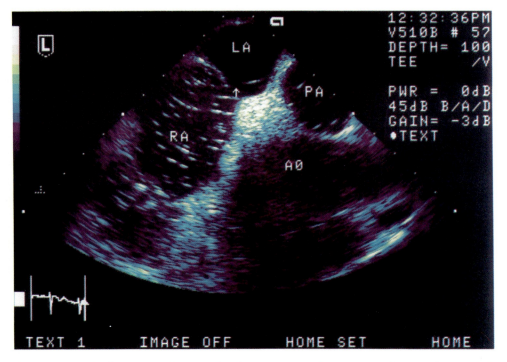

Figure 12-21C: Contrast injection in the longitudinal plane confirms a right-to-left shunt (arrow). LA = left atrium; RA = right atrium; PA = pulmonary artery; AO = aorta.

Ventricular Septal Defect

Ventricular septal defects (VSD) are common congenital abnormalities. Most frequently, the defect occurs in the membranous portion of the interventricular septum and may vary in size from a small opening to virtual absence of the intraventricular septum. The most common type of defect lies below the crista supraventricularis. Clinical sequela of the VSD depends on size and the subsequent development of pulmonary vascular resistance. Smaller defects may close spontaneously, while the larger defects may cause pulmonary hypertension and congestive heart failure. Associated lesions include right ventricular outflow obstruction, both infundibular or valvular, and aortic regurgitation. Because left ventricular pressures are greater than right ventricular pressures, there is a systolic left-to-right shunt through the VSD. However, in a patient who previously had a loud murmur and thrill who has a decrease in the murmur, one should suspect the development of pulmonary hypertension with reduction in the left-to-right shunt size. Patients with VSDs are at risk for bacterial endocarditis which will occur on the downstream side of the jet lesion, which will be on the right ventricular side of the VSD. Frequently, they can be seen adequately by transthoracic echo and color flow Doppler. Continuous wave Doppler interrogation through the defect will provide the left ventricular to right ventricular pressure gradient. Assuming that there is no left or right ventricular outflow obstruction, left ventricular systolic pressure should be equal to aortic systolic pressure. Thus, the right ventricular systolic pressure can be estimated by the formula: (aortic systolic pressure) − (VSD gradient) = RV systolic pressure.

Fig. 12-22.

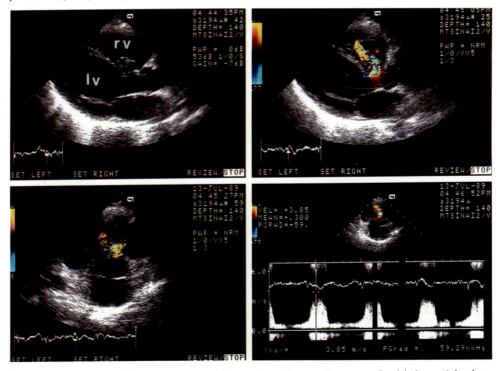

Figure 12-22: Multiple sequence transthoracic echocardiogram of a high ventricular septal defect (VSD). The upper left-hand figure demonstrates a development of an aneurysm in the area of the VSD, this may herald closure of the defect. The upper right-hand corner and lower left-hand corner demonstrate color flow through the VSD in long axis and short axis views, respectively. The lower right-hand frame demonstrates a VSD gradient of 60 mm, which yielded an estimated right ventricular (rv) systolic pressure of 50 in this patient with aortic systolic pressure of 110 (110 mm Hg of aortic pressure—60 mm Hg VSD gradient = 50 mm Hg RV systolic pressure).

Fig. 12-23.

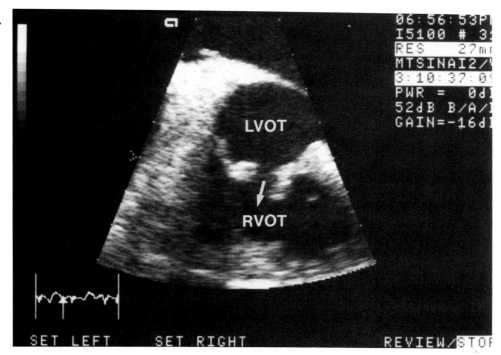

Figure 12-23A: A high membranous ventricular septal defect is seen separating the left ventricular outflow tract (LVOT) from the right ventricular outflow tract (RVOT) below. The two remaining edges of the defect were fluffy and irregular, consistent with endocarditis in this patient with a high fever and positive blood cultures.

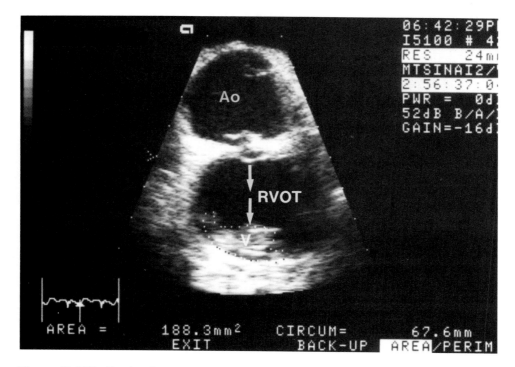

Figure 12-23B: Further interrogation of the right ventricular outflow tract (RVOT) revealed a vegetation (V) measuring 1.88 cm^2 due to the jet lesion. Ao = aorta.

Fig. 12-23. (cont'd)

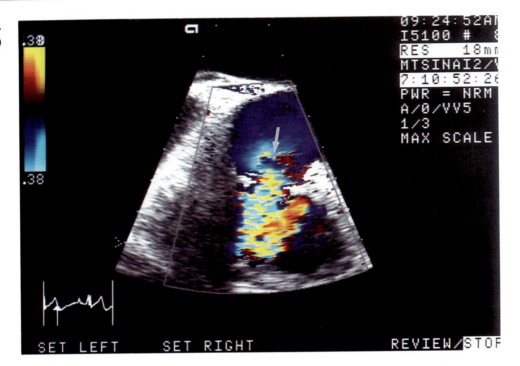

Figure 12-23C: Color Doppler confirms left-to-right shunt through the ventricular septal defect.

Fig. 12-24.

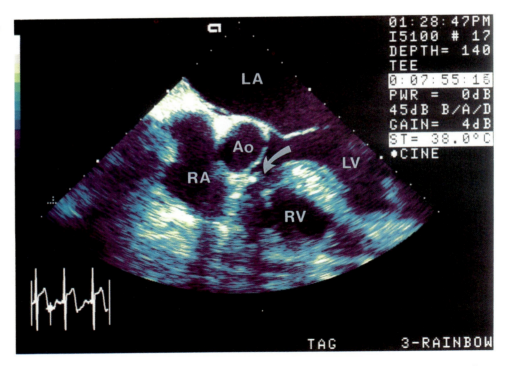

Figure 12-24A: A ventricular septal defect (arrow) in the transverse modified five-chamber view. LA = left atrium; LV = left ventricle; Ao = aorta; RA = right atrium; RV = right ventricle.

Fig. 12-24.
(cont'd)

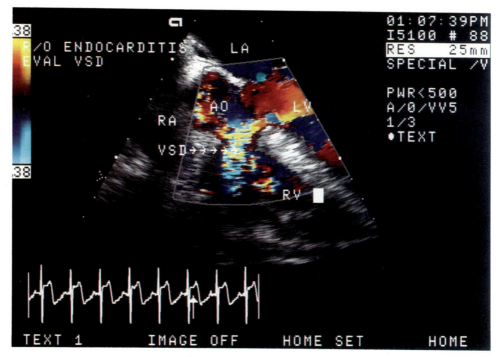

Figure 12-24B: Color flow confirms left-to-right shunt through the ventricular septal defect (VSD). LA = left atrium; RA = right atrium; RV = right ventricle; AO = aorta.

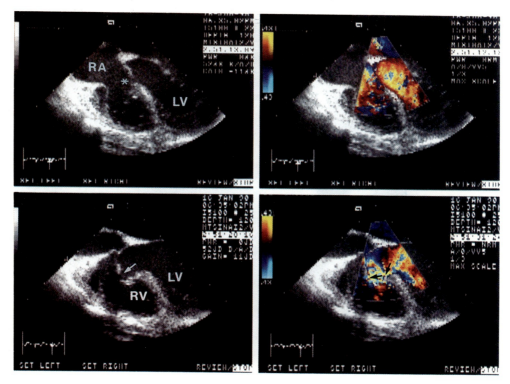

Figure 12-24C: During diastole, the excursion of the septal leaflet of the tricuspid valve (asterisk, upper left frame) prevents shunt flow (upper left). However during systole, the ventricular septal defect bulges from the left into right ventricle (RV, lower left), with shunting (arrows, lower right frame).

Fig. 12-25.

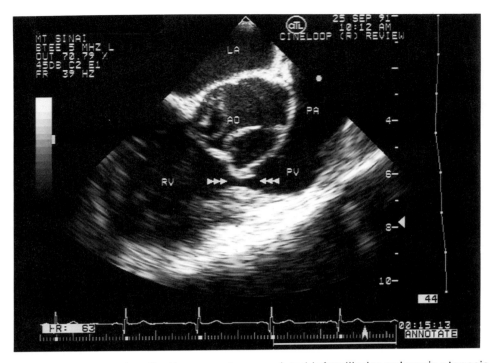

Figure 12-25: Occasionally, there may be associated infundibular pulmonic stenosis (arrows point to a conus obstruction). This would tend to reduce the left-to-right shunt and increase right ventricular (RV) pressures. LA = left atrium; PA = pulmonary artery; AO = aorta; PV = pulmonary valve.

Ebstein's Anomaly

Normally, the three leaflets of the tricuspid valve are attached to the annulus fibrosus; however, in Ebstein's disease, the posterior and frequently the medial leaflets originate in the right ventricle, towards the apex. The anterior leaflet is usually attached from its normal annular origin. The distorted tricuspid anatomy results in "ventricularization" of the atrium or "atrialization" of the ventricle, with part of the ventricle incorporated into the atrium. The remaining right ventricle is underdeveloped and may be associated with an atrial septal defect or a patent foramen ovale. Clinically, patients develop right ventricular failure and atrial or ventricular arrhythmia's (5–10% have Wolff-Parkinson-White syndrome, type B). Classic echocardiographic features include an apically displaced septal tricuspid valve leaflet and right ventricular dysfunction. Surgical revision is dependent on the extent of the free anterior leaflet, which can be repaired and residual right ventriclar function.

Fig. 12-26.

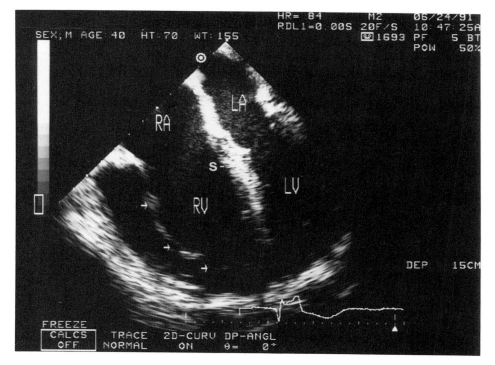

Figure 12-26: Transverse four-chamber view demonstrating the elongated anterior leaflet (asterisks), which originated from the annulus. The septal leaflet (S) originated 2.5 cm more apically than the septal mitral leaflet (normally <1 cm). LA = left atrium; LV = left ventricle; RA = right atrium; RV = right ventricle.

Fig. 12-27.

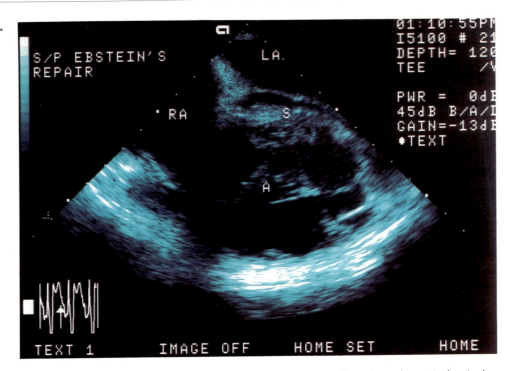

Figure 12-27A: Systolic frame demonstrating poor coaptation of an elongated anterior leaflet (A) and redundant, diminutive septal (S) leaflet causing significant tricuspid regurgitation. LA = left atrium; RA = right atrium.

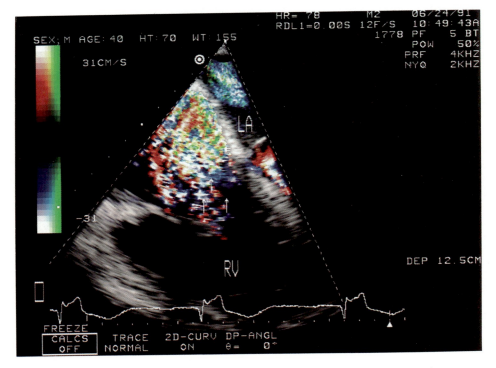

Figure 12-27B: Severe tricuspid regurgitation in Ebstein's anomaly.

Endocardial Cushion Defect

Failure of the channel between the atria and ventricles to partition results in a range of defects that may include ostium primum atrial septal defects of various sizes, ventricular septal defects, and cleft mitral valve.

Fig. 12-28.

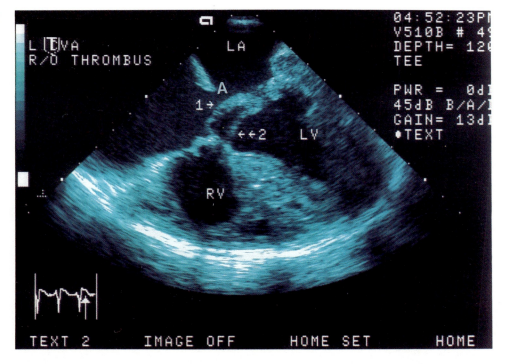

Figure 12-28: Transverse four-chamber view demonstrating an atrial septal defect (A) (ostium primum) and the two sections (numbered 1 and 2) of a cleft anterior leaflet of the mitral valve. Both the mitral and tricuspid leaflets originate at the same plane. There was only a small ventricular septal defect. LA = left atrium; LV = left ventricle; RV = right ventricle.

Cor Triatriatum

Cor triatriatum, "heart with three atria," is a rare congenital anomaly in which the left atrium is divided by a fibromuscular diaphragm into posterior and anterior chambers. The membranous structure is a remnant of the common pulmonary vein which failed to resorb. The membrane can obstruct blood flow from the posterior to anterior chambers, creating symptoms similar to mitral stenosis.

Fig. 12-29.

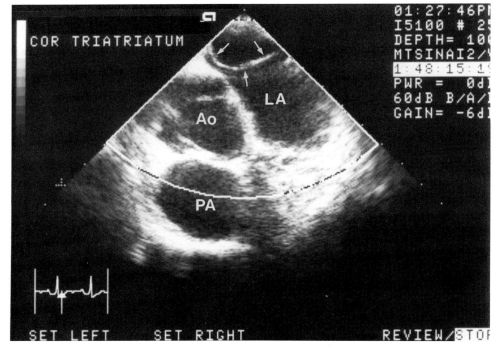

Figure 12-29: Basal transverse plane demonstrating membrane (arrows) separating the left atrium into two chambers. Ao = aorta; LA = left atrium; PA = pulmonary atrium.

Fig. 12-30.

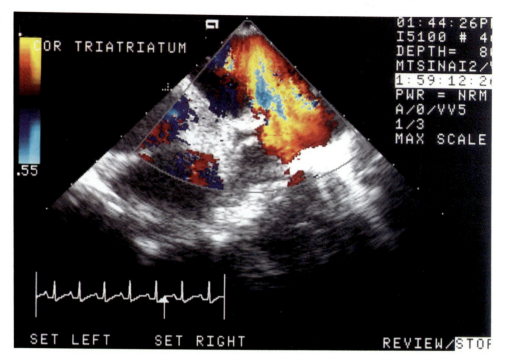

Figure 12-30: Turbulent color Doppler flow confirms the obstruction created by the membrane.

Transposition of the Great Vessels

Anatomically, transposition of the great vessels means that the aorta originates from the morphologic right ventricle, while the pulmonary artery arises from the morphologic left ventricle. In "corrected transposition," there is L loop (left ventricle on the right side, the morphologic right ventricle on the left side) and L transposition (the aortic valve is anterior, superior, and to the left of the pulmonary valve). Patients may have associated congenital lesions, such as subvalvular pulmonic stenosis or ventricular septal defects or arrhythmias.

Fig. 12-31.

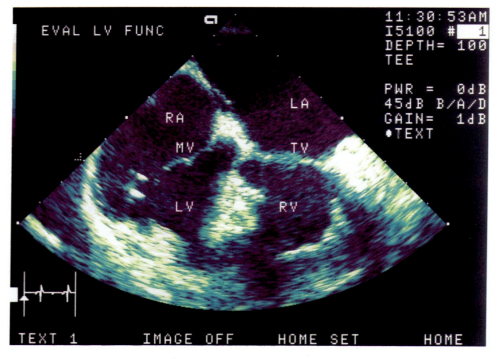

Figure 12-31: The right atrium (RA) empties through the mitral valve (MV) into an anatomical left ventricle (LV); the left ventricle (LA) into the morphologic right ventricle (RV). TV = tricuspid valve.

Fig. 12-32.

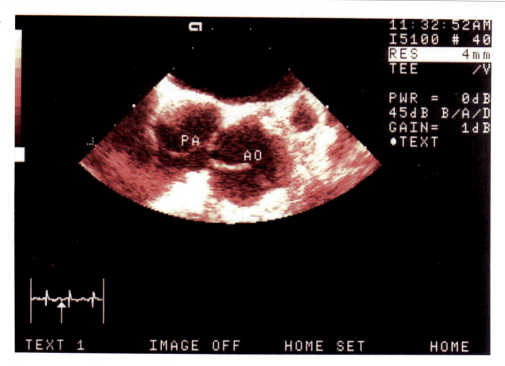

Figure 12-32: The aorta (AO) is superior, anterior, and to the left of the pulmonary artery (PA).

13

Intraoperative Application of Transesophageal Echocardiography

*Allen Mogtader, M.D.,
Theresa Guarino, R.N.,
Martin E. Goldman, M.D., and
Bruce P. Mindich, M.D.*

Introduction

Various echocardiographic modalities are used intraoperatively to examine the heart and great vessels at three specific stages of the cardiac surgical procedure: baseline, weaning from cardiopulmonary bypass, and post-bypass (Table 1). Two-dimensional ultrasound imaging can be performed epicardially and/or transesophageally to assess cardiac anatomy and function. The addition of color flow Doppler mapping and contrast echocardiography permits evaluation of flow characteristics within the cardiac chambers and great vessels.

Transesophageal and epicardial imaging are complementary rather than alternative techniques.[1,2] Epicardial echocardiography examines the heart from its anterior surface in contrast to transesophageal imaging, which views the cardiac structures from a retrocardiac position within the esophagus. The transesophageal examination is, therefore, constrained by the lumen of the esophagus and by its anatomical relationship to the heart, as well as being restricted by the number of imaging planes afforded by transducer technology. Although placement of the epicardial transducer within the chest cavity is limited by the extent of the surgical incision, the probe may be placed directly on the region of interest by the surgeon. Epicardial imaging provides unobstructed examination of the left ventricular outflow tract, whereas with transesophageal echocardiography (TEE), this area may be obscured by a calcified or prosthetic valve. While a mitral prosthesis may shadow into the left ventricle if the TEE approach is used, epicardial imaging can assess the left ventricle from multiple planes. TEE, on the other hand, is superior to

Table 1
Echocardiographic Imaging Periods

I. Baseline Study
  A. Definition of anatomic abnormalities
    1. Precise definition of pathoanatomy
    2. Detection of unsuspected coexisting lesions
    3. Identification of potential sources of embolization, i.e., aortic plaque, cardiac thrombus
  B. Assessment of cardiac function
  C. Planning the operative approach
II. Weaning from Cardiopulmonary Bypass
  A. Detection of retained intracardiac air
  B. Assessment of cardiac function
  C. Initial evaluation of the surgical procedure
III. Post Cardiopulmonary Bypass
  A. Evaluate the adequacy of the procedure
  B. Assess for potential complications
  C. Assess cardiac function and determine etiology of hemodynamic compromise

epicardial echocardiography for assessment of the left ventricular apex, aorta, left atrium and appendage, and atrioventricular valves, and for continuous monitoring of left ventricular function. However, in certain individuals, transgastric cross-sectional imaging cannot be readily obtained, and in patients with esophageal pathology, TEE may be contraindicated. Epicardial imaging affords an alternative approach to the assessment of left ventricular function and cardiac pathology. Thus, surgeons should be familiar with both imaging modalities.

Intraoperative Transesophageal Procedure

The transesophageal probe is inserted following endotracheal intubation, prior to sternotomy. Baseline evaluation, performed prior to the initiation of cardiopulmonary bypass, is extremely valuable in planning the optimal surgical approach. Baseline imaging will either confirm the preoperative diagnosis, uncover unsuspected lesions, or provide new data on the severity of regurgitant lesions, possibly resulting in modification of the surgical approach. Additionally, baseline imaging will define pathoanatomy and ventricular function in patients who are too unstable to undergo complete preoperative evaluation. The identification of atherosclerotic changes in the aorta, i.e., aortic plaque and/or thrombus, is helpful in choosing the site for aortic cannulation, aortic cross-clamping, and construction of proximal anastomoses in coronary bypass grafting, thereby reducing the risk of perioperative stroke due to embolization of atherosclerotic debris.[3-8] In addition, the identification of intracardiac thrombus prior to surgical manipulation can potentially prevent neurological injury (Fig. 13-1).

The transgastric TEE short axis view is excellent for beat-to-beat monitoring of left ventricular chamber size and function throughout the perioperative period and particularly useful during the critical phase of weaning the patient from bypass, facilitating immediate pharmacological, volume, or mechanical

Fig. 13-1.

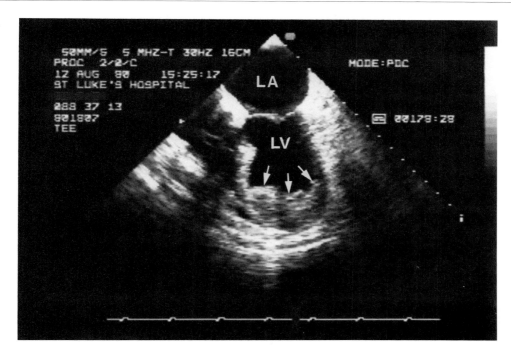

Figure 13-1: Baseline four-chamber transverse TEE view demonstrating left ventricular (LV) thrombus (arrows). LA = left atrium.

intervention. Global left ventricular dysfunction due to an abrupt change in the hemodynamic burden placed on the ventricle is not an uncommon occurrence following valvular surgery or repair of congenital lesions. The appearance of a new segmental wall motion abnormality, on the other hand, may indicate insufficient regional myocardial perfusion. This finding alerts the surgeon to a potential compromise of the coronary circulation due to such factors as coronary artery embolus, mechanical compression of a graft or native coronary artery, or incomplete revasculariztion. Rapid identification of the problem can result in myocardial salvage. Also, at this stage, inadequate valve repair, paravalvular leaks, and residual regurgitant lesions are readily apparent, expediting the appropriate response before cardiopulmonary bypass is discontinued. Importantly, during the weaning process, TEE detection of retained intracardiac air (Figs. 13-2A,B) facilitates prompt evacuation.[9-11]

Postoperative evaluation, performed after the discontinuation of cardiopulmonary bypass but prior to chest closure, enables the surgeon to evaluate the adequacy of the procedure with the patient in an unassisted physiological state. This instantaneous feedback can result in important modifications to the surgical procedure prior to chest closure. If a problem is identified, cardiopulmonary bypass can be reinstituted and further surgical intervention performed, thereby avoiding potential postoperative morbidity and mortality related to an inadequate surgical result.

Throughout the imaging periods, both transesophageal and epicardial modalities are affected by the electrocautery which produces a "pinwheel" artifact pattern from radiofrequency interference, obscuring the underlying image (Fig. 13-3). Additionally, structures such as the Swan-Ganz catheter, left atrial line, cannulation catheters, or even the surgeon's finger[12] (Fig. 13-4) may be visualized within the heart.

Fig. 13-2.

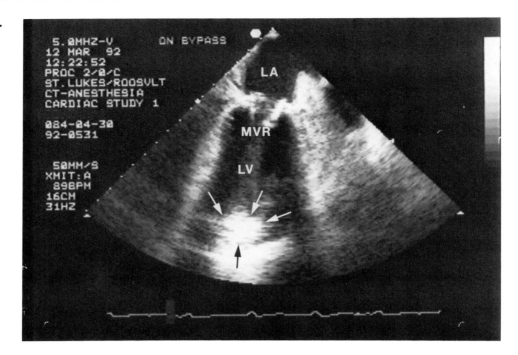

Figure 13-2A: Two-chamber apical view demonstrating retained intracardiac air during weaning from cardiopulmonary bypass following mitral valve heterograft insertion. Sequestered air (arrows) is highly echogenic and appears in the left ventricle (LV) at the apex (longitudinal plane). LA = left atrium; MVR = mitral valve replacement.

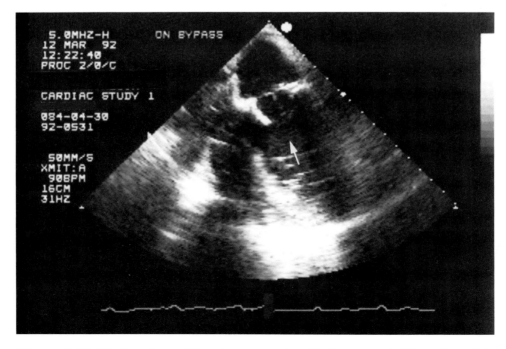

Figure 13-2B: The breakup of the air-pocket, visualized as microbubbles (arrow) in the left ventricular cavity, is achieved by cardiac manipulation and direct needle puncture of the left ventricle.

Fig. 13-3.

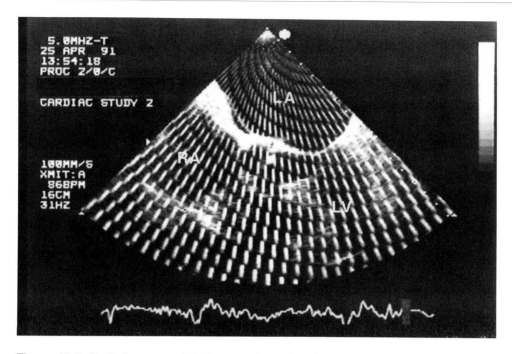

Figure 13-3: Radiofrequency interference from the electrocautery producing a "pinwheel" artifact obscuring the underlying two-dimensional image. LA = left atrium; LV = left ventricle; RA = right atrium.

Fig. 13-4.

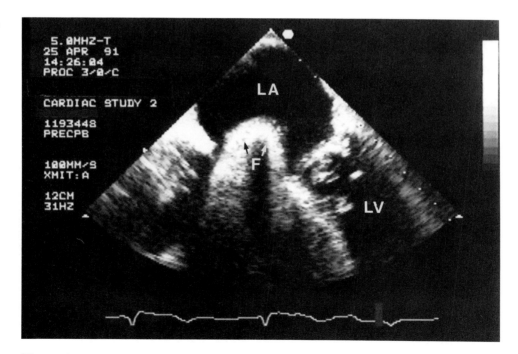

Figure 13-4: Four-chamber view demonstrating the surgeon's index finger (F) (arrows), which was inserted through the right atrium, displacing the interatrial septum. LA = left atrium; LV = left ventricle.

Mitral Valve Evaluation

The mitral valve apparatus is a complex structure composed of the annulus, anterior and posterior leaflets, chordae tendineae, and papillary muscles. Derangement of any of these components may result in valve dysfunction. The techniques of mitral valve reconstruction[13,14] incorporate complete analysis of the component parts to determine the type of repair necessary to restore valve competency and function. Intraoperative TEE allows the surgeon to assess the mitral apparatus under physiological conditions prior to the initiation of cardiopulmonary bypass to determine whether repair is feasible. Annular dilatation, prolapse, or flail anterior vs. posterior leaflet, regurgitant jet direction, elongated or ruptured chordae tendineae, and papillary muscle dysfunction are clearly defined, (Figs. 13-5A–C). Lesions less amenable to mitral valve reconstruction are readily identified. These include severe rheumatic disease involving the anterior leaflet, unrepairable fusion of the leaflets and chordae tendineae, and extensive calcification of the posterior mitral valve annulus.

The ability to objectively evaluate surgical results intraoperatively enables the surgeon to be more aggressive with valve repair techniques. Residual regurgitation following mitral valve repair is easily detected, (Figs. 13-6A–D). If more than mild regurgitation is present, revision of the repair can be immediately undertaken. Potentially, the severity of residual mitral regurgitation can be underestimated with color flow Doppler mapping due to jet orientation, to alterations in hemodynamic status, and to limited imaging planes. Therefore, the degree of residual mitral regurgitation should be assessed at physiological loading conditions comparable to those of daily living. If arterial systolic pressure (afterload) and ventricular preload are low, an underestimation of regurgitation severity is possible. Therefore, hemodynamic manipula-

Fig. 13-5.

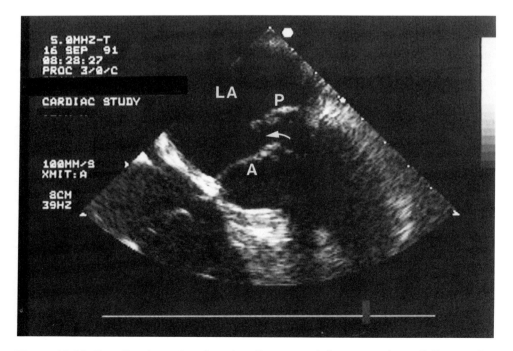

Figure 13-5A: Baseline four-chamber view (transverse) demonstrating a flail posterior mitral valve leaflet (P) (arrow). A = anterior leaflet; LA = left atrium.

Fig. 13-5. (cont'd)

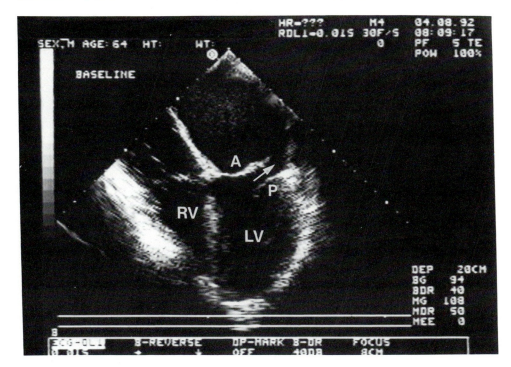

Figure 13-5B: Baseline four-chamber view demonstrating a flail anterior (A) mitral valve leaflet (arrow). LV = left ventricle; RV = right ventricle.

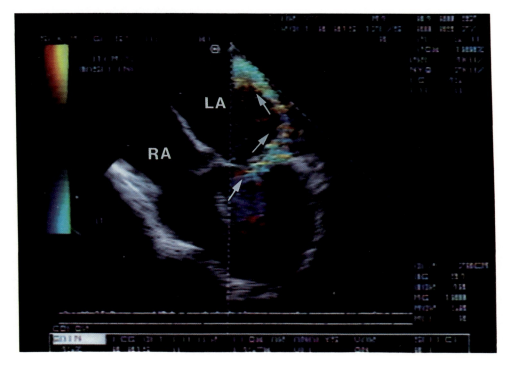

Figure 13-5C: Color flow Doppler representation of a posterolaterally directed mitral regurgitation jet (arrow) corresponding to Figure 5B.

Fig. 13-6.

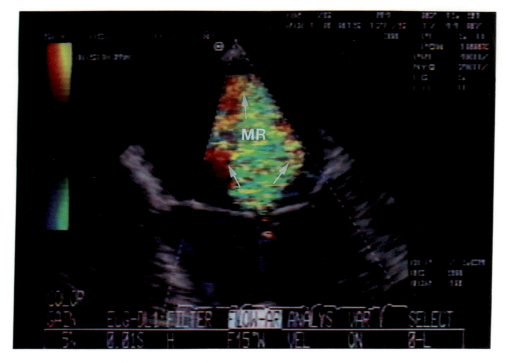

Figure 13-6A: Baseline transverse four-chamber view in a patient with mitral regurgitation (MR). Color flow Doppler imaging during systole demonstrates moderate mitral regurgitation (arrows).

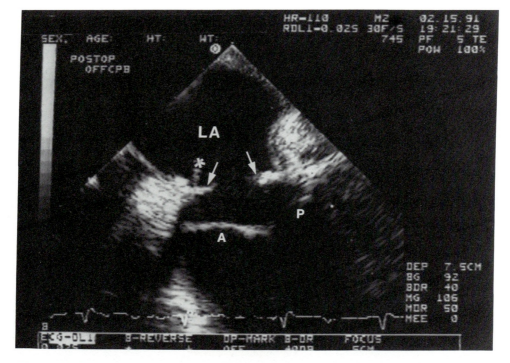

Figure 13-6B: Post-procedure image of mitral valve repair with insertion of a Carpentier-Edwards ring (arrows), in the mitral valve annulus. A suture is seen in the anterior mitral annular region (asterisk). The posterior mitral valve leaflet (P) is not clearly visualized due to shadowing from the prosthetic ring. A = anterior mitral valve leaflet; LA = left atrium.

Fig. 13-6. (cont'd)

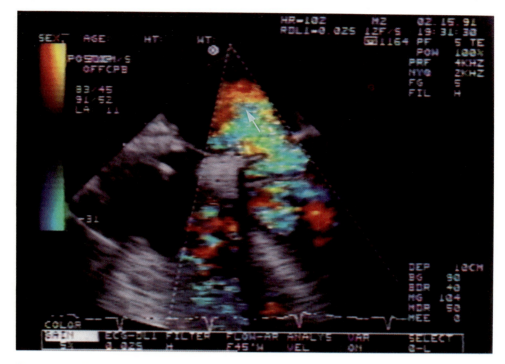

Figure 13-6C: Post-procedure Doppler color flow image in the same view during systole demonstrating significant residual mitral regurgitation (arrow).

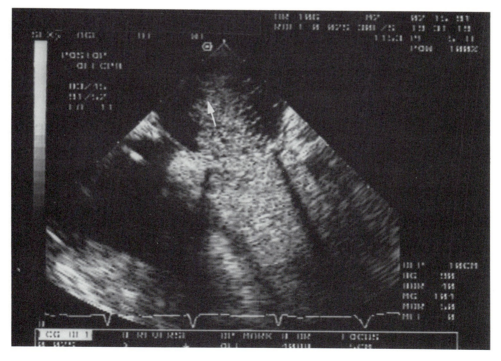

Figure 13-6D: Post-procedure two-dimensional "contrast" echocardiogram in the same view also demonstrates significant residual mitral regurgitation (arrow). "Contrast" microbubbles are produced by injecting agitated saline directly into the left ventricle.

tion with volume loading and/or vasopressors as well as complete left atrial interrogation are vital for accurate assessment of mitral valve repair. By providing additional imaging planes, biplane or multiplane TEE technology is particularly helpful in determining the extent and location of regurgitant lesions.[15] Contrast echocardiography[16] (injection of agitated saline producing echogenic microbubbles to evaluate blood flow characteristics) is complementary to color flow Doppler in clarifying the severity of residual mitral regurgitation (Fig. 13-7A,B).

A relatively rare complication following mitral valve repair with insertion of a Carpentier-Edwards ring is systolic anterior motion of the mitral leaflets.[17,18] The anterior displacement of the anterior leaflet into the left ventricular outflow tract can result in hemodynamic compromise secondary to outflow tract obstruction or severe mitral regurgitation. This finding is easily detected on post-repair imaging (Fig. 13-8).

Patients with severe aortic stenosis and concomitant moderate mitral regurgitation often present a clinical dilemma. Replacement of both the aortic and mitral valves increases operative complexity, morbidity, and mortality. With relief of aortic stenosis, the degree of mitral regurgitation may diminish dramatically, particularly in patients with an anatomically normal mitral apparatus.[19] Tunick and colleagues[20] report a decrease in the severity of significant mitral regurgitation in 12 of 13 patients (92%) following aortic valve replacement for aortic stenosis. On the other hand, Adams and Otto[21] report that a clinically significant decrease in mitral regurgitation is not always seen after relief of aortic stenosis. In their series, only 11 of 21 patients (52%) had a decrease in mitral regurgitation following successful relief of aortic stenosis (aortic valve area >0.8 cm² and a 50% increase in aortic valve area). The authors conclude that the decision to perform concurrent mitral valve surgery

Fig. 13-7.

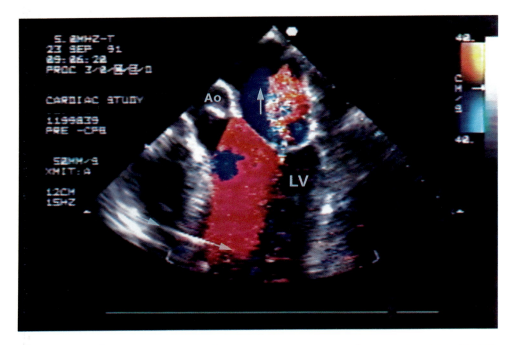

Figure 13-7A: Five-chamber view. Comparison of color flow Doppler (A), and contrast echocardiography (B) demonstrating mitral regurgitation (MR) (arrow). Note the similarity of jet area by the two methods. Agitated saline producing echogenic microbubbles (contrast) is injected through a needle placed transseptally into the left ventricle (LV).

Intraoperative Application of TEE • 359

Fig. 13-7.
(cont'd)

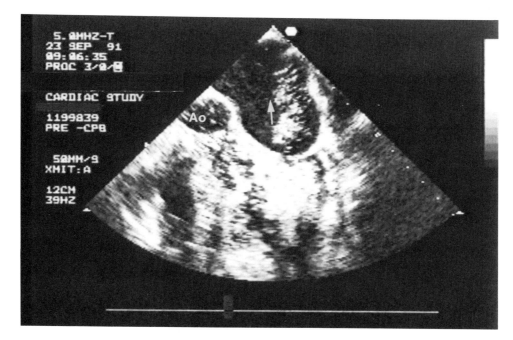

Figure 13-7B: Ao = aorta.

Fig. 13-8.

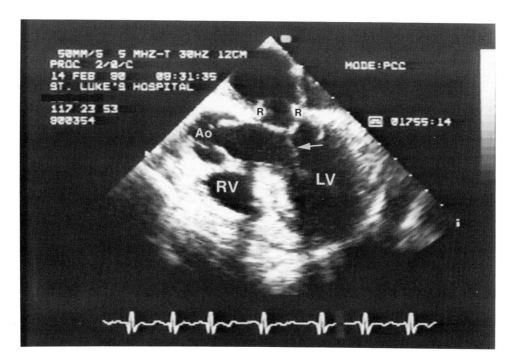

Figure 13-8: Post mitral valve repair with a Carpentier-Edwards ring (R). TEE horizontal plane left ventricular outflow tract view demonstrating mitral leaflet systolic anterior motion. LV = left ventricle; RV = right ventricle; Ao = aorta.

must be carefully considered in each individual patient. If TEE detects significant residual mitral regurgitation following aortic valve replacement, the mitral valve can be repaired or replaced before the patient leaves the operating suite.

The severity of mitral regurgitation at the time of surgery can be quite different from that detected at cardiac catheterization. Ischemia, catheter orientation, volume status, and afterload can alter the angiographic assessment of mitral regurgitation. Intraoperative TEE is useful in guiding the operative management of patients with ischemic mitral regurgitation. Sheikh and colleagues[22] report a change in operative approach in 27 of 246 patients undergoing surgery for ischemic heart disease based on intraoperative TEE imaging; 22 patients originally scheduled to undergo coronary bypass grafting and mitral valve surgery had bypass surgery alone, whereas five patients originally scheduled to undergo isolated coronary bypass surgery required additional mitral valve surgery. Thus, patients were spared an unnecessary mitral valve operation that is associated with a higher operative mortality, while those with unsuspected significant mitral regurgitation were treated appropriately.

Tricuspid Valve Evaluation

Tricuspid regurgitation may be present in 10% to 50% of patients with severe mitral regurgitation or stenosis.[23] Although functional tricuspid regurgitation may diminish spontaneously after mitral valve operation, the presence of significant tricuspid regurgitation increases postoperative morbidity and mortality.[24] Intraoperative ultrasonic measurement of the tricuspid annulus and determination of the degree of tricuspid regurgitation prior to the initiation of bypass enables the surgeon to decide objectively whether tricuspid repair is indicated.[25,26] The severity of residual tricuspid regurgitation immediately after correction of the left heart lesion or following tricuspid repair can be assessed with TEE before chest closure. If significant residual tricuspid regurgitation is present, correction should be undertaken.

Prosthetic Valve Evaluation

TEE is an excellent modality to assess prosthetic valve function. With epicardial echocardiography, mitral regurgitation can be masked by left atrial shadowing produced by the metallic components of the prosthesis. Because TEE images from a retrocardiac position, shadowing from a mitral valve prosthesis is directed into the left ventricle. Therefore, normal "intrinsic" mechanical valve regurgitation versus prosthetic paravalvular regurgitation (Figs. 13-9A–D) is easily differentiated by TEE. Bioprosthetic valves do not have any intrinsic regurgitation characteristics. During weaning from cardiopulmonary bypass, small, low-velocity jets may be detected with leaflet closure. However, any jet that extends back into the left atrium is considered abnormal. Whenever a prosthetic valve is implanted in a patient with a severely calcified annulus[27] or replaces a previously implanted dysfunctional prosthesis, the incidence of paravalvular regurgitation increases. Complete chamber interrogation is vital for accurate assessment of paravalvular regurgitation in these patients. Furthermore, prosthetic valve dysfunction, such as disc

Fig. 13-9.

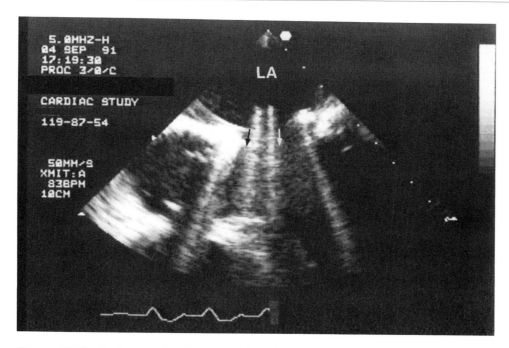

Figure 13-9A: Post-procedure four-chamber view demonstrating normal diastolic excursion (arrows) of a bileaflet St. Jude mechanical valve in the mitral position. Both leaflets are clearly visualized. LA = left atrium.

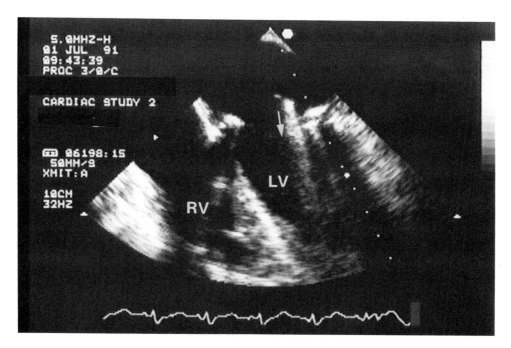

Figure 13-9B: Post-procedure four-chamber view demonstrating normal diastolic excursion (arrow) of an Omniscience single tilting disc mechanical valve in the mitral position. RV = right ventricle; LV = left ventricle.

Fig. 13-9. (cont'd)

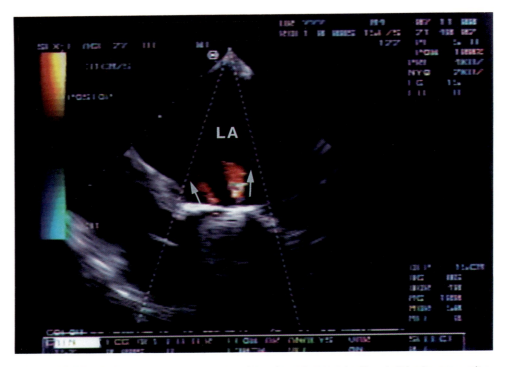

Figure 13-9C: Post-procedure four-chamber view demonstrating intrinsic regurgitation characteristics of an Omniscience mechanical valve. Two small jets (arrows) are seen at the major and minor orifice closure points during systole.

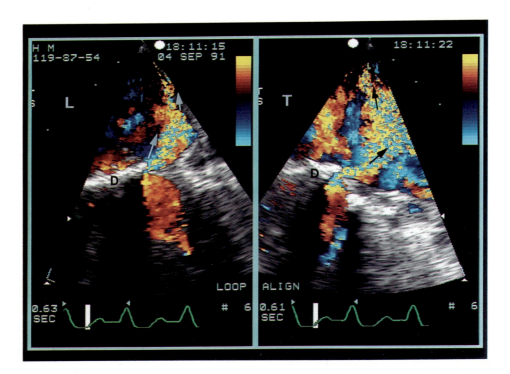

Figure 13-9D: Biplane TEE representation of a paravalvular regurgitation jet (arrows) in a patient with a mitral Omniscience prosthetic disc valve (D). Transverse plane (T, right side) demonstrates a larger regurgitant jet than the longitudinal plane (L, left side).

impingement from residual chordae tendineae or suture, or disc sticking is easily detected.

Monoplane TEE evaluation is limited in patients with both an aortic and a mitral valve prosthesis. Both prostheses shadow the left ventricular outflow tract, preventing detection of possible aortic regurgitation and subaortic obstruction. Epicardial echo and/or multiplane TEE provide clearer views of the left ventricular outflow tract, thereby eliminating these problems.

Aorta, Aortic Valve, Left Ventricular Outflow Tract Evaluation

In patients with aortic valve endocarditis, TEE imaging has been shown to be superior to conventional transthoracic imaging for the diagnosis of aortic annular abscess, vegetation, torn prosthetic leaflet, satellite lesions on the mitral valve, and intracardiac fistula.[28,29] However, some patients are too ill to permit preoperative TEE assessment. Furthermore, due to the progressive nature of the infectious process, cardiac pathology may change from the last preoperative evaluation to the time of surgery. Therefore, in this patient subset, intraoperative TEE imaging is especially valuable for the assessment of native and prosthetic aortic valve and root involvement (Figs. 13-10A,B). Knowledge of precise pathoanatomy is extremely helpful in guiding surgical management prior to the institution of cardiopulmonary bypass in these highly complex situations.

TEE is the imaging technique of choice for the diagnosis and classification of acute aortic dissection.[30-33] Intraoperative TEE is an accurate diagnostic tool for evaluating hemodynamic instability during anesthetic induction and allows the surgeon to evaluate potential ongoing anatomical changes immediately preceding repair of the defect. The intimal flap, true and false lumens, entrance and exit sites, presence or absence of coronary artery involvement, presence of pericardial effusion or tamponade, and the presence and severity of aortic regurgitation can be readily evaluated (Figs. 13-11A–C). Aortic regurgitation often complicates aortic dissection or aneurysm as a result of annular dilatation or distortion. Repair of the aortic lesion alone may result in a significant decrease in or elimination of aortic regurgitation obviating the need for aortic valve replacement.

Native aortic valve repair procedures for both stenotic and regurgitant lesions are being performed to avoid the inherent complications of prosthetic valves.[34,35] We routinely use intraoperative echocardiography to assess valve mobility, coaptation, and the severity of residual aortic regurgitation following aortic valve reparative surgery.

Intracardiac Shunts

Intraoperative echocardiographic imaging allows the surgeon to evaluate congenital heart lesions as well as acquired defects secondary to endocarditis or myocardial infarction. Shunt flow from atrial septal defects, ventricular septal defects, and fistulous tracts can be evaluated. A patent foramen ovale or unsuspected atrial septal defect may be present in patients with mitral disease and left atrial enlargement. The identification of significant shunting through the patent foramen ovale may alter the operative approach from left atrial entry to right atrial entry to include closure of the patent foramen ovale.

Fig. 13-10.

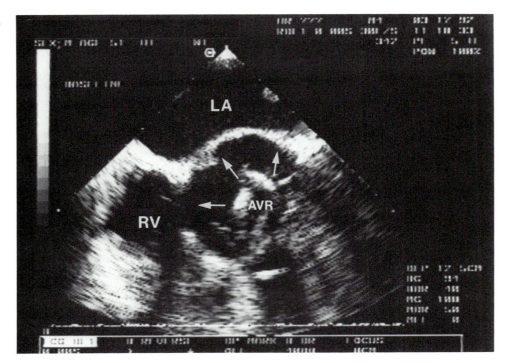

Figure 13-10A: Baseline imaging in a patient with a mechanical aortic valve (AVR) and a clinical diagnosis of infective endocarditis revealed an echolucent paravalvular area in the left coronary sinus interpreted as an abscess (arrows). LA = left atrium; RV = right ventricle.

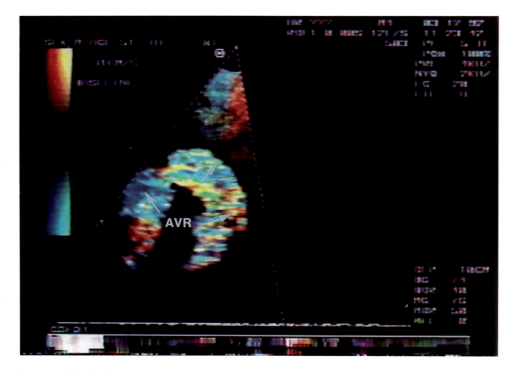

Figure 13-10B: Corresponding color flow Doppler mapping demonstrated continuous flow (arrows) throughout the cardiac cycle in this region. AVR = aortic valve replacement.

Fig. 13-11.

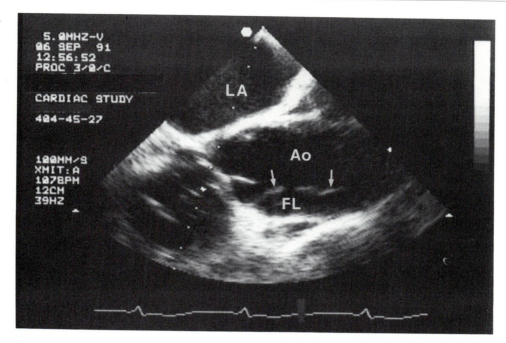

Figure 13-11A: Longitudinal plane of the aortic root and proximal ascending aorta demonstrating aortic dissection with intimal flap (arrows). FL = false lumen; LA = left atrium; Ao = aorta.

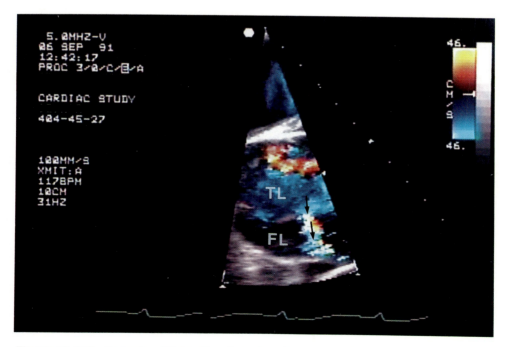

Figure 13-11B: Corresponding color flow Doppler demonstrating systolic flow from the true lumen (TL) into the false lumen (FL) confirming the presence of the entrance site (arrows).

Fig. 13-11.
(cont'd)

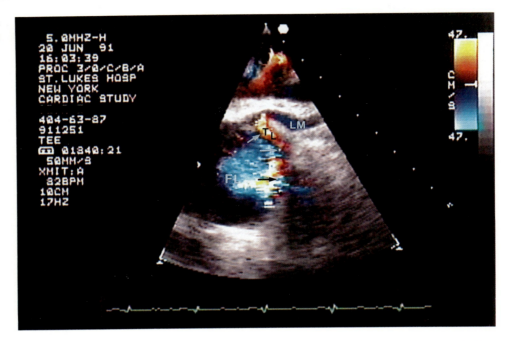

Figure 13-11C: Transverse plane at the aortic root demonstrating false lumen (FL) enlargement during diastole, leaving only a rim of true lumen (TL) from which the left main (LM) coronary artery arises.

Additionally, in surgery involving partial excision of the atrial septum, i.e., atrial myxomectomy, TEE is used to evaluate the repaired septal defect. In patients having extensive cardiac tumor invasion undergoing complex operative reconstruction, echocardiography can confirm complete intracardiac tumor excision and can exclude an intracardiac communication or valvular insufficiency.

Various surgical approaches have been used to alleviate left ventricular outflow tract obstruction and mitral insufficiency in patients with hypertrophic cardiomyopathy.[36,37] For the majority of surgical patients with hypertrophic cardiomyopathy, septal myomectomy is the procedure of choice. Mitral valve replacement should be reserved for those patients who are severely symptomatic, have significant elevation of left ventricular outflow gradient, have severe mitral regurgitation, or fail to improve after septal myomectomy.[38] The associated immediate complications of iatrogenic ventricular septal defects, complete heart block, and aortic or mitral insufficiency usually occur in 1% to 3% of patients undergoing septal myomectomy.[37] Intraoperative post-bypass TEE allows the surgeon to inspect the area of myomectomy and assess for the presence or absence of an iatrogenic ventricular septal defect and/or residual mitral regurgitation. In addition, the presence of residual outflow tract obstruction can be assessed by two-dimensional imaging and the residual pressure gradient measured by continuous Doppler in the transgastric five-chamber view or transesophageal two- or four-chamber views.

Impact of Intraoperative Echocardiography

Intraoperative echocardiography[39,40] has been shown to affect surgical outcome and can alter surgical decision-making and technique. A review of our first 1630 consecutive patients evaluated with intraoperative echo demonstrated new information obtained in 256 (16%), alteration in the planned operative procedure occurred in 261 (16%), and a therapeutic change was indicated in 127 (7.8%).[41] Also, based on intraoperative echo findings, an immediate reoperation was performed in 36 patients (2.2%). Similarly, Sheikh and co-workers[42] reported immediate reoperation in 10 of 154 patients (6%) based on unsatisfactory operative results detected on post-bypass imaging. Stewart and colleagues,[43] in a series of 100 patients undergoing valve repair for mitral regurgitation, reported eight cases of unsatisfactory results detected on post-repair intraoperative epicardial imaging. Six of these patients had immediate reoperation, whereas the other two required reoperation at a later date.

Real-time two-dimensional imaging, along with either contrast or color flow Doppler, provides an objective anatomical and physiological view of cardiac performance thereby eliminating much indecision and subjectivity involved in surgical decision-making. In our series,[41] 367 of 1630 patients (22.5%) directly and immediately benefitted from intraoperative echocardiographic findings.

Conclusion

Intraoperative echocardiography is an invaluable adjunct to cardiac surgery. Baseline and postsurgical imaging facilitates appropriate staging of the operation and immediate assessment of the procedure, ensuring the best possible outcome. Monitoring of ventricular function, particularly in patients with low ejection fraction, facilitates prompt intervention when necessary. Potential future development of TEE including multiplane imaging, 3-D reconstruction, and real-time ejection fraction monitoring as well as myocardial perfusion contrast echocardiography will be important contributions to improve surgical outcome. The more comfortable surgeons and anesthesiologists are with understanding, performing, and interpreting intraoperative echocardiograms, the greater the benefit to their patients.

Bibliography

1. Mitchell MM, Sutherland GR, Gussenhoven EJ, et al: Transesophageal echocardiography. *J Am Soc Echo* 1:362–377, 1988.
2. Stumper O, Kaulitz R, Steeram N, et al: Intraoperative transesophageal versus epicardial ultrasound in surgery for congenital heart disease. *J Am Soc Echo* 3:392–401, 1990.
3. Marshall WG, Barzilai B, Kouchoukos NT, Saffitz J: Intraoperative ultrasonic imaging of the ascending aorta. *Ann Thoracic Surg* 48:339–344, 1989.
4. Barzilai B, Marshall WG, Saffitz JE, Kouchoukos NT: Avoidance of embolic complications by ultrasonic characterization of the ascending aorta. *Circulation* 80(Suppl I):I-275–I-279, 1989.
5. Hosoda Y, Watanabe M, Hirooka Y, et al: Significance of atherosclerotic changes of the ascending aorta during coronary bypass surgery with intraoperative detection by echography. *J Cardiovasc Surg* 32:301–306, 1991.
6. Ribakov GH, Katz ES, Galloway AC, et al: Surgical implications of trans-

esophageal echocardiography to grade the atheromatous aortic arch. *Ann Thorac Surg* 53:758–763, 1992.

7. Wareing TH, Davila-Roman VG, Barzilai B, et al: Management of the severely atherosclerotic ascending aorta during cardiac operations. *J Thorac Cardiovasc Surg* 103:453–462, 1992.
8. Blauth CI, Cosgrove DM, Webb BW, et al: Atheroembolism from the ascending aorta. *J Thorac Cardiovasc Surg* 1103:1104-1112, 1992.
9. Rodigas PC, Meyer FJ, Haasler GB, et al: Intraoperative 2- dimensional echocardiography: ejection of microbubbles from the left ventricle after cardiac surgery. *Am J Cardiol* 50:1130–1132, 1982.
10. Oka Y, Inoue T, Hong Y, et al: Retained intracardiac air: transesophageal echocardiography for definition of incidence and monitoring removal by improved techniques. *J Thorac Cardiovasc Surg* 91:329–337, 1986.
11. Diehl JT, Ramos D, Dougherty F, et al: Intraoperative, two-dimensional echocardiography guided removal of retained intracardiac air. *Ann Thorac Surg* 43:674–675, 1987.
12. Kronzon I, Tunick PA, Schrem SS, Yarmush L: Fingerlike mass in the left atrium. *J Am Soc Echo* 4:75, 1991.
13. Carpentier A: Cardiac valve surgery: the "French correction." *J Thorac Cardiovasc Surg* 86:323–337, 1983.
14. Galloway AC, Colvin SB, Baumann FG, et al: Current concepts of mitral valve reconstruction for mitral insufficiency. *Circulation* 78:1087–1098, 1988.
15. Yoshida K, Yoshikawa J, Yamaura Y, et al: Assessment of mitral regurgitation by biplane transesophageal color Doppler flow mapping. *Circulation* 82:1121–1126, 1990.
16. Mindich BP, Goldman ME, Fuster V, et al: Improved intraoperative evaluation of mitral valve operations utilizing two-dimensional contrast echocardiography. *J Thorac Cardiovasc Surg* 90:112–118, 1985.
17. Krenz H, Mindich BP, Guarino T, Goldman ME: Sudden development of intraoperative left ventricular outflow obstruction: Differential and mechanism. An intraoperative two-dimensional echocardiographic study. *J Cardiac Surg* 5:93–101, 1990.
18. Grossi EA, Galloway AC, Parish MA, et al: Experience with twenty-eight cases of systolic anterior motion after mitral valve reconstruction by the carpentier technique. *J Thorac Cardiovasc Surg* 103:466–470, 1992.
19. Mindich BP, Guarino T, Lazar S, et al: The surgical fate of mitral regurgitation associated with severe aortic stenosis: an intraoperative echo study (abst). *JACC* 13:72A, 1989.
20. Tunick PA, Gindea A, Kronzon I: Effect of aortic valve replacement for aortic stenosis on severity of mitral regurgitation. *Am J Cardiol* 65:1219–1221, 1990.
21. Adams PB, Otto CM: Lack of improvement in coexisting mitral regurgitation after relief of valvular aortic stenosis. *Am J Cardiol* 66:105–107, 1990.
22. Sheikh KH, Bengston JR, Rankin S, et al: Intraoperative transesophageal Doppler color flow imaging used to guide patient selection and operative treatment of ischemic mitral regurgitation. *Circulation* 84:594–604, 1991.
23. Cohen ST, Sell JE, McIntosh CL, Clark RE: Tricuspid regurgitation in patients with acquired, chronic, pure mitral regurgitation. II. Nonoperative management, tricuspid valve annuloplasty, and tricuspid valve replacement. *J Thorac Cardiovasc Surg* 94:488–497, 1987.

24. King RM, Schaff HV, Danielson GK, et al: Surgery for tricuspid regurgitation late after mitral valve replacement. *Circulation* 70(Pt 2):I-193-I-197, 1984.
25. Goldman ME, Guarino T, Fuster V, Mindich B: The necessity for tricuspid valve repair can be determined by two-dimensional echocardiography. *J Thorac Cardiovasc Surg* 94:542–550, 1987.
26. Czer LSC, Maurer G, Bolger A, et al: Tricuspid valve repair. *J Thorac Cardiovasc Surg* 98:101–111, 1989.
27. Dhasmana JP, Blackstone EH, Kirklin JW, Kouchoukos NT: Factors associated with periprosthetic leakage following primary mitral valve replacement: with special consideration of the suture technique. *Ann Thorac Surg* 35:170–178, 1983.
28. Gussenhoven EJ, van Herwerden LA, Roelandt J, et al: Detailed analysis of aortic valve endocarditis: comparison of precordial, esophageal and epicardial two-dimensional echocardiography with surgical findings. *J Clin Ultrasound* 14:209–211, 1986.
29. Daniel WG, Mugge A, Martin RP, et al: Improvement in the diagnosis of abscesses associated with endocarditis by transesophageal echocardiography. *N Engl J Med* 324:795–800, 1991.
30. Erbel R, Mohr-Kahaly S, Rennollet H, et al: Diagnosis of aortic dissection: the value of transesophageal echocardiography. *Thorac Cardiovasc Surg* 35(special issue 2):126–133, 1987.
31. Schippers OA, Gussenhoven WJ, van Herwerden LA, et al: The role of intraoperative two-dimensional echocardiography in the assessment of thoracic aorta pathology. *Thorac Cardiovasc Surg* 36:208–213, 1988.
32. Erbel R, Engberding R, Daniel W, et al: Echocardiography in diagnosis of aortic dissection. *Lancet* 1(8636):457–461, 1989.
33. Simon P, Owen AN, Havel M, et al: Transesophageal echocardiography in the emergency surgical management of patients with aortic dissection. *J Thorac Cardiovasc Surg* 103:1113–1118, 1992.
34. Mindich BP, Guarino T, Goldman ME. Aortic valvuloplasty for acquired aortic stenosis. *Circulation* 74(Suppl I):I-130-I-135, 1986.
35. Cosgrove DM, Rosenkranz ER, Hendren WG, et al: Valvuloplasty for aortic insufficiency. *J Thorac Cardiovasc Surg* 102:571–577, 1991.
36. Walker WS, Reid KG, Cameron WJ, et al: Comparison of ventricular septal surgery and mitral valve replacement for hypertrophic obstructive cardiomyopathy. *Ann Thorac Surg* 48:528–535, 1989.
37. Krajcer Z, Leachman RD, Cooley DA, Coronado R: Septal myotomy-myomectomy versus mitral valve replacement in hypertrophic cardiomyopathy: ten-year follow up in 185 patients. *Circulation* 80(Suppl I):I-57-I-64, 1989.
38. McIntosh CL, Maron BJ: Current operative treatment of obstructive hypertrophic cardiomyopathy. *Circulation* 78:487–495, 1988.
39. Lazar HL, Plehn J: Intraoperative echocardiography. *Ann Thorac Surg* 50:1010–1018, 1990.
40. Maurer G, Siegel RJ, Czer LSC: The use of color flow mapping for intraoperative assessment of valve repair. *Circulation* 84(Suppl I):I-250-I-258, 1991.
41. Goldman ME, Guarino T, Zadeh B, et al: Impact of intraoperative echo in open heart surgery: a study of 1630 consecutive cases over 8 years (abstr). *JACC* 19:55A, 1992.

42. Sheikh KH, de Bruijn NP, Rankin S, et al: The utility of transesophageal echocardiography and Doppler color flow imaging in patients undergoing cardiac valve surgery. *J Am Coll Cardiol* 15:363–372, 1990.
43. Stewart WJ, Currie PJ, Salcedo EE, et al: Intraoperative Doppler color flow mapping for decision-making in valve repair for mitral regurgitation: technique and results in 100 patients. *Circulation* 81:556–566, 1990.
44. Daniel WG, Shroder RE, Nonnast-Daniel B, et al: Conventional and transesophageal echocardiography in the diagnosis of infective endocarditis. *Eur Heart J* 8(Suppl):287–292, 1987.
45. Erbel R, Rohmann S, Frexler M, et al. Improved diagnostic value of echocardiography in patients with enfective endocarditis by transesophageal approach: a prospective study. *Eur Heart J* 9:43–53, 1988.
46. Mugge A, Daniel WG, Frank G, Lechtlen PR: Echocardiography in enfective endocarditis: reassessment of prognostic implications of vegetation size determined by the transthoracic andthe transesophageal approach. *J Am Coll Cardiol* 14:631–638, 1989.
47. Shiveley BK, Gurule FT, Roldan CA, et al: Diagnostic value of tranesophageal compared with transthoracic echocardiography in infective endocarditis. *J Am Coll Cardiol* 18:391–397, 1991.

Index

Aging, aortic plaque, 192
Air-pocket, intraoperative TEE, 352
Aneurysm
   coronary artery disease, 213
   ventricular septal defect, 336
Anticoagulation, left atrium, 262
Aorta
   aortic dissection, 162–182
   normal descending, 162
Aortic dissection, 159–182
   case history, 177–179, 181
   false lumen, 163–182
   intimal flap, 164, 168
   proximal aorta, 164, 166
   true lumen, 163–182
   types of, 159–161
Aortic evaluation, intraoperative TEE, 363
Aortic leaflet excursion, 108
Aortic orifice area, planimetry, 111
Aortic plaque, 183–201
   aging, 192
   blood stasis, 185
   buckled aorta, 199
   calcium in, 186
   cerebral embolus, 200
   heterogenous nature, 187
   laminar, 191
   laminar plaque, 186
   mobile thrombus, 190
   nodular, 189
   sessile plaque hemorrhage, 188
   thrombus, 187
   transient ischemic attack, 190
   ulcerated, 188
Aortic regurgitation, 113–120
   aortic valve prolapse, 115
   M-mode, 26
   short axis plane, 114
   transverse plane, 113
Aortic stenosis, 109, 111
Aortic valve
   basal view, 27
   endocarditis, 121–127
   intraoperative TEE evaluation, 363
   M-mode, 26
   prolapse, 108–109
   prosthesis, 128–136
   stenosis, 105–112
Aortic valve disease, 105–145
   aortic regurgitation, 113–120
   aortic valve endocarditis, 121–127
   aortic valve prosthesis, 128–136
   aortic valve stenosis, 105–112
   bicuspid aortic valve, 137–146
Ascending aorta
   with aortic regurgitation, 120
   transverse plane, 32
Ascending aortic dissection, type of, 161

Ascites, right atrium, 293
Atrial fibrillation
    Doppler velocity, 39
    left atrium, 251–253
    mitral stenosis, 39–40
    right atrium, 283
Atrial flutter, left atrium, 254
Atrial septal aneurysm, patent foramen ovale, 332–333
Atrial septal defects, 303–326
    endocardial cushion defect, 343
    ostium primum, 303–304
    ostium secundum, 303, 327
    sinus venosus, 303

Ball valve, mitral valve replacement, 72–77
Balloon pump, aortic plaque, 199
Basal view, 7, 24, 26–29
Basic views, TEE, 1–32
Bicuspid aortic valve, 137–146
    congenital aortic stenosis, 137
Blood stasis, aortic plaque, 185
Biplane imaging, 3, 5, 11
Buckled aorta, aortic plaque, 199

Calcified segment, coronary artery disease, 211
Calcium, in aortic plaque, 186
Cardiac transplantation, right atrium, 280
Carpentier-Edwards ring, intraoperative TEE, 356, 359
Central venous pressure catheter, right atrium, 287–288
Cerebral embolus, aortic plaque, 200
Chiari network, right atrium, 285
Congenital heart disease, 303–347
    aortic stenosis, 137
    atrial septal defect, 303–326
    cor triatriatum, 344–345
    Ebstein's anomaly, 341–342
    endocardial cushion defect, 343
    microbubbles, 305, 306
    "negative contrast" effect, 313
    patent foramen ovale, 307, 310, 327–335
    secundum atrial septal defect, 307–310
    transposition of great vessels, 346–347
    ventricular septal defect, 336–340
Cor triatriatum, 344–345
Coronary artery disease, 209–232
    aneurysm, 213
    calcified segment, 211
    coronary flow enhancement, 212
    horizontal plane, 211
    ischemic heart disease, 220–232
    saphenous veins, 218–219
    stenotic lesion, 212, 215
    transverse, short axis, 210
    transverse plane, 29
    ventricular tachycardia, 216
Coronary flow enhancement, coronary artery disease, 212

Descending aorta
    longitudinal plane, 31
    transverse plane, 30
Descending aortic dissection, type of, 161
Diastole, aortic valve, 106, 107
Diastolic doming, tricuspid regurgitation, 154
Diastolic frame, mitral stenosis, 35
Diastolic motion, mitral valve, 36
Disc valve prosthesis, mitral valve replacement, 78–88
Distal aortic dissection, type of, 161
Doppler velocity, atrial fibrillation, 39
Doppler wave, mitral valve stenosis, 38
Dyspnea, left atrium, 235, 241

Ebstein's anomaly, 341–342
    tricuspid regurgitation, 342
Edema, right atrium, 293
Effusions, pericardial disease, 297–301
Electrocautery radiofrequency interference, intraoperative TEE, 353
Emergency room TEE, 160
Endocardial cushion defect
    atrial septal defect, 343
    congenital heart disease, 343
Endocarditis, aortic valve, 121–128
Endocarditis, mitral valve, 63–71

Endocarditis, tricuspic valve, 155–158
Eustacian valve, right atrium, 284
Examination techniques, 1–32

False lumen
 aortic dissection, 163–182
 intraoperative TEE, 366
Fibrillatory wave, left atrium, 252–253
Fibrin strand, left ventricle, 110
Flail, intraoperative TEE, 354–355
Fossa ovalis, patent foramen ovale, 329

Great vessels, transposition of, 346–347

Heterogenous nature, of aortic plaque, 187
Heterografts, mitral valve replacement, 90–100
Hockey stick configuration, tricuspid regurgitation, 153
Hypertension, tricuspid regurgitation, 153
Hypertrophic cardiomyopathy, left ventricular outflow obstruction, 205
Hypotension, left atrium, 243

Image orientation, 5, 8
Imaging periods, intraoperative TEE, 350
Imaging planes, 3–8
Interatrial septum, tricuspid regurgitation, 150
Intimal flap, aortic dissection, 164, 168
Intra-atrial septal aneurysms, left atrium, 272–275
Intracardiac shunt, intraoperative TEE, 363–366
Intraoperative application, of transesophageal echocardiography, 349–370
Intraoperative TEE
 air-pocket, 352
 aorta evaluation, 363
 aortic valve evaluation, 363
 Carpentier-Edwards ring, 356, 359
 electrocautery radiofrequency interference, 353
 false lumen, 366
 flail, 354–355
 impact of, 366–367
 intracardiac shunt, 363–366
 left ventricular outflow tract evaluation, 363
 mitral graft heterograft, 352
 mitral regurgitation, 355–356
 mitral valve evaluation, 354–360
 Omniscience valve, 361–362
 procedure overview, 350–354
 tricuspid valve evaluation, 360–363
Intraoperative transesophageal procedure, 350–353
Ischemic heart disease, coronary artery disease, 220–232
Isovelocity area, mitral valve, 37

Laboratory equipment, for TEE laboratory, 2
Laminar plaque, 191
 aortic plaque, 186
Left atrial appendage, 25, 244–265
 left atrium, 249
 mitral valve, 41
Left atrium, 233–275
 anticoagulation, 262
 atrial fibrillation, 251–253
 atrial flutter, 254
 Doppler flow, pulmonary vein, 267
 dyspnea, 235, 241
 fibrillatory wave, 252–253
 hypotension, 243
 interatrial septal aneurysm, 272–275
 intra-atrial septal aneurysms, 272–275
 left atrial appendage, 244–265
 left atrial myxomas, 233–243
 left atrial thrombus, 244–265
 mediastinal tumor, 242, 271
 mitral annulus calcification, 240–241
 mitral regurgitation, 237, 270
 myxoma, 235–241
 pectinate muscle, 246–247

pedunculated myxoma, 239
pulmonary vein, 266–271
sarcoma, 242
sinus rhythm, 248
syncope, 235
tachycardia, 254
transducer, 249
transthoracic echo abnormality, 238
Left ventricular outflow obstruction, 203–207
hypertrophic cardiomyopathy, 205
mitral valve opened, 204
subaortic membrane, 206–207
Left ventricular outflow tract evaluation, intraoperative TEE, 363
Lipoma, right atrium, 279, 281, 293
Longitudinal plane, 6, 24, 25
Lumen, false, intraoperative TEE, 366

Mass, right atrium, 277–295
Mediastinal hematoma, pericardial disease, 301
Mediastinal tumor, left atrium, 242, 271
Membrane, cor triatriatum, 344–345
Microbubble, congenital heart disease, 305, 306
Mitral annulus calcification, left atrium, 240–241
Mitral graft heterograft, intraoperative TEE, 352
Mitral regurgitation, 40, 42–60
intraoperative TEE, 355–356
left atrium, 237, 270
severity quantification, 47
Mitral short axis, 11, 14
Mitral stenosis, 33–42
Mitral valve
anterior leaflet, aortic regurgitation, 116
prolapse, 60–62
Mitral valve disease, 33–104
mitral regurgitation, 43–60
mitral stenosis, 33–42
mitral valve endocarditis, 63–71
mitral valve prolapse, 60–62
mitral valve repair, 101–104
mitral valve replacement, 72–100
Mitral valve endocarditis, 63–71
Mitral valve evaluation, intraoperative TEE, 354–360
Mitral valve opened, left ventricular outflow obstruction, 204
Mitral valve prolapse, 60–62
Mitral valve repair, 101–104
Mitral valve replacement, 72–100
ball valves, 72–77
disc valve prosthesis, 78–88
heterografts, 89–100
transthoracic apical view, 72–73
Monoplane imaging, 3
Multiplane probe, 3, 8, 31, 137, 171
Myxoma, left atrial, 235–241

"Negative contrast" effect, congenital heart disease, 313
Nodular aortic plaque, 189

Omniscience valve, intraoperative TEE, 361–362
Ostium primum, atrial septal defect, 303–304
Ostium secundum, atrial septal defect, 303

Pacemaker, right atrium, 286–287
Patent foramen ovale, 20, 327–335
atrial septal aneurysm, 332–333
congenital heart disease, 307, 310
fossa ovalis, 329
septum, 328
Valsalva maneuver, 330–331
Patient preparation, for examination, 2–3
Pectinate muscle
left atrium, 246–247
right atrium, 282
Pedunculated myxoma, left atrium, 239
Pericardial disease, 297–301
effusions, 297–301
hematoma, 301
mediastinal hematoma, 301
pleural effusion, 300

Personnel, for TEE laboratory, 2
Physiological mitral regurgitation, 45
Planimetry, mitral valve, 41
Plaque, aortic, 183–201
Pleural effusion, pericardial disease, 300
Pressure half-time, mitral valve, 42
Prolapse, mitral valve, 60–62
Prostheses, aortic valve, 128–136
Protocol, imaging, 4–5
Proximal aorta, dissection, 161, 164
Pulmonary artery, 28–30
  bifurcation, 29
  color flow Doppler, 30
Pulmonary veins, left atrium, 266–271
Pulmonic stenosis, ventricular septal defect, 340

Radiofrequency interference, electrocautery, intraoperative TEE, 353
Regurgitation, aortic, 113–121
Regurgitation, mitral, 43–60
Renal cell carcinoma infiltrate, right atrium, 295
Right atrial appendage, 17
Right atrial inflow view, 16–17
Right atrium, 15–17, 277–295
  ascites, 293
  atrial fibrillation, 283
  cardiac chamber overview, 278
  cardiac transplantation, 280
  central venous pressure catheter, 287–288
  Chiari network, 285
  edema, 293
  eustacian valve, 284
  lipoma, 279, 281, 293
  pacemaker, 286–287
  pectinate muscle, 282
  renal cell carcinoma infiltrate, 295
  septum, 278
  superior vena cave, 287, 290, 291
  thrombus, 283
  transverse plane, 15
  tricuspid annulus, 289
Right ventricular inflow, 15, 15–20, 18

Saphenous veins, coronary artery disease, 218–219
Sarcoma, left atrium, 242
Secundum atrial septal defect, congenital heart disease, 307–310
Septum
  patent foramen ovale, 328
  right atrium, 278
Sessile plaque hemorrhage, aortic plaque, 188
Sinus rhythm, left atrium, 248
Sinus venosus, atrial septal defect, 303
Standard views, 9–32
  basal, 24–3
  four-chamber, 18–21
  longitudinal plane, 6, 24
  mitral short axis, 11–14
  right ventricular inflow, 15–18
  transverse, 7
Stenosis, coronary artery disease, 212, 215
Subaortic membrane, left ventricular outflow obstruction, 206–207
Subvalvular apparatus, mitral valve, 36
Subxiphoid five-chamber view, 13
Subxiphoid longitudinal plane, 11–13
Subxiphoid position, mitral valve, 37
Subxiphoid transverse plane, 9–10
Subxiphoid view, 9–13
Superior vena cave, right atrium, 287–291
Syncope, left atrium, 235
Systole, aortic valve, 106, 107

Tachycardia, left atrium, 254
Thoracic aorta, 28–32
Thrombus
  aortic plaque, 187, 190
  left atrial, 243–265
  right atrium, 283
Transducer, left atrium, 249
Transducer manipulation, 5, 8
Transducer probe tip, 8
Transesophageal echocardiography
  aortic dissection, 159–182

aortic plaque, 183–201
aortic valve disease, 105–145
basic views, 1–32
congenital heart disease in adults, 303–347
coronary artery disease, 209–232
examination techniques, 1–32
intraoperative applications, 349–370
left atrium, 233–275
left ventricular outflow obstruction (nonvalvular), 203–207
mitral valve disease, 33–104
performance steps overview, 2
pericardial disease, 297–301
right atrial masses, 277–295
standard views, 9–32
tricuspid disease, 147–158
Transesophageal procedure, intraoperative, 350–353
Transient ischemic attack, aortic plaque, 190
Transmitral pulsed Doppler flow, 22, 23
Transposition of great vessels, 346–347
Transthoracic echo abnormality, left atrium, 238
Transvalvular gradient, in subxiphoid, 112
Transverse plane, five-chamber view, 23
Tricuspid annulus, right atrium, 289
Tricuspid disease, 147–158
 tricuspid regurgitation, 147–154
 tricuspid valve endocarditis, 155–158
Tricuspid regurgitation, 147–154
 diastolic doming, 154
 dilated right atrium, 149
 Ebstein's anomaly, 342
 hockey stick configuration, 153
 hypertension, 153
 interatrial septum, 150
 right ventricular inflow view, 148–149
 systolic pressure, 152
Tricuspid valve, 18
Tricuspid valve endocarditis, 155–158
Tricuspid valve evaluation, intraoperative TEE, 360–363
Tricuspid valve leaflet excursion, ventricular septal defect, 339
True lumen, aortic dissection, 163–182

Ulcerated aortic plaque, 188

Valsalva maneuver, 18, 330–331
 patent foramen ovale, 330–331
Variants, normal, 105–112
Vegetations, mitral valve endocarditis, 64–71
Vena cava, 19
Ventricular outflow tract, ventricular septal defect, 337
Ventricular septal defect, 336–340
 aneurysm, 336
 congenital heart disease, 336–340
 pulmonic stenosis, 340
 tricuspid valve leaflet excursion, 339
 ventricular outflow tract, 337
Ventricular tachycardia, coronary artery disease, 216
Views, basic, 1–32

Wave form reversal, diastolic compliance abnormality, 22